I0891176

Psychology Revivals

Clinical Lectures on Diseases of the Nervous System

Originally published in 1991 as part of the *Tavistock Classics in the History of Psychiatry* series, this re-edition of J-M. Charcot's *Clinical Lectures on Diseases of the Nervous System* provides a unique opportunity to examine the work of one of the last century's most controversial and admired physicians. Widely esteemed for his work in neuropathology, Charcot was also an innovator in the study of hysteria, making important contributions to its study in both women *and* men.

The *Clinical Lectures* reproduced here are especially important for two key reasons. First, they provide insight into Charcot's often neglected study of male hysteria, especially traumatic shock, as well as, hysteria among children. Secondly, they give an opportunity to examine his clinical method and style. His presentations and scholarly compilations greatly influenced an entire generation of French and other physicians interested in the study of the 'unconscious' during the turn of the century.

The introduction, which precedes the work, places the volume in its social, political and historical context. It highlights the key features of the historiographical debate surrounding Charcot, which ranges in scope from the social and intellectual history of the Third Republic through that of early psychoanalysis. It then proceeds with an examination of the key themes – both substantive and methodological – underlying Charcot's researches, providing both a general *entrée* into the history of medicine and society in this period, as well as an *explication du texte* which carefully analyses the lectures themselves.

Clinical Lectures on Diseases of the Nervous System

J-M. Charcot

Edited with an introduction by
Ruth Harris

Routledge
Taylor & Francis Group
LONDON AND NEW YORK

First published in 1991
by Routledge

This edition first published in 2014 by Routledge
27 Church Road, Hove, BN3 2FA

Simultaneously published in the USA and Canada
by Routledge
711 Third Avenue, New York, NY 10017

Routledge is an imprint of the Taylor & Francis Group, an informa business

Publisher's Note
The publisher has gone to great lengths to ensure the quality of this reprint but points out that some imperfections in the original copies may be apparent.

Disclaimer
The publisher has made every effort to trace copyright holders and welcomes correspondence from those they have been unable to contact.

A Library of Congress record exists under ISBN: 0415057388

ISBN: 978-0-415-73191-1 (hbk)
ISBN: 978-1-315-84948-5 (ebk)
ISBN: 978-0-415-73192-8 (pbk)

CLINICAL LECTURES
ON
DISEASES OF THE NERVOUS SYSTEM

BY

J-M. CHARCOT

Edited with an Introduction by

Ruth Harris

TAVISTOCK/ROUTLEDGE
London and New York

First published in 1991
by Routledge
11 New Fetter Lane, London EC4P 4EE

Simultaneously published in the USA and Canada
by Routledge
a division of Routledge, Chapman and Hall Inc.
29 West 35th Street, New York, NY 10001

Printed in Great Britain by Antony Rowe Ltd

British Library Cataloguing in Publication Data

Charcot, J-M.
Clinical lectures on diseases of the nervous system.
(Tavistock classics in the history of psychiatry)
1. Man. Nervous system. Diseases
I. Title II. Harris, Ruth *1958–* III. Series
618.8

Library of Congress Cataloging in Publication Data

Charcot, J-M. (Jean Martin), 1825–1893.
[Leçons sur les maladies du système nerveux. English]
Clinical lectures on diseases of the nervous system / J-M.
Charcot; edited by Ruth Harris.
p. cm. — (Tavistock classics in the history of psychiatry)
Reprint. Originally published: London: New Sydenham Society, 1878.
Translation of: Leçons sur les maladies du système nerveux.
Includes bibliographical references.
1. Nervous system—Diseases. I. Harris, Ruth, *1958–*
II. Title. III. Series.
[DNLM: 1. Nervous System Diseases. WL L466 1878a]
RC346.C4613 1991
616.8—dc20
DNLM/DLC 90–8472
for Library of Congress CIP

ISBN 0–415–01732–7

CONTENTS

ACKNOWLEDGEMENT

I would particularly like to thank Mark Micale and Bernard Brais for allowing me to consult and cite unpublished work. I am grateful to Roy Porter who was an understanding and helpful editor.

INTRODUCTION

Ruth Harris

In the last fifteen years, Jean-Martin Charcot has emerged as one of the most paradoxical and controversial figures in the history of medicine. Neurologists who esteem his great clinical contributions in the neurosciences tend to write in embarrassed tones about his 'unscientific' forays into the realms of hysteria and hypnotism, characterizing this work as the less successful element of an otherwise impressive *œuvre*.[1] As one medical historian of the subject has perceptively remarked, 'Charcot, charged with sins, entered into purgatory',[2] a dark limbo from which he has not yet entirely emerged. From the moment of his death, pupils and associates dissociated themselves from his analysis of hysteria, some rebelling openly when it seemed that he was barely cold in his grave.[3]

The critical reappraisal has not yet stopped. On the contrary, fresh interpretations have only added to the controversies surrounding his work. In the last decade or so, critics, particularly feminist historians, have examined Charcot's complex evaluation of the quintessentially 'feminine malady' of hysteria by focusing on his ambiguous relationship to his female patients.[4] Their work, as well as that of others such as the art historian and philosopher Georges Didi-Huberman, has begun to unravel the significance of his medical diagnoses for the politics and representation of gender in the early Third Republic.[5] Not surprisingly, their remarks have often been critical, as they seek to unmask this progressive paragon, the great 'Napoléon des névroses', as a man led astray by ambition and the desire for self-aggrandizement. Most of their accusations centre on his depiction of *grande hystérie*, and the way in which he exploited the mental woes and physical debility of the women under his care.

Still other interpretations of Charcot's work stress the link between his interest in hysteria and the politics of anti-clericalism, a convincing argument which suggests that even the specific content of his diagnoses, as well as their popular and medical presentation, were significantly conditioned by extra-scientific concerns.[6] Equally, psychoanalysts either extoll or condemn him, treating him not as an object of historical study in his own right, but rather as a precursor of their discipline, examining his work for the positive or negative influence it may have had upon the young Freud.[7]

As is so often the case, a revision of the revisionism is already under way. Other historians seem eager to fling themselves into the mêlée and give what they consider a more balanced appreciation. For them, *grande hystérie* in women was only a small fragment of Charcot's studies. They offer a view that weighs up methodological and clinical preoccupations with the more explicitly ideological and political elements in his work.[8] Against the feminist stress on the maltreatment of women patients, they contrast Charcot's open-mindedness, his willingness to investigate and expand upon the importance of hysteria in men. His preoccupation with the subject is seen as strong evidence of a thorough and effective attempt to strike the final blow against the uterine interpretation of the disease. Placing their analyses squarely within an historical context, they stress his 'progressive' character within the contemporary medical world.

All of these approaches are important for understanding the volume being reprinted here, as it concentrates heavily on the topic of hysteria, with fifteen of the twenty-five lectures dealing with cases in women, men and children.[9] Four out of the five appendices, collected and edited largely by his disciples, elaborate on the same theme, adding a clinical richness to the expositions presented in the lectures themselves. In the course of these presentations, Charcot provides no systematic overview of his theoretical and clinical preoccupations, preferring instead an episodic rendition of case studies. Such an approach seemed particularly well-suited to his 'nosological method'. As the translator of this volume, Thomas Savill, explained in a footnote, this approach entailed not merely a more rigorous classification of disease, 'but ... the clinical method of investigation in its widest sense'. It was an orientation which began at the patient's bedside and ended in the dissecting chamber, in Charcot's words, with 'animated living shapes [and] concrete realities',[10] which all could recognize and confirm. The job of the physician was the slow building up of a clinical picture and the careful teasing out and differentiation of symptoms and syndromes. Easy generalizations were eschewed and caution advised, a case-by-case approach which fitted in well with the nature of the public lecture.

In this volume, which comprises lectures given between 1882 and 1885, the most significant pieces deal with hysteria in men, particularly as it related to the consequences of trauma and shock. Here Charcot supplied several important statements on the unacknowledged, but none the less widespread, impact of the disease on otherwise robust artisanal men. Where hysterical women were involved in the discussion, they were generally (although not always) included to provide a contrast with men suffering from the malady. The work also presents an important and interesting departure in medical thinking by emphasizing hysteria in both female and male children.

If these lectures are the highlights of the volume, there is much else of interest. We are plunged into the public arena of Charcot's lecture hall at the Salpêtrière and a particular *fin-de-siècle* medical culture, enabling us to observe the ways he transmitted his knowledge through a unique rhetorical style and visual presentation. We have stories of spiritualist séances more reminiscent of Edgar Allen Poe than of scientific lectures; a woman with a paralysed arm who was suddenly, almost miraculously, cured during the course of the lecture and proved it by rapturously shaking hands with a congratulatory audience; elaborate instruments which unmasked malingerers and revealed the sufferings of 'true' hysterical patients; and, finally, any number of hypnotic experiments that showed human beings as unconscious automata acting upon Charcot's experimental commands. We begin to grasp, in sum, what constituted *the* model for a specialist in the diseases of the nervous system in Paris in the last decades of the century when science and art, and what seemed a dose of medical magic, all combined to produce a unique experience.

Charcot, the Salpêtrière and the medical profession

These lectures on the nervous system were delivered when Charcot was approaching the zenith of his powers, fame and influence. Charcot at this time had an international reputation; esteemed by the leading lights of Parisian medicine, he was to become a virtual dictator within his own neurological speciality. The public adored and abhorred him, flocking in extraordinary numbers to hear his public lectures. He came to receive almost every honour, professional and other, that the French state could bestow. The first lecture printed here, indeed, is the inaugural lecture he delivered after his installation as Professor of the Diseases of the Nervous System in 1882. This award was a tribute to two decades of work in the field as well as the result of an equal amount of political and medical infighting.

Charcot had scientific as well as political credibility and knew how to exploit both. He became the exemplar of the new Gambettist Republican order to which men of the lower-middle classes could aspire through merit. Gambetta came to power in 1882 and promised a Republican regime based on the political and social incorporation of the lower-middle and professional classes. After the intellectual conservatism of the Second Empire, and the threat of a monarchical restoration in the 1870s, the new regime ushered in a new political era which promised, and indeed delivered, the means of social advancement and recognition for men like Charcot.

The favoured narrative of Charcot's life, as well as his lectures, seems to have had a well-staged quality. He, as much as anybody, laid enormous stress on his humble origins – he was born on 29 November 1825, the son of a skilled but scarcely eminent carriage-maker – a point which is important for his self-creation as a *grand maître* whose life and work were the proud embodiment of meritocratic values. By 1882, the year of his special appointment as Professor at the Salpêtrière Hospital, he was clearly and unquestionably a 'Great Man', a position which he set out self-consciously both to enjoy and to perpetuate.[11]

Moreover, Charcot was the perfect embodiment of the new prestige associated with the medical profession, which seemed to have truly come into its own under the Third Republic. The medical press dominated the world of academic periodicals. Scientific advance seemed assured (if sometimes haltingly introduced) by the contemporary discoveries and therapeutic applications of Louis Pasteur's work in microbiology.[12] The prominence of physicians in Republican politics suggested that, after years of opposition under the Empire, they had finally won an important voice in the nation's affairs. Finally, the law regulating medical practice and education, passed on 30 November 1892, promised the gradual elimination of the *officiers de santé*, the medical profession's longstanding, and less well-trained, competitors, who had provided a large share of the medical treatment in France. The law of 1892 assured, if not physicians' monopoly over healing, then a greatly expanded legal basis on which to build.[13]

Charcot was the paragon of this professionalizing process. He was, however, more than a medical man at the forefront of the drive for specialization and scientific medicine. He was also hostile to what he regarded as superstition and religious dogma, characteristics which both placed him in an older tradition of enlightened learning and underscored his particular credentials in one of the more actively anti-clericalist moments in French history. Above all, he was a cultivated man, a repository, as his home seemed to indicate, of the humanist literary and artistic values within the Western tradition. He lived in an impressive house on the Boulevard St Germain and acquired a reputation as a host and collector. He demonstrated an eclectic and knowledgeable taste for Classical, Renaissance and northern European paintings, and even modelled his bookcases on those in the Library of the Medici in the Convent of San Lorenzo in Florence. He showed his refinement through his knowledge of the classics and of Shakespeare, and was well-known for his reading knowledge of several languages. At home, he welcomed men from politics, the arts and letters, and enjoyed a private clientele of the highest order, including the son of the Pasha Bey of Tunis and the grand dukes of Russia.[14]

Clearly, he was a far cry from the quacks and charlatans who had been the targets of many a nineteenth-century satirist. This is not to suggest, however, that he was not a focus for adverse literary comment, or that he was not at times condemned as the embodiment of a new kind of scientistic charlatanism. For example, he figures prominently, and not always in a flattering light, in the *Journal of the Goncourt Brothers* and as the redoubtable, perhaps even sinister, physician in Daudet's *Les Morticoles.*[15] In his final work, Roger Martin du Gard characterized him as a man ruthlessly insensitive to the pain and anguish of his patients and so enamoured of his scientific mission that he dispensed with ethical proprieties when presenting them to the public.[16]

Whether extolled or criticized, Charcot was a model Third Republic Man. The regime sought social legitimacy in a political world in which kings, queens and emperors were finally swept from the scene. To replace them, the Republic self-consciously created its own heroes, constantly wary of the possibility of de-stabilization from the right; there was, after all, a precedent for the Republican vision being attacked and destroyed by the forces of reaction. A craze for new street names, busts, statues and plaques established a growing pantheon of exceptional men whose achievements epitomized the greatness of French genius in general, and of Republicans in particular.[17]

It is only in understanding this search for legitimacy that the contemporaneous Charcot cult can be properly put into perspective. When he was photographed in Napoleonic pose, hand tucked into his jacket, the association was too clear to be overlooked. The constant comparisons with Caesar and Danton, the descriptions of his imperious temperament, were both part of the way contemporaries viewed him and integral to the myth-making process itself, linking him to classical greatness on the one hand and French Republican 'genius' on the other. The statue by Falguière, the medallion by Vernon and the marble bust by Dalou at the Academy of Medicine were all part of the memorialization process in which the Third Republic specialized. Doctors were not the only figures to be commemorated in this way, but they benefited especially from a veritable wave of 'statumania', which meant that they were placed on the city's streets and in and around its public buildings in ways that hitherto had been inconceivable.

Despite his extraordinary celebrity when in his fifties, Charcot's career was hardly meteoric. After the *lycée* he went to the Paris Faculty of Medicine, and proved himself to be neither an exceptional student nor a brilliant young physician, although he was able to secure sufficient patronage to qualify as an *interne* (the French term for a house physician) at the Bicêtre Hospital. He ultimately gained an academic post as *agrégé* (a winner in the French system of competitive examinations), but only after 1860 and then not on his first try. His career advanced in a traditional fashion, relying on the aid and support of powerful patrons to assure his promotion, a system of professional association which he, in turn, used to dominate Parisian neurology at the zenith of his own career in the 1880s.[18]

During the Second Empire, his major patron was P-F-O. Rayer, a leading figure in pathological anatomy and laboratory research who helped form his protégé's intellectual universe as well as promote his professional development. Charcot inherited his patron's belief in the importance of pathological anatomy and was influenced by his association with the *Société de Biologie*. Nominated by Rayer to this important scientific society, he encountered at its meetings many of the key medical scientists of his generation. Rayer also provided an introduction to Achille Fould, a Jewish banker and financier, who became the first in a long line of famous private patients who ultimately launched Charcot into the highest echelons of Parisian political and social life.[19]

In this early period, Charcot's research focused on general questions of internal medicine, rather than on the diseases of the nervous system. His 1854 doctoral dissertation distinguished gout from rheumatism, and other work concentrated on diseases of the aorta, on typhoid, typhus and plague. It was only after 1862, when he was made head physician at the Salpêtrière at the already advanced age of thirty-seven, that he began to develop the interests that led to international renown.

From then on, his fame was inextricably associated with his institutional fief and, in the later parts of his career, Charcot and the Salpetrière were almost synonymous. The oldest parts of the hospital had been converted from an arsenal where gunpowder was stored, hence the derivation of Salpêtrière from saltpetre. The hospital had been founded by the great seventeenth-century philanthropist, Saint Vincent de Paul, to imprison women, prostitutes, 'debauched girls' and female adulterers.[20] From the 1680s onwards, other buildings were continually added to contain the aged, the insane, the socially marginal and even some children when the Salpêtrière became an asylum in the tradition of the *hôpital général* of the Old Regime. During the seventeenth and eighteenth centuries, the Salpêtrière was the largest institution of its kind in

Europe, and housed from five to eight thousand women and girls when Paris had only half a million inhabitants. It specialized in the guardianship of the incurable, and contained an assortment of insane, aged, deformed and beggar women, as well as serving as a prison for criminal women and prostitutes.

When Charcot took over, his interests in the sick population were extremely wide-ranging. Rather than being discouraged by the enormity of the clinical population, he was inspired by the richness of the pathological material on offer. As he says in the first lecture in this volume, the Salpêtrière was a 'living pathological museum', an 'inexhaustible' source of raw data waiting to be exploited.[21] He and his colleague Vulpian spent long hours in wards examining the chronic patients, and statistics indicate that they may have performed as many as 800 autopsies in a single year.[22] It was during this period that Charcot did his most memorable neurological work, examining the diseases of old age, paraplegias relating to cancer, cerebral localizations, Charcot's malady and the Charcot–Marie amyotrophy.[23] This work gained him a permanent place in the historical annals of the neurosciences and also helped shape his attitude to the study of hysteria.

For research physicians, then, the Salpêtrière was a treasure trove. However, as an institution whose role was ostensibly to tend to the sick, conditions were far from ideal; there was, for example, only one doctor for approximately 500 patients.[24] Some argue that, by the time of the early Third Republic, the asylum had become more of a vast community, a hospital that had lost many of its Bastille-like qualities.[25] Perhaps a more accurate assessment would be that the Salpêtrière was little different from other large-scale Parisian institutions of its kind which were often custodial rather than curative in orientation.

The physicians who worked in these public facilities were overwhelmed by the number and often abject and impoverished state of charges who, while they found long-term refuge from the vicissitudes of Parisian life, could not hope to receive individual treatment. There is no denying that, at least in the elaboration of the diagnosis of *grande hystérie*, Charcot and his associates were most concerned with patients who demonstrated dramatic symptoms. It is possible to suggest that the flamboyance of the hysterical subjects, especially in the early years of their study, was in part generated by the extraordinary difficulty of winning the attention of the hard-pressed physicians in any other way. In a sense, then, the institutional structure of the Salpêtrière played an important part in generating the symptoms that Charcot then built into his general theory of the illness.

From the very beginning of the century, the Salpêtrière played a key role in the study of the insane, with the *aliénistes* (the term used to describe those physicians who tended *les esprits aliénés*) of the French School regularly working in wards containing women who suffered from mental illness. However, Charcot was not himself an alienist by training, and it has often been argued by contemporaries and later biographers that he 'plunged into full hysteria' only after 1870, and then only by a chance reorganization of the ward headed by the alienist Docteur Delasiauve when an attempt was made to separate the hysterical from the epileptic subjects.[26] It was this exercise, so these arguments maintain, which first led him to form a greater interest in a subject he had hitherto little explored.

To suggest, however, that it was only administrative serendipity which led him to the study of hysterical women ignores the important political backdrop which made the subject particularly congenial. In the 1860s Charcot was a Republican member of the opposition and shared with other medical colleagues the hope that the 'liberal' empire would permit a greater openness in educational and scientific initiatives.[27] But change was limited by strong opposition from conservative officials and especially from the Catholic clergy who were wary of the increasingly materialistic bent of scientific research in the life sciences. In this respect, mental pathology was singled out for attention because it raised serious questions about the philosophical viability of the doctrine of free will. Controversies flared up over medical theses, particularly the growing contention of young medical students that free will was an outmoded 'metaphysical' concept, and that medicine ought to provide a rigorous deterministic and physiological account of human agency.[28] The result was a campaign of official harassment of medical and scientific societies, which continued through to the fall of the Empire and the subsequent years of the so-called 'regime of moral order'.

However, the avant-garde of the medical profession did progress in these years, with a new set of professors appointed to the reconstituted Paris Faculty of Medicine. This effective purge not only gave Charcot his chance as Professor of Pathological Anatomy, it also resulted in an advance to positions of authority by several long-standing allies, many of whom hailed from the *Société de Biologie*.

This new group wanted to establish laboratory medical science within the Faculty and improve clinical teaching. Above all, they wanted more money and better facilities to compete successfully with German science. Identifying themselves as medical and scientific patriots, they argued that the defeat of France during the Franco-Prussian War of 1870–1 was a product of German educational superiority which needed to be countered on all levels.[29] Charcot, in particular, was vividly aware of the value of this line of reasoning and addressed the matter in the first lecture of this book. He firmly believed that the progress of 'nerve pathology' was largely being made in France and, if the government did not support his work, the lead would pass to Germany: 'ought she not to continue the work, or should she leave other countries to make advances in her domain?'[30]

The reshaping of institutions was only part of the push towards establishing the ascendancy of the new brand of medical man. Almost as important was the foundation of journals promoting the novel vision of medical education, particularly *Le Progrès Médical*, which established itself as the profession's gazetteer and watchdog. *Le Progrès* became associated with the new trends which the young generation endorsed with enthusiasm, and it promoted Charcot as one of *the* leading figures in the avant-garde, an educational and progressive advocate of student rights. From being a virtual unknown, he became a key medical figure in a matter of a few years. As late as 1874, his lectures were attended only by a select group of interns and other physicians; yet a few years later they were an essential part of Parisian intellectual life.[31] *Le Progrès Médical* is particularly important for this discussion, as the lectures contained in this volume appeared in editions during the early 1880s.

The eminence, therefore, which Charcot achieved in the 1880s was the product of many contributing influences which had as much to do with the changing educational and political climate as with the quality of his scientific work. Moreover, in addition to links with educational reform, he was also associated with the successful anti-clericalist movement to secularize the hospitals by laicizing the nursing staff. This initiative was part of a greater institutional reform movement from which the Salpêtrière, with Charcot at its head, benefited greatly. With his anti-clerical acolyte, D-M. Bourneville, elected to the municipal council, Charcot was granted the facilities he had been requesting for a decade – more beds, better salaries for ancillary staff, improved bathing facilities, as well as laboratories, a museum, a new lecture hall, and more besides. It is not surprising, therefore, that he went out of his way in his inaugural lecture to thank the 'Municipal Council of the City of Paris, and also ... the Administration of Public Assistance, whose prompt and liberal aid has rendered possible a scheme which, without it, would have encountered obstacles well-nigh insurmountable'.[32]

However, the increasingly successful anti-clericalism was not confined solely to the administrative and political arena, but also spread into Charcot's research programme. While the initial interest in hysteria may well have come from his intimate and novel contact with the hysterics on the ward of the *épileptiques simples*, he rapidly expanded the scope of his enquiry to forge a scientific link between their symptomatology and the history of epidemic mental pathology as a whole. In devising his portrait of *grande hystérie*, Charcot proposed a picture of feminine disinhibition which, as will be seen, was overtly and unceasingly compared with convulsive religious episodes.

It was not only in his elaboration of *grande hystérie* that Charcot's research work demonstrated anti-clericalist credentials. In the series of retrospective diagnoses attempted in his art-historical works,[33] he constantly reiterated the opinion that the visions and ecstasies of saints in past ages were nothing more than undiagnosed hysteria which, in the modern age, would be treated rather that revered. Building on an older tradition within mental medicine, he and his disciples focused on a long catalogue of episodes which included the convulsionaries of the eighteenth century, many examples of demonic possession, and contemporary instances of excessive religious enthusiasm.[34]

D-M. Bourneville produced one particularly interesting case in the genre, writing about Louise Lateau, a young Belgian woman who became a noted stigmatic in the 1870s, bleeding from wounds on hands and feet, and even occasionally from the forehead. For the

Catholic physicians who examined her and subjected her to a battery of rigorous physiological tests (in order to ferret out any simulation), she represented a possible candidate for beatification.[35] Her suffering was an awesome miracle, her ability to perceive blessed objects and to speak in eloquent French while in an ecstatic trance a sign of divine intervention. But for the anti-clerical Bourneville, she was no more than an hysteric whose sufferings were the result of nervous illness, an interpretation which tended to pathologize both the woman and her religious utterances in a single medical stroke.[36]

Anti-clericalism, therefore, pervaded the early years of Charcot's study of mental disturbance and figured prominently in the 1880s. His appointment as Professor of Diseases of the Nervous System in 1882 must be seen in the context of this movement. While Charcot may not have had the direct patronage of the new premier, Gambetta, as some have suggested – the discussion of the chair's creation preceded the politician's election – it none the less seems clear that the appointment was heavily supported by his friend Paul Bert, erstwhile Professor of Physiology at the Sorbonne and later Gambetta's Minister of Public Instruction. Their shared anti-clericalist commitment and dedication to the reformist educational programme made them powerful allies. In his inaugural lecture, Charcot went out of his way to acknowledge his debt and nail up his political colours by also thanking 'the Chamber that originated the project, the Minister of Public Instruction who promoted it, and my colleagues of the Faculty who, consulted as to the advisability of its creation, returned a favourable verdict, giving me thereby a proof of their estimation . . .'.[37]

Charcot's hysteria

Female hysteria, male hysteria: an introduction

In the *Clinical Lectures*, Charcot began the demonstration of his views on male hysteria, a subject in which he intended to break radically with past medical tradition. From classical times, hysteria had commonly been associated with adult women and adolescent girls; it was a disease of the uterus which could erupt during puberty and afflict women throughout their lives, certainly until the menopause. This is not to suggest that the discussion of hysteria had not moved on from the time of the Greeks. As Mark Micale has shown,[38] the medical view of the disorder changed in the early modern period with the introduction of new models of mental illness centring on the nervous system. None the less, it remained an essentially female malady. Writers in the eighteenth century, for example, noted the occasional appearance of the 'vapours' in men, but, by and large, men were more commonly associated with hypochondria, while women were designated as hysterics.

As the debate continued in the nineteenth century, alienists argued over the precise seat of the disorder, some opting for a neurophysiological account, others for a more traditional uterine interpretation. The systematic break with these earlier studies came with the work of Pierre Briquet who published the *Traité Clinique et Thérapeutique de l'Hystérie* in 1859. Using a wealth of clinical case studies, he insisted that hysteria was 'une *névrose* de l'encéphale' which occurred in both sexes.[39] Despite a few criticisms on small points, Charcot was deeply indebted to Briquet's work, regarding it as an important scientific treatise which had vastly improved the state of knowledge in the field. His own work on female hysteria began in 1872, leading to the formulation of *grande hystérie* by 1876; the study of the male variant followed shortly after, beginning in 1878 and lasting until his death in 1893.[40]

In his studies, Charcot sought an accurate clinical foundation in much the same way as he did with, say, spinal affections. He tried to ground the affliction in the nervous system and to identify physical signs which could not be simulated, to localize paralyses, contractures, anaesthesias and hyperaesthesias so that hysteria – the lying, mocking, Protean disorder – could be finally illuminated and permanently enshrined in an unchangeable clinical nosology.

But hysteria was not so easily confined and, although a neurologist, Charcot was obliged to turn half-alienist both to understand its many permutations and to treat it. He repeatedly demonstrated his debt to his psychiatric colleagues and to the issues that preoccupied them, assimilating, as I will show, their discussion of hereditarian degeneration in relation to the study of hysteria. Moreover, he collaborated closely with the most notable psychiatric clinician of the era, Valentin Magnan, on sexual pathologies, an area in which a distinction between the neurologist's and alienist's viewpoints can scarcely be discerned.[41] In turn, the alienists seemed keen to accept his account of hysteria. There is no sense in which one perceives any feeling of invasion from a hostile 'neurological' camp, and the many hysterical 'stigmata' which Charcot's study of the disorder provided were rapidly incorporated into their analyses.[42] There was, in sum, a considerable and constant interchange between these two kinds of medical practitioner.

The portrait that he eventually developed of *grande hystérie* showed the feminine mind and body in spasms of uncontrollability.[43] Although recognizing important deviations from the norm, he reduced the disorder to 'four periods [which] succeeded each other in the complete attack with mechanical regularity'.[44] The patient began with *la période épileptoide*. In the *phase tonique* (suggesting elasticity) of this stage, she exhibited the first unrestrained movements of legs and arms followed by a loss of consciousness. As the patient moved along the crisis, she displayed respiratory loss, pallor and then flushing of the face. These symptoms were succeeded by rigidity in the body and limbs. The hysteric then erupted into the *phase clonique* (implying spasmodic movements) of the epileptoid period, with arms and legs oscillating and the body racked by generalized seizures. After a brief respite, the most dramatic period, that of the *grands mouvements*, began. At this juncture, the intensity of the circular gyrations resembled the gymnastic contortions of acrobats (hence the term, *la période de clownisme*). Physical extravagance was followed by another period of emotional intensity, the so-called stage of the *attitudes passionnelles*, when the patient was subject to both sad and happy hallucinations, acting out fantasies in which she was often the object of attention. It was in this period that poses of erotic seduction were transformed into those of religious ecstasy (here represented in similar terms to sexual orgasm) and the attitude of the crucifixion – expressions which most strikingly captured the connection between hysteria and religious iconography. Finally, during the *période terminale*, the subject regained consciousness, screaming in agony as the cramps which had overtaken her body were released. An attack of this kind took about a quarter of an hour, although the more heavily afflicted could continue for up to a day.

There is no denying that, in public perception, *grande hystérie* was associated with women. However, the *Clinical Lectures* was the first of a series of writings in which Charcot expanded the discussion to include the examination of men as victims of the disease, using case studies from the Salpêtrière's new *service des hommes*, which, like many other facilities, was established in 1882.[45] Why this emphasis? Clearly it was underpinned by the scientific conviction that the seat of the disorder lay in the nervous system rather than the womb. This motivation, however, was also supported by a broader ideological commitment to tearing aside all superstitions and misconceptions about the disease.[46] In more specific terms, it led Charcot to examine the role of trauma and shock in producing hysterical symptoms among men in the workplace. Trauma was a key issue, especially where cases of compensation were involved. The study of nervous shock enabled him to reflect on the 'diseases of civilization' to which the urban environment – big machines, city crime, congested streets, intoxicants and poisons – contributed.

In order to stress the way he was flouting tradition, Charcot consistently emphasized the masculine appearance of his subjects. This is an important polemical point which he underscored by citing cases of modest and respectable men from the artisanal working classes. We have, for example, a '34-year-old ... blacksmith, father of four children';[47] a shop assistant, once a cooper, 'a big man, strong and well developed';[48] a metal gilder and a locksmith;[49] an apprentice baker;[50] and a 'vigorous, well-built navvy'[51] – all men, except for the adolescent baker, whose apparent normality and robust masculinity defy the common conception of the decadent aesthete tormented by hysterical inner turmoil and crisis:[52]

> One can conceive that it may be possible for a young effeminate man, after excesses, disappointments, profound emotions, to present hysterical phenomena, but that a vigorous artisan, well built, not enervated by high culture, the stoker of an engine for example, not previously emotional, at least to all appearance, should, after an accident to the train, by a collision or running off the rails, become hysterical for the same reason as a woman, is what surpasses our imagination.[53]

In focusing on such men, Charcot implied that it was indeed remarkable that they should be struck with hysteria. At the same time, he proposed two opposing representations of the working-class and upper-class man which were crucial to his analysis. The richer, educated male was seen as more susceptible to emotional distress and the debilitating effects of civilization and its refinements than was his poorer counterpart. Indeed, there is a scattering of evidence which suggests that Charcot was more inclined to label his private patients as neurasthenic, rather than hysterical.[54] This diagnosis, at least in the 1880s, tended to taint the sufferer with an illness of privilege, a disease of overworked nerves common among the professional classes, or of nervous frailty associated with genteel Victorian women who underwent Weir Mitchell's rest-cure.[55] In contrast, the working-class male was considered both more physically robust and emotionally simple, if not downright callous, attributes more appropriate to his occupational and cultural position. Charcot leaves no doubt as to what kind of a man he is speaking of when he presents us with an engraving[56] of an agricultural labourer from the Dordogne who 'has looked after sheep, attended fairs, and slaughtered animals',[57] and who is now employed in the Parisian abattoirs. He is pictured here with a rumpled waistcoat, baggy trousers, no cravat and sporting a large and lushly-grown moustache with unkempt hair. Indeed, this man is of an even lower social status than the artisans mentioned above; he is without skill, a migrant worker who has made his way to one of the dirtiest of Parisian trades. Charcot even alludes to his 'red-bloodedness' by describing what he considers the man's disgusting habit of drinking the blood of slaughtered animals to give himself extra strength.

In knocking down stereotypes about hysteria, Charcot is keen to make another qualification, noting that adult men are more commonly afflicted by the malady than boys going through the stages of puterty.[58] Once again, this suggestion went against received wisdom; after all, as children and adolescents were more impressionable they ought to have been more susceptible. They were not, and he concluded that hysteria was associated exclusively neither with the young or the adolescent – although, as will be seen, he does cite some interesting cases – nor with men of a particularly feeble or refined nervous disposition.

Even more than with women, male hysteria was associated with heredity. When examining the work of a young physician named Auguste Klein,[59] Charcot pointed to the fact that twenty-three out of thirty of the cases examined inherited a tendency to the disease from their mothers through *similar* heredity, a designation which suggests that the maternal infirmity was passed on directly to the son. This qualification was important; men might become hysterical but the disease itself had feminine origins and could be traced to the female line in the genealogy of the man's family.

In this regard, Charcot shared the pervasive late-nineteenth century preoccupation with the theory of degeneration which marked many branches of medicine and particularly psychiatry. Alienists had been at the forefront in developing this approach to mental disturbance, insisting that psychophysiological weaknesses were incorporated into the hereditary make-up of the individual and were transmitted to offspring.[60] Unlike Klein, however, the majority did not emphasize the importance of 'similar heredity' – the simple transmission of like to like – but rather the complicated inheritance of constitutional weakness.[61] In fact, Charcot's own investigations into the hereditarian background of his subjects did not always bear out Klein's interpretation. A wealth of nervous complaints, temperamental eccentricities, and organic diseases were seen to indicate a pathological terrain which nurtured any number of hysterical symptoms. In such cases, the exact nature of the disorder or the timing of its appearance were never pre-determined.

So convinced was he by the theory of degeneration that Charcot seemed frustrated when hereditary antecedents could not be rooted out. When examining the six cases of male hysteria, he finds Rig.., the shop assistant, to have had a father who suffered from 'nervous attacks'[62] and a mother who died of an epileptic fit. Gil.., a metal gilder, had a nervous, tubercular mother and a paralytic and violent father.[63] The locksmith Gui.. had an 'inveterate drunkard' for a father,[64] while the youth Mar.. had a dissipated grandfather of a 'very violent character'.[65] Ly.., a mason, had an alcoholic father and a mother who had 'hysterical attacks' and died of tuberculosis.[66] Of the group, Charcot was most clearly satisfied and intrigued with his investigation of Ly..'s hereditary history; going back into the generations, he discovered that 'we have very important antecedents – four hysterical individuals and an inebriate in one family!'[67] Finally, Pin.., a mason, had an 'inebriate father', a mother who might have died of rheumatism, while 'one of his sisters . . . [was] subject to frequent nervous attacks'.[68] In Charcot's view, it was not surprising that with such a host of lurking disorders, these men with innate morbid tendencies developed hysteria after traumatic episodes.

Trauma, the hysterical man and the dangers of the workplace

While concerned to demonstrate the existence of cases of *grande hystérie* in men, Charcot spent more time in this volume examining a wider range of cases in which convulsive seizures were not apparent. His concern is with accidents and the apparent production of an hysterical contracture, often several days after an insignificant injury. He noted that the effect of trauma, especially on the psychic realm, operated in ways which had not yet been fully explored and produced symptoms often more severe than those 'due to an organic lesion'.[69]

In his exploration of this theme, he contrasted a woman and a man with similar experiences of accidents. She fell ill after an 'insignificant wound on the back of the hand'[70] when she broke a pane of glass, while he was wounded when a 'bar of iron heated to a white heat touched his forearm and left hand'.[71] Neither incident was serious, but both developed extreme symptoms. Charcot was more interested in the man; the female patient's reaction was somehow deemed less remarkable, as the fact that she was a confirmed hysteric necessarily made her prone to all manner of symptoms. The thirty-five-year-old blacksmith manifested distinct signs of creeping paralysis in his arm and physiological deterioration. Here was a rare case where morbid heredity was seen as playing no role – 'no moral emotion can be ascertained as the actual cause of the complaint . . .'[72] – allowing Charcot to drive home a point which he had hinted at earlier on. He argued that hysteria in men could afflict even those who seemed the least susceptible, that some unspecified psycho-physiological process could occur which, as in this instance, was able to produce extremely painful hysterical contractures.

The main body of his analysis of male hysteria continues in the last two hundred pages of the work. Charcot enthusiastically garners the evidence and at the beginning of Lecture 18 on 'Six Cases of Hysteria in the Male' sets out the wider medical issues, citing both the work of French colleagues as well as the English and

American literature on the subject of 'railway-spine'. Many have written on the economic and social implications of the train, the unification of markets, the increasing centralization of the French state and society, and the invasion of regional cultures.[73] With its noise, velocity and power, the train was the symbol of the industrial age and became a potent metaphor for both progress and the forces of disorder which modernity had unleashed. It is not perhaps surprising that in his novel, *La Bête Humaine*, Émile Zola coupled his portrait of a savage murder, executed by a man tainted by morbid heredity, with an account of a cataclysmic train crash. In characteristically dramatic fashion, Zola used the train as a metaphor for a society out of control, a wild animal without human direction:

> Now out of control, the engine tore on and on ... The boiler was full of water, the newly stoked furnace was white-hot, and for the first half-hour the pressure went up wildly and the speed became terrifying ...
>
> What did the victims matter that the machine destroyed on its way? Wasn't it bound for the future, heedless of spilt blood? With no human hand to guide it through the night, it roared on and on, a blind and deaf beast let loose amid death and destruction.[74]

Railways and the accidents they caused were important to the discussion of male hysteria. The term 'railway-spine' was coined by John Eric Erichsen, Professor of Surgery at University College Hospital, London, who in 1866 published a series of lectures 'on certain obscure injuries of the nervous system commonly met with as the result of shocks to the body received in collision on railways'.[75] His work, and subsequent revisions, was influential in putting forward the view that concussions to the brain and spinal cord during railway accidents caused organic lesions responsible for a variety of symptoms, many of which occurred long after the actual accident.

These studies were produced when litigation over rail accidents was becoming more common in England. The early days of rail travel, the intense velocity, the jerking motion, and the sometimes frightening derailments, were seen as responsible for severe and persistent symptoms of injury which Erichsen defined as 'concussion of the spine'. At issue were large sums of money, as litigants and their attornies used Erichsen's work to prove that their injuries deserved compensation. Erichsen maintained, despite the ambiguity and paucity of evidence from post-mortem examinations, that an actual pathological transformation of the tissue occurred, even if it was only molecular in nature.

His views were contested by the men Charcot cited at the start of his own discussion, such as the Englishman Herbert Page, surgeon to the London and North-West Railway, who published his *Injuries of the Spine and Spinal Cord Without Apparent Mechanical Lesion* (1885). Using evidence from 234 of his own cases, Page insisted that the majority of the injuries experienced were the result of 'nervous shock'.[76] He asserted that it was very rare for damage to the spinal cord to occur without harm being done to the spinal apparatus around it, and when such disturbances did happen clear clinical symptoms could be identified. Page's work was seen as an important legal counterweight to Erichsen, and was further endorsed by such medical men as J. J. Putnam in North America.

While Page used his own work to promote a case against compensation, Charcot employed the Englishman's findings to press for the recognition that hysterical reactions were real, painful and debilitating, and hence worthy of legal acknowledgement. In his view, 'railway-spine' or 'railway-brain' were further instances of hysteria in men. He opposed, therefore, the creation of a separate class of 'traumatic neuroses' which was favoured by Oppenheim and the German School,[77] arguing that these illnesses were no different to other kinds of hysterical phenomena which could be observed either in the clinic or produced experimentally, particularly through hypnosis. Like other neurotic conditions, therefore, the impact of 'nervous shock' involved 'not ... an organic lesion, but simply ... a dynamic alteration', although the effects of such disturbances were often very dramatic and harmful to the subject.[78]

Charcot regarded sympathetically the demand for compensation and even went so far as to acknowledge that a patient with a broken leg might be less harmed – despite a three to four month convalescence – than another victim 'with an outburst of nervous symptoms' who could be prevented from working 'for six months, a year, or more'.[79] When examining and trying to treat one such victim whose hysterical hip disease meant he could not work, he supported the decision of the company in question to give the man a pension for life.[80]

Charcot's analysis did not focus only on the effects of railway accidents, but rather on any number of cases in which extreme nervous shock seemed to produce hysterical symptoms. But railway accidents were clearly the best examples and most often preoccupied medico-legists and jurists.[81] Their complexities often involved several medico-legal interventions over successive years to determine the state of the patient. One such case involved a man named Monsieur T.. who was in a train crash near St Omer in 1883. The car rolled off the tracks, jerked along, and then brusquely halted, with the result that T.. was flung about inside, hurt his chest, but did not lose consciousness. Although able to get home on his own, he did so in a 'state of *stupor* and of intellectual *cloudiness* ... in a manner which was automatic and semi-conscious'.[82]

Such a sequence of events was fairly common. A train crash involving neither serious physical injury nor a loss of consciousness was followed by a series of seemingly willed and directed activities all accomplished while in a state of nervous shock. T.. suffered a wide range of intellectual and nervous troubles after this accident. The first medical prognosis was extremely vague; T.. might become a raving lunatic or fully recover his intellectual faculties, a conclusion which was of little help to T.., who found himself partially incapacitated.

While thus recognizing that accidents had potent psychophysiological effects, Charcot was also keen to demonstrate that some victims were more susceptible than others to nervous symptoms. Although they might have had the *appearance* of robust working-class health, deeper investigation could well uncover a wealth of irregularities, especially tendencies to shyness, terror and rage. For example, two of the subjects, Rig.. and Gil.., were somnambulists as children, a symptom of a self-induced *état second* which indicated hysteria.[83] Anyone who tended to 'waking unconsciousness' was clearly seen as more prone than others to nervous disorders. Equally, we are told that Rig.. and Pin.. were both timid; Gil.. 'dreaded the darkness';[84] Gui.. 'became very cowardly, [and] was never able to remain alone in a room without experiencing a sentiment of fear'.[85] Mar.. was 'subject to paroxysms of anger'[86] and two others were notably unintelligent.

Working-class people, it seemed, were also more prone to hysteria because of the dangerous and debauched nature of their *manière de vivre*. For example, Charcot discovered that the mason Ly.. was a drinker who admitted imbibing 'five or six little glasses of brandy per day, in addition to a considerable quantity of wine',[87] a habit he may well have inherited from his drunken father. Although the metal gilder Gil.. was a good workman and an accomplished musician, such achievements were more than vitiated by his 'sexual excesses, his need to masturbate', and his 'irresistible impulse towards women'.[88] Gui.. shared this tendency towards debauchery and danced the night away with girls he met in the Parisian *bals*. Although sexual excess was not supposed to figure importantly in Charcot's vision of hysteria, it is certainly clear that in these instances he saw such habits as contributing to the male hysterical personality.[89]

Most of the sufferers had both unfortunate heredity and bad habits of some kind, but it was the series of accidents, and the extreme fright associated with them, which brought on the hysterical symptoms. Rig.. cut open his arm with a razor, and was so frightened that he 'fell to the ground, deprived of sensation and movement'. But even more terrifying was an accident at work when a barrel nearly fell on him, causing him a 'slight wound of the left hand'. Once again he lost consciousness, and then 'was disturbed by fearful dreams', with the first attack of *grande hystérie* appearing ten days later, followed by the whole range of physiological and emotional symptoms.[90] All of these men, then, might very well *seem* robust and emotionally stable, but the onset of the disorder accentuated any latent tendency towards womanly feelings and disturbances.

In examining 'nervous shock' Charcot sought kindred psycho-physiological phenomena as a means of understanding the pathological implications. He considered that it was similar to the hypnotic state in which 'the *mental spontaneity*, the *will*, or the *judgement*, is more or less suppressed or obscured, and suggestions become easy'.[91] To put it another way, when people were scared to death, their intellectual and moral capacities were overwhelmed by the rush of terror, turning them into unconscious automata which were prey to the most terrifying suggestions. In the appendix, we have a striking case of another man who demonstrated this process.

After being in a road accident, he was unconscious for five or six days. He awoke in a state of '*traumatic retrograde amnesia*',[92] having no memory of what had happened to him and with paralysis in his legs. In the course of his convalescence, he came to believe, erroneously, that the lower part of his body had been crushed; he had, in sum, been affected by a profound and overpowering autosuggestion which made his recovery difficult. Terror had erased memory and will, a psychological state which found analogues in somnabulism, or in periods of acute intoxication produced by alcohol and drugs.

What general characteristics do these cases share? Doctors were vividly aware of the dangers of the workplace and its ability to cause any number of ailments. In studying degeneration, they recognized the importance of mercury and lead poisoning in disturbing the physiological equilibrium.[93] Alcohol occupied an important place in contemporary medical discussion, and was particularly associated with certain trades. For example, carters were seen as especially prone to drunkenness, often being tipped with wine and absinthe rather than money. Metal workers often drank alcohol from sheer thirst, while construction workers punctuated their day by visits to the café. In the case of Gui.., for example, Charcot seems to attribute his fall to the possibility of mild intoxication.[94]

Indeed, throughout the volume, Charcot is alive to the disturbing effects of the work environment on the mental and physical health of the Parisian man. The building trades were notoriously dangerous, with men falling and breaking limbs, crushing skulls and never fully recovering their former personalities. So important was a blow to the head that it was commonly accepted as a reason for diminished responsibility in criminal cases.[95] It was one of the many instances in which a medical diagnosis matched lay perception, and those whose personalities were irrevocably changed after such incidents were accepted as being likely to suffer from eccentricity at best and violent outbursts at worst.

Industrial accidents were not the only dangers facing working-class men in the city, as some male hysterics were the victims of violence. Gil.. was stabbed '*in the head*'[96] and this traumatic episode ultimately resulted in convulsive attacks and hemianaesthesia. His extreme melancholia led him to commit suicide, a fate from which Charcot sought to learn by performing an autopsy. The lack of any discernible organic lesion made him conclude that his diagnosis of hysteria had indeed been accurate. The young baker's apprentice Mar.. was also attacked on the street, lost consciousness and, although there was no sign of a wound, developed all kinds of psychological symptoms, especially 'horrible nightmares, which torment him to the present time'.[97] Gui.. also received a violent blow from a knife after one of his nocturnal expeditions, a fright which later produced horrifying visions of a 'monster in human form coming towards him'.[98] In his case, trauma followed trauma when, fixing a balcony, he fell and knocked himself unconscious. Despite the seeming return of mental and physical health, Charcot then found strong hysterical stigmata.

How do these examples of male hysteria compare to the female variety? How is an analysis of gender and social role incorporated into Charcot's account of the disorder? First, both men and women developed hysterical symptoms after trauma and accident. We observe, for example, the case of Henriette A——, a laundress, who was hit on the head by a falling shelf. Although not hurt physically, she was emotionally agitated and the next day slipped and fell, ultimately developing a paralysis in the right arm. In the sequence of events and symptoms which Charcot described, Henriette's reaction differed little from the men described above. With only trifling irregularities in her medical history, she succumbed to a bout of hysteria which Charcot was able to cure very quickly, so quickly in fact that at the end of the lecture she was able to go 'round among the audience vigorously shaking them by the hand, desirous of proving how real was the recovery they had just witnessed'.[99] Women too would be frightened by rabid dogs, robbers in the streets and cadavers of murdered women, all traumatic episodes which differed little from those described by men who had taken fright in other, comparable instances.[100]

But while women were as prone to the effects of trauma as men, the nature of many of the accidents which plagued them tended to be of a rather different kind. The focus on the workplace in the episodes of male hysteria must be contrasted with the higher tendency among women to suffer other kinds of *moral* shocks; they were far more likely than men to be the victims of romantic and domestic distress than their male counterparts.[101] When, for example, discussing a woman with hysterical mutism who could not speak after the first interrogation when accused of infanticide, Charcot used the information provided by his colleague Paul Brouardel – Dean of the Faculty of Medicine and Professor of Legal Medicine – to delve deeply into her background. Not only had the woman given birth, but she had also wrapped the dead child up, labelled it 'cheese', and presented it to the priest whom she claimed was the father. While her claims were rapidly dismissed, the details of her wayward life and sexual fantasies (as they were considered) were seen by Charcot as an integral part of the clinical story.[102]

Another case, not included in this volume, involved a woman who had slapped her seven-year-old son and developed a paralysis of the hand. Was it the force of the blow that caused the symptom, or rather the feelings of shame and suffering which the mother felt at her uncontrolled anger? Charcot preferred the second explanation, providing a vivid example of the effects of emotional trauma potentially associated with motherhood.[103] In both these instances, then, particular episodes directly related to the woman's place and women's emotions were deemed relevant to the clinical story. Such details of the lives of hysterical men were generally not as complete.

Perhaps the most striking difference in the account of hysteria in the two sexes is the rarity in men of the stage of *attitudes passionnelles*. In women, the stylized portrayal of eroticism, the sexual imagery and the discussion of past romantic woes were thoroughly reported. Fear, shock and terror were all cited as possible reasons for the appearance of hysterical symptoms in men, but rarely disappointment, abandonment or betrayal. There are numerous accounts of nightmares and hallucinations, but no attempt made to decode or understand these visions of assassins, brigands and monsters. The fullest account of an hallucination is given in the discussion of the mason Ly.., who re-enacts the terror of a quarrel with a colleague in which he calls him 'scoundrel' and 'Prussian', the latter a term of abuse which had become popular after the defeat and Commune of 1870–1.[104] However, such phenomena had no bearing on the therapy for either men or women, but were rather seen as mere symptoms, perhaps even insignificant ones, in the larger clinical tableau.[105]

Children, adolescents and parents: authority and psychic isolation

Children were especially important to Charcot's discussion of hysteria. In these cases, we have the clearest view of the psychology of his therapy, in which he gave forceful orders and managed patients, as well as their often uncooperative and, in his view, overly solicitous families, to gain results. Unlike cases of adult hysteria, he had more positive prognoses for the young and concentrated less on the hereditarian and incorrigible aspects of the disorder, especially in children who had not reached the age of puberty.[106] He intervened forcefully and unselfconsciously used his authority in an attempt to hasten a cure.

In perhaps one of the most striking literary efforts in the volume, Charcot examines the effects of spiritualism on a family. Children's minds were seen as especially susceptible to the destabilizing effects of spiritualist experiments, sparking off dangerous latent tendencies which would otherwise have lain dormant. Such alarm was expressed forcefully by Gilles de la Tourette, the editor of this lecture, who was to become a key figure in a much broader campaign against spiritualism and its debilitating consequences.[107] As Charcot's acolyte, he would argue that spiritualist séances produced dangerous suggestions and acted as important *agents provocateurs* of the disease. Charcot's contribution here, therefore, has two aims: to examine the effects of hysteria on the family and to demonstrate generally,

> the danger, especially in those predisposed to this class of disease, of superstitious practices ..., the danger of ... a love of the marvellous – a love that has such a remarkable hold on the minds of children.[108]

Charcot's account is more reminiscent of a gothic horror story than a clinical lecture, and is set in an isolated military penitentiary in Brittany, where life was dark and dreary and the duties dull and monotonous. The parents' hereditary history provided clues of potential mental disorder, the father having suffered an extended episode of delirium, the mother having a 'neurotic disposition'. The adolescent Julie was particularly susceptible because of her mother's dangerous addiction to 'spiritualistic séances', during which the girl was encouraged by her misguided parents to act as a medium. According to Charcot, it was when she was instructed to communicate with the spirit of one Paul Denis that she began to develop hysterical signs 'which were characterized chiefly by clownish acts'. So bad did her condition become that she underwent the ordeal twenty to thirty times a day, whereupon François, the youngest child, also began to have pains and hallucinations of 'lions and wolves'. Jacques, the middle child, was next to fall to the attack, and he too was overtaken by visions of 'brigands and assassins whom he wished to strike'.[109] It is important to note that the adolescent female medium was the one held responsible for setting off her brothers' attacks.

The parents brought their afflicted children to the Salpêtrière where isolation from each other was prescribed, although conditions in the hospital made it difficult to keep the two boys completely apart. The message of the treatment was clear; any interference from the parents would bring on further difficulties, countermanding the authority of the physicians and undermining the effect of the 'firm hand ... calm demeanour, and much patience' of the guardians on the wards.[110] The key to the treatment was the moral and psychic dimension, with the parents excluded until there was a significant improvement in the children's condition.

This saga was interrupted in the next lecture by the story of another case which illustrates well Charcot's belief in 'isolation' for the treatment of hysteria. In his view, a major weapon in his therapeutic arsenal was the power of his own personality. He tells the remarkable story of an anorexic girl of thirteen or fourteen years brought to him on the brink of death. Of all the many cases in the *Clinical Lectures*, this one most unselfconsciously recorded his heroic triumph over both misguided parents and the patient herself. Unlike the impoverished patients in the hospital, or the more modest clients of the polyclinic, the girl came from a well-to-do family. Despite the family's stringent objections (the father uttered '*malédictions*' against Charcot's intervention), he maintained that her only hope was for the parents to leave her alone. She was then put in the care of a patient nun (a surprising guardian considering Charcot's anticlericalism, but one which demonstrates that even he was sometimes obliged to rely upon the experience of the nursing orders) and subjected to his firm, intractable directions. For

Charcot, the cure lay in his making the girl realize that he was in absolute control, a view confirmed, so he tells us, by the patient's own significant confession:

> 'As long as papa and mamma had not gone – in other words, as long as you had not triumphed (for I saw that you wished to shut me up), I was afraid that my illness was not serious, and as I had a horror of eating, I did not eat. But when I saw that you were determined to be master, I was afraid, and in spite of my repugnance I tried to eat, and I was able to, little by little.'[111]

The final example of this kind of case which taught the same lesson involved a Russian Jewish child attending a gymnasium. Unlike the older hysterical men from the working classes, this adolescent had all the characteristic signs of his privileged background and, moreover, showed what Charcot saw as the particular Jewish tendency towards neuropathic conditions. Although avowedly opposed to anti-semitism, he believed that Jews were more prone than others to nervous illness, a view which tended to reinforce, rather than undermine, common stereotypes of the Jew as a wandering and persecuted minority afflicted by the need for constant adaptation and assimilation.[112] In this instance Charcot acknowledged the young man's intelligence, but noted that he suffered from pallor and headaches, symptoms which suggested mental overwork. The destructive influence of his father was outlined when Charcot pointed out that the child regularly had his attacks around six o'clock in the evening, that is, about the time his father asked him how he was feeling.[113] In Charcot's view the father's enquiry was the suggestion that set off the nervous crisis.

In all these cases Charcot clearly recognized the powerful effect that parents could have on children, and, with a certain psychological canniness, showed a perceptive understanding of the situation. He made no attempt, however, to probe further into the nature of the family dynamics at work and understand the children's reactions, but rested content with substituting his own more forceful authority for that of the parents. His therapeutic regime was deliberately firm and even coercive and, in these instances, he believed his strategy was eminently successful.

Charcot's method

Pathological anatomy, 'dynamic' disorders and the hystericized body

Charcot's analysis of trauma and shock sought to understand the emotional states which might produce hysterical reactions. Although he came closer than his predecessors to thinking about the nature of such unconscious mechanisms, his account was still hardly psychodynamic. Rather, he provided a classical medical account of neurophysiological disinhibition likened to hypnosis, drunkenness or drugged oblivion. From our contemporary perspective, such an approach may suggest the poverty of Charcot's investigations. However, his concentration on, and highlighting of, the phenomena of trauma and shock – and their association with somnambulism – provided an important spur to other researchers more interested in the emotional aspects of hysteria.

Charcot laid out his particular methodological preferences in the first lecture in this volume. Above all, he wished to uncover the organic *siège* [seat] of disease through the techniques of pathological anatomy, hoping to determine the localized origins of motor and perceptual malfunctions. Much of his most renowned work was based on an attempt to correlate clinical symptoms with traces of diseased tissue discovered during post-mortem examinations. However, he soon realized that neurological examination on its own was insufficient, and he introduced new clinical techniques and theories to account for extravagant symptoms which seemed to have no organic, or localized, origins. As he noted, in the sphere of nervous illness, lesions were often strikingly elusive:

> But you are aware, gentlemen, that there still exists at the present time a great number of morbid states, evidently having their seat in the nervous system, which leave in the dead body no material trace that can be discovered. Epilepsy, hysteria, even the most inveterate cases, chorea, and many other morbid states ..., come to us like so many Sphynx, which deny the most penetrating anatomical investigations.[114]

Charcot refused to be defeated by this circumstance. Instead, he professed, as an article of faith, that the numerous 'functional' disorders which still eluded his search were none the less 'governed, in the same way as other morbid conditions, by rules and laws, which attentive and sufficiently numerous observations always permit us to establish'.[115] He believed, moreover, that some day the source of the dynamic lesion would be discovered, as he stated after inducing hysterical mutism in an hysterical woman during somnambulism: 'it is in the grey cortex of the cerebral hemispheres that we must seek for the dynamic lesion whence emanate the symptoms in question.'[116]

In Charcot's eyes, there was no doubt that hysteria was a 'real' illness. Blocked in the search for an organic seat of the disorder, he turned his classificatory and observational skills instead to the shifting and changing symptoms of the disease, hoping to discover patterns and sequences that would help him pin it down. He was equally concerned to separate the wheat of genuine hysterics from the chaff of simulators who merely pretended to be sick. Such an effort had an obvious scientific rationale. But it was also, at least in part, aimed at fending off criticisms from often sceptical colleagues who believed that many of the symptoms and maladies Charcot discovered were the result of a powerful personality which tempted patients to simulate merely to gain his attention.[117]

Charcot's defence against such accusations was to stress the rigour of his clinical methods and his determination to unmask simulators through physiological tests which, in his view, could not be deceived. Employing an apparatus to measure movement during the cataleptic state of hypnosis – the second stage of the four stages of *grand hypnotisme* in which the subject performed remarkable feats defying normal physiology – he instructed patients to stretch out their arms. Those who simulated would get tired, their exhaustion demonstrated through muscle strain and uneven respiration. In contrast, 'real' cataleptic subjects remained in a state of restful stillness, unaware of the severe physiological demands placed upon them.[118]

When, for example, he examined a young Jewess from St Petersburg suffering from a 'facial tic non-doloureux', he compared her condition to a long-time hysteric whose symptoms were far more convincing. While the older woman demonstrated a 'very rapid quivering, some 200 times per minute',[119] the younger produced a spasm when invited to do so, which disappeared when a small pad was put on her eye: 'there is a personal influence in the matter which gives us material for much thought.'[120]

This comment indirectly challenged his detractors by showing Charcot's willingness to accept the reality of suggestion. He explained her behaviour by implying that she simulated 'for the worship of art for its own sake'. Her pleasure in playing this part derived from her ability to fool the 'physicians of St Petersburg, then those of Paris, next the Faculty of Vienna, and thus to make a tour through the whole of Europe ...' Charcot alone, through his experiments, was able to unmask her deception by obliging her to sit on an electric machine with uncovered eyes until she 'displayed evident signs of fatigue'. Showing some compassion when a 'genuine nervous storm seemed imminent', he finally decided not 'to push the experiment further' and released her from her torment.[121]

Seen in this light, Charcot's fascination with the 'stigmata' of hysteria is more clearly understandable. Unable to localize hysteria during autopsy, he remained committed to a programme of mapping in which zones of the body were noted and visual fields measured to demonstrate their difference from symptoms that were due to organic disturbance. The primary examination focused on the so-called hysterogenic zones, which were 'more or less circumscribed regions of the body, pressure on which, or simple rubbing, produces the symptoms of an aura, which may be followed, if you persist, by an hysterical attack'.[122] Charcot introduced a schematic drawing from the *Iconographie Photographique de la Salpêtrière* to show the disc-like points which could both spark off and contain a full-blown hysterical attack.[123]

A further significant aspect of Charcot's vision of the disease was his emphasis on the phenomenon of '*ovarie*',[124] an aspect of his work which shows a somewhat paradoxical attitude towards the older uterine interpretation of hysteria. Indeed, he chided his forebear, P. Briquet, for his seeming reticence, even prudery, in failing to recognize the importance of ovarian hyperaesthesia as a key stigma of the disease. Briquet, in his view, was too concerned to dissociate hysteria from the uterus and hence from traditional associations with feminine sexual voraciousness. Although Charcot was hardly an 'exclusive partisan of the old doctrine, which placed the point of departure of the hysterical malady entirely in the genital organs',[125] he none the less believed strongly in the key role played by ovarian hypersensitivity as a sign of hysteria.

Unlike previous physicians, however, Charcot asserted that it was not the ovaries themselves but the nerve bundles behind them which, when compressed, set off an hysterical seizure, and for this reason he opposed surgical techniques such as ovariotomy as both harmful and misdirected.[126] Yet, although he set out to change radically the characterization of the disorder by giving it a neurological foundation, he none the less came close to reproducing the traditional vision of the 'raging womb', and hence reinforced the conventional image of hysteria as a feminine disease. Moreover, even in this series of lectures which laid heavy stress on the existence of hysteria in men, he did little to sever the link between the disease and a vision of female sexual lubricity and indelicacy.[127]

The hysterogenic zones were transferred to the male anatomy virtually without change, except, of course, for the ovarian phenomena. When discussing the locksmith Gui.., however, Charcot showed that men demonstrated a similar sensitivity by touching 'the testicle and the course of the right spermatic cord reaching to the groin of the right side'. As with women, the stages of the attack began with a 'well-defined painful *aura*' which moved into the epigastric region and then to the throat, producing the 'feeling of constriction' of which the women patients also complained.[128] Gui.. too lost consciousness, a symptom which began the epileptoid stage. We see the man with his arms outstretched and his body in rigid contracture, producing the well-known 'arc of circle backwards', which was followed by similar movements forwards and to the side.[129] Gui.. is pictured naked as he flails about the bed, moving in a 'manner that fully justifies the denominaton of *clownism*':[130] 'Gui..'s attacks differ in absolutely nothing from those which we observe each day in hystero-epileptic patients of the female sex.'[131]

The hysterical attack was the most obvious sign of the disease, but Charcot was not satisfied with only dramatic symptomatology. Instead he also searched unendingly for evidence of what he considered the key symptom of hemianaesthesia. He demonstrated how young women remained insensitive to the most intense faradization – a form of treatment with electric current – losing their sense of feeling not only on the skin, but also in the 'muscles and nerve trunks'. The young Russian Jewish student was presumed to be an hysteric when there was a 'loss of sensation to pricking, to cold, and to faradization on the right side'.[132] This loss of sensibility, in sharp contrast to the hyperaesthesia of the hysterogenic zones, was most strikingly illustrated by the disturbance of the visual field, a symptom which Charcot held to be particularly important.[133] Through a series of diagrams,[134] he mapped out a disturbance which was 'most interesting to the physician. The patient can neither simulate nor exaggerate it, and not uncommonly it is very accentuated, although the troubles of general sensibility may be but little marked'.[135] Different kinds of symptoms abounded, such as cloudiness, colourblindness or the substitution of one colour for another. Once again, these functional disorders were not revealed by the ophthalmoscope: 'they are exclusively dynamic troubles, as they are called.'[136]

Finally, a similar desire to map and chart can be seen in the drawings representing regions of paralysis and insensibility.[137] By comparing organic and hysterical paralysis, Charcot once again sought a means of localizing both, pointing to their dissimilarities and hence to the importance of the diagnostic task he had undertaken. He showed symptoms caused by the destruction of nerve and muscle in one, and the uncanny, but not identical, resemblance in the other. In Lecture 20, for example,[138] he contrasted the cases of two men who had suffered accidents, the cab-driver Porcz– who injured his right shoulder, and the navvy Deb– who damaged the left shoulder. Porcz– suffered from symptoms apparently due to a hysterical reaction, while Deb–'s were similar but more readily traceable to a physical lesion. A diagram mapping the loss of sensibility in both subjects demonstrated that the apparent similarity between the two was deceptive.[139] Deb– suffered a rupture of his bronchial plexus with a loss of movement and sensibility down to his hands. Moreover, he had lost his tendon reflexes and his muscles had atrophied.

In contrast, mapping Porcz–'s anaesthesia demonstrated a different, and less severe, clinical picture: 'we have here unquestionably one of those lesions which escape our present means of anatomical investigation, and which, for want of a better term, we designate *dynamic* or *functional* lesions.'[140] The distinction was highly significant. Not only did the neurologist have the benefit of an accurate diagnosis, he could also offer Porcz– a much better prognosis. Deb–'s paralysis would stay with him for life, while Porcz–'s condition, with the proper therapeutic attention, might well leave him altogether. Nor was this the only case in which Charcot demonstrated the clinical value of such distinctions. He tells of one instance in which a painful hysterical contracture in the leg was ended by an amputation, a disastrous intervention which this sort of investigation might avoid.[141]

Metals, magnets and hypnosis

From the earliest days of his investigation of hysteria, Charcot was particularly interested in an experimental approach, no doubt inspired, like many others of his generation, by the methodological dicta of the widely influential Claude Bernard.[142] Charcot willingly and sometimes audaciously experimented on human subjects, as the *Clinical Lectures* demonstrates. Of particular use to him was hypnosis, which became one of his most important techniques in two distinct but interrelated areas. First, it provided a means of investigating psychophysiological conditions which, in his view, prepared the ground for hysterical symptoms. Patients under hypnosis displayed intense suggestibility and were able, in this state of unconscious automatism, to reproduce hysterical symptoms such as contractures and hemianaesthesias. Second, hypnosis was a therapeutic tool. Although wary of indiscriminate use, which he thought might provoke latent hysterical susceptibilities in otherwise normal subjects, Charcot none the less recommended the technique for alleviating symptoms.[143]

While Charcot's exposition of his views on hypnotism were hailed as unquestionably scientific and untainted by past charlatanry, the fact remains that he was indebted to an older, and less scientifically-respected, tradition through the work of the neo-mesmerist Victor Jean-Marie Burq.[144] On the medical fringe, Burq was allowed by Claude Bernard, then president of the *Société de Biologie*, to investigate the therapeutic value of metals and magnets for hysterical symptoms.[145] He also worked in Charcot's ward on a group of female hysterics and demonstrated that several physical agents, including magnets, metals, and electric currents (a technique often used in the *Clinical Lectures* to try and restore sensibility and movement) had a positive effect on hysterical symptoms of all varieties. Such investigations also produced results that even Burq had not anticipated. He found, for example, that when sensation was restored to one side of a hemianaesthesiac's body, the other side tended to lose it. Like the magnets themselves, the body seemed to have an innate polarity, and the 'law of transfer' was thus established.

In his 1882 address to the *Académie des Sciences*,[146] Charcot dissociated himself and his hypnotic investigations from this older tradition, making a distinction between his own 'scientific' study and older 'occult' interpretations. But, even in this volume, the remnants of Burq's approach periodically appear. For example, in discussing an hysterical woman who developed a rigid contracture in the left leg after she toppled down a dozen stairs, Charcot suggested the application of a magnet 'or of agents of the same kind to bring about a transference of the contracture to the opposite side . . .'. He then concluded that it would be 'possible . . . at the end of a large number of such transfers' to make the contracture completely disappear.[147] A magnetic treatment was also used on the similarly afflicted young Jewess.[148] In still another instance involving a man with a contracture of the arm, Charcot recounted how the patient was treated outside the Salpêtrière by Dr Burq's method and how his 'hands and fingers [were] covered with plates and rings of copper'.[149]

While Charcot was, then, deeply indebted to Burq's investigations – using his work in understanding the phenomena of transfer, particularly where anaesthesias and contractures were concerned – he determined to elaborate his own version of *grand hypnotisme*. For Charcot, hypnosis was a symptom of hysteria, a physiological state of mental impoverishment in which free will and moral sense were obliterated. While some other Parisian neuropathologists maintained that people susceptible to hypnosis possessed heightened rather than diminished mental capacities, Charcot remained convinced that hypnosis was a pathological condition and one that should be induced only in an attempt to improve the already afflicted subject.[150]

Charcot's description of hypnosis involved three distinct phases – catalepsy, lethargy and somnambulism. In the first state, the subject was deemed to be completely at the mercy of the experimenter, who could abolish sensibility (that is, the operator could hit or pinch the subject with no sensation of pain), and heighten muscular rigidity in a way that enabled some to stand with out-stretched and unflinching arms for twenty-five minutes. This state was the one in which the apparatus described above was used in order to determine if the subject was simulating. It was also the state in which 'certain phenomena of suggestion are easily obtained', when 'unconscious cerebration' produced automatic and purely mechanical actions. The cataleptic subject was the '*human machine*, in all its simplicity, dreamt of by De la Mettrie'.[151] The second, lethargic, state had an opposite effect, making the subject like a 'cadaver before *rigor mortis*',[152] with a muscular tonicity causing physical defencelessness and psychic inertia.

The final state was somnabulism, in which the subject obeyed all the commands of the operator and executed acts upon waking without any conscious awareness or memory. This state was particularly important for Charcot because it enabled him to reproduce symptoms artificially and thus investigate the mental conditions surrounding hysteria. For example, in Lecture 21, he put the female hysteric Gruez– into a somnambulic trance 'by means of slight pressure exercised on the eyeballs for a few seconds'. He then explained that she was relatively new to hypnotism and might resist his suggestions, as indeed initially she did. When told that her right hand was paralysed, she replied, 'but no, … you are mistaken'.[153] Despite her resistance, Charcot triumphed, and eventually the woman produced the paralysis.

In the case of Pin.., a similar experiment also worked successfully. Although the man's paralysis was already on the mend, Charcot none the less reproduced the symptom during hypnosis to prove his point to the audience: '"You believe yourself cured," I said to him, with an accent of entire conviction, "it is an error; you are not able to raise your arm, nor to bend it, nor to move the fingers …" The experiment succeeded marvellously …'[154] Realizing perhaps that his public might be disturbed by his willingness to render ill a patient he was meant to cure, Charcot remarked: 'I was not anxious on this account, … for I know from long experience, that *what one has done, one can undo*.'[155]

Literary illusion and the visual sense

Although a physician and research scientist, much of Charcot's success came from his dexterous use of literary allusion and art-historical reference in his works and lectures. He built on old medical and natural-historical traditions which paid careful attention to literary style and rhetorical form, knowing full well that such care was essential to making his views known to a wider audience.[156] Indeed, there were moments when he seemed quite carried away by the power of a well-turned phrase, as when he discussed the sad case of the patient D.., a victim of breast cancer, whose repeatedly unsuccessful operations and horrible disfigurement led him, before her eyes, to suggest that the cancer ward should be inscribed with Dante's words on the gates of hell.[157] He presumed on the knowledge of the audience and did not give the quotation – 'abandon hope all ye who enter here' – making his meaning clear to all listeners except the patient who was thereby spared hearing his hopeless prognosis.

In a similar manner, when examining the possibility of simulation in a case of hysterical mutism, he could not resist the temptation to demonstrate his literary breadth, quoting an episode in Molière's *Le Médecin malgré lui* as a perfect example of malingering:

> Sganarelle: 'What is the matter? What pain is it that you feel?'
> Lucinde: (*replying by signs, carrying her hand to her mouth, to her head, and to her chin*) 'Han, hi, hon, han.'
> Sganarelle: 'Eh! what do you say?'
> Lucinde: (*continuing the same gestures*) 'Han, hi, hon, han, han, hi, hon. . . .'[158]

Such allusions were an essential part of his lecturing method, establishing a common, and privileged, bond of educated cultural discourse. Moreover, he used this comic example for a practical effect, contrasting the literary simulation with the more serious example of the infanticidal mother who became hysterically mute and aphonic after an official interrogation: 'not the least sound, no hin, hi, hon, han; not the least unnecessary gesture.'[159]

This style of presentation became even more effective through his use of visual materials. By now it is a virtual cliché to talk about Charcot's visual sense, the way in which his clinical diagnosis was influenced by his penetrating gaze and artistic sensibilities. All who attended his lectures were struck by the strong visual effect produced by his expositions, no one more than Sigmund Freud who, in an article in 1893, remarked: 'he was not a reflective man, not a thinker: he had the nature of an artist; he was, as he himself said, a "*visuel*", a man who sees.'[160]

Charcot was not only a man who loved seeing, identifying and distinguishing between symptoms and placing them in a correct classificatory scheme. He was also one who loved to be seen, to present his observations in an individual and sometimes quite dramatic fashion, particularly during his Tuesday public lectures. These orchestrations have become the subject of much attention in recent years, as the 1887 Salon painting by Brouillet makes the rounds of the exhibition halls and begins to hold a prominent place in the history of psychoanalysis.[161] The painting shows Charcot during one of his lessons on hypnotism before an enthralled male public. We see one of the famous '*vedettes*' of the hysterical performances, Blanche Wittman, alluringly décolletée and ready to go into an hysterical seizure (her left hand is already in contracture) with the nursing supervisor of the Salpêtrière, Mlle Bottard, poised to lay the patient on the cot. The painting reinforces Charcot's reputation as a clinician, giving him a commanding and impressive presence. He addresses the audience, and does not even have to look at the patient in order to explain what is happening to her, so well does he know the progress of the malady. The painting, however, also gives much away, showing the suggestive influence of Charcot on his subject, who willingly, it seems, performs her role in sequence with the progress of his lecture, to ensure that those watching appreciate fully the point that the *maître* is making.

How important were these artistic representations? Do they only figure prominently in the extravagant portrait of *grande hystérie*? All agree that Charcot resorted to theatricality and drama, but was this only a small part of a more sober, scientific totality? I would argue that in all aspects of his work, visual imagery and dramatic display were central to the originality of his clinical method. It was Charcot's confidence and authority over his subjects that made him so impressive and gained him public and professional attention. His willingness to present certain cases to the public, even when doing so brought on serious symptoms in the patient, reinforced his reputation as a tenacious and inexorable scientific investigator. For example, in discussing the hysterical origin of the rhythmical chorea, he recognized that the patient would erupt before the audience because of her distress at the public exposure: 'It will not be necessary for us to intervene, for the emotion that she has experienced at finding herself before so many people in the lecture room will save us the trouble of provoking an attack.'[162] Similarly, he sometimes admitted that symptoms had not been alleviated in order to preserve them for public view. In presenting a case of a woman with an hysterical contracture, he suggested that the technique of chloroformization could have proven whether the disorder resulted from hysteria and indeed might have offered some relief. Instead of doing this, however, he took no action because 'we feared a perturbation which would have prevented you from studying this deformity *de visu*'.[163]

This preference for visual example led Charcot to fill his volume with pictures, many of which were photographs. Charcot favoured photography because, as his associate Albert Londe, director of the service in the 1880s, asserted: 'the photographic plate is the real retina of the scholar.'[164] Those at the Salpêtrière depended on photography to present what was in their view an accurate account of pathology unmediated by the inexactitude of language or the subjective creativity of the artist.

The photographs produced, however, were hardly transparent reflections. Like all artistic creations, their power derived from the selection of particular subjects in particular positions and with particular symptoms. The enthusiasm for photography was underpinned by a scientistic belief that this most up-to-date technology provided the exact mirror of nature which had eluded earlier generations. However, even Charcot himself sometimes seemed ambivalent about its function, one moment stressing the objectivity of the method, the next speaking proudly of 'artistic'[165] merits in a way that suggests that he believed in the mutually reinforcing effects of 'true' art and 'true' science.

The Salpêtrière was a 'pathological museum', and Charcot wished to preserve the myriad specimens contained within its walls by capturing them for posterity. Photography provided an important tool in the clinical laboratory which helped him compile an unparalleled scientific archive, a museum within the museum. Above all, photography was an essential teaching tool, capturing moments on the wards which students would otherwise have missed. For example, in Lecture 18 he used a sequence of photographs of Gui.., whose hysterical attack differed virtually not at all from those of women.[166] If there was any scepticism on the part of the audience, then these 'reproductions' of flailing limbs in an hysterical male should have convinced them.

The photographs of Gui.. are matched by others which display symptoms of a more specifically neurological kind. Almost all the subjects are represented without clothing,[167] except for an adolescent girl, a woman, and a more elderly man who are shown with their loins covered by pieces of material. The man afflicted by Erb's disease is shown in only his shoes and socks, the front and back views having no consideration for his privacy nor any regard for the confidentiality of the doctor–patient relationship. The faces are clearly displayed, and no attempt is made to isolate the facial distortions in order to hide the identities. In the discussion of rhythmical chorea, Charcot presents the last eleven photographs of a sequence of forty-eight showing the jerking movements and almost primitive dancing steps of a diseased woman, a disturbing picture of disinhibition which Charcot himself admits became a 'most distressing infirmity[,] preventing the patient from following any occupation, and obliging her to live apart from the world by reason of the fear which these attacks inspire in those around, and the sentiment of repulsion which these unfortunates feel themselves the object'.[168]

These photographs are unselfconsciously invasive and even by the standards of the day stretched to the limit the ethical proprieties seen to govern professional relations between doctor and patient.[169] Charcot was accused of exploiting the 'hospitality' of the hospital by using individuals who could neither pay for their treatment nor select their physician. In the photographs of one famous young hysterical woman, Augustine, a clearly erotic tone was struck, with this beautiful adolescent appearing in poses of semi-nude contracture which were strikingly alluring, if not downright seductive.[170] It is important to note that these patients were from the poorer classes of Paris; the faces and bodies of Charcot's private clientele never became part of the *Iconographie Photographique* or of the *Clinical Lectures*.

In this area, Charcot's responsibility as a discreet healer clashed with the strong desire to transmit his knowledge. For him, science revealed deformed nature, and the body's nudity may have been essential for the full exposition of its contortions; moreover, facial tics and contractures were the key to diagnosis. There is also a way in which the nude takes on an almost privileged position in his scientific *œuvre*, in much the same way as it did in the *beaux-arts* tradition.[171] At the same time, his work differed from this tradition; rather than presenting an ideal of academic and classic perfection, it sought to represent a deformed opposite, while sometimes partaking of orthodox conventions and practice. For example, when examining a case of hysterical hip disease, Charcot placed next to the patient a nude artist's model 'who is accustomed to pose for painters, and whom we have instructed to imitate as much as possible (after careful study) the attitude of the patient'.[172]

Charcot's appreciation of the visual was not limited to photographs. His most famous artistic/medical collaborator was Paul Richer. Charcot himself was adept with the pencil and crayon, but Richer was truly accomplished, his sketches providing some moving portraits which encompassed both the clinical symptomatology and the emotional reality of physical and mental distress. In this he was within an important visual tradition which examined the insane and the sufferers of nervous affliction by focusing on their contorted physiognomies and contracted limbs.[173] In the *Clinical Lectures* we have a variety of such drawings, especially images of hands in which Richer specialized.[174] Hands, always a challenge to the artist, were even more so in these instances where the exact angle of a crooked finger, or an extended thumb, or a splayed wrist, were seen as key elements in making an accurate diagnosis.

Conclusion

Was Charcot unique in *fin-de-siècle* medical culture and society? I would answer in the affirmative, and suggest that his brilliance derived from the peculiar acuity of his visual sense and inimitable expository style, which made otherwise esoteric neurological arguments into both fashionable discourse and tantalizing intellectual challenge.

There is no denying that Charcot's vision of hysteria and hypnotism was both radical and influential. The delineation of *grande hystérie* among women was itself a major undertaking, an attempt to find and promote a novel and impressively documented neurophysiological account of hysteria. As I have suggested, this vision of hysteria – removed from the womb and conceived of as a diffuse functional disorder – none the less reinforced the most extreme and ancient characterizations of the disease of feminine disinhibition. Clearly the *grandes hystériques* were a minority, the exceptional cases in a myriad examples with less severe symptoms. However, these women – Blanche Wittman and Augustine, for example – provided a public perception of what Charcot's hysteria meant.

As we have seen, hysteria at the Salpêtrière was much more than this. Charcot liked to break down conventions, and he sought to do so in his study of male hysteria. His work in this field was felt keenly in the medical community.[175] Contemporaneous with the *Clinical Lectures*, and for some time after his death, the study of male hysteria was all the vogue, with doctors discovering cases in men that were almost as extravagant as any in the women at the Salpêtrière. If Charcot had shown a certain reticence in discussing and describing the personal and sexual difficulties of his male subjects, then those around him were far less hesitant, as they eagerly sought a psychological understanding of the origins of the disease and concentrated less systematically on determining the physiological stigmata which were so central to Charcot's delineation.

How can we judge Charcot's willingness to study the problem of male hysteria? We can safely presume that his interest in the subject derived from a desire, both scientific and polemical in origin, to sweep away any lingering superstitions about the disease as an exclusively feminine malady. But his work took him in other directions and, perhaps most progressively, led him to consider the reality of traumatic disorder arising from the pace and nature of life in a crowded, dangerous and fast-paced city.

However, Charcot's discussion of working-class male hysterics can hardly be seen as unproblematic. His views of the working-class male, despite all his qualifying remarks, had, I think, the effect of 'feminizing' his subjects. The surface appearance of robust masculinity was belied by the ready transfer of symptoms from the feminine body to the masculine one. Charcot devised a portrait of *grande hystérie* in women and merely transposed the same symptoms, albeit with shades of difference, to the men whom he observed. Rather than liberating these patients, Charcot seemed to stigmatize them in a way not dissimilar to the tainting process observed in his characterization of women. In his discussion of such men he mixed an obvious sympathy for their plight with a strong draught of disapproval for the way they and their forebears carried on the business of life, which often included immorality, sexual excess and drunkenness. I think it important that it was the working-class man – even though of respectable artisan status – rather than his middle-class counterpart who was more readily diagnosed in this fashion.

Charcot's elaboration of male hysteria suggests many questions about notions of masculinity and their relationship to class in the *fin de siècle*. Much more work is needed to understand the characteristics attributed to the male hysteric, the neurasthenic and the homosexual. What did they have in common and how did they diverge? Clearly, the interpretations changed with the decades, but all three designations figured prominently in medical and popular discussions in the last few decades of the century. Men of all classes were prone to nervous and sexual 'affliction', conditions that were perceived as somehow inextricably bound up with the toils of modern life and the price it exacted.

Charcot's investigation of male hysteria, as well as the many other contemporaries who examined similar cases, became important for the later elaboration of psychoanalysis. Perhaps most significantly, this work provided an important beginning for the larger exploration of shell shock, *traumatisme de guerre*, during the First World War. More work needs to be done on how male hysteria was metamorphosed in such a way that it acquired a new name, one which, once again, was gender-based. As Showalter has suggested, the experience of the trenches meant that literally millions of men were obliged to undergo the feelings of powerlessness more commonly associated with women's place and sphere.[176] The war itself, the enormity of the carnage and the collapse of a whole system of masculine values of heroism and valour, necessarily played a key role in this transformation.

A note on the French text

The *Clinical Lectures on Diseases of the Nervous System* was regarded as an important text and was the third volume (published in 1890) of the never-finished *Œuvres Complètes*. It was compiled by some of Charcot's most devoted and well-respected students and included noted neurologists, some of whom did their first significant scientific work under his tutelage: Babinski, Bernard, Féré, Guinon, Marie and Gilles de la Tourette.

These lectures occupy a special place in Charcot's work. They were first published in *Le Progrès Médical* between 1882 and 1885 and represented the sober, academic lectures performed on Friday. They differed significantly from those presented on Tuesday, during which Charcot sought to give his audience a greater sense of the difficulties of clinical diagnosis. In the Tuesday lectures (*leçons du mardi*), Charcot engaged in often long conversations (*interrogations*) with the patients, and demonstrated surprise and even confusion as he tried to reach an accurate diagnosis.[177] He sought to deal with patients who were not always cooperative, and reserved some of his most dramatic performances for this impromptu setting. It is important to note that even in these spontaneous presentations Charcot prepared as much as possible, providing such fluent expositions that his audience could not help but suspect a careful rehearsal of the material.[178] The published product was far from perfect, however. Charcot told Freud that they contained many technical errors, having been recorded by young, inexperienced physicians (Colin and Blin) who tried to keep up with his rapid expository style. Clearly, the stenographer's art was not as accurate as that of the photographer.[179]

In contrast, we know less about the process of compilation which marked the Friday presentations. We can, perhaps, make some educated guesses. These were 'official' texts, incorporated into the *Œuvres Complètes*. This third volume was used for translation both by Savill and by Freud, a task which doubtlessly meant that the latter was intimately aware of its contents.[180] Perhaps such familiarity explains Freud's fascination with the concept of trauma which Charcot spent several lectures elucidating.[181]

In contrast to the Tuesday lectures, the *Clinical Lectures* were compiled by his older, more trusted disciples, and seemed to have had his full endorsement. If the impromptu lectures of Tuesday showed the signs of preparation, then the Friday presentations made no claim at all to spontaneity. There is no evidence of wavering, no interruptions, no suggestion of uncooperative patients, although, even here, he sometimes suggests that the audience might observe some reticence among those subjected to hypnosis. Formality did not mean, however, that Charcot disposed of the dramatic, as the reading of these texts amply demonstrates.

A note on the translator and the translation

Charcot had important connections with English medicine. The first volume of the *Clinical Lectures on Diseases of the Nervous System*, containing some classic lectures on female hysteria, were published by the New Sydenham Society in 1877 and translated by George Sigerson, who followed up this work with another volume in the 1880s. Other works on senile and chronic diseases as well as cerebral and spinal diseases, translated respectively by Hack Tuke and Baugh Hadden, followed soon after. The connection between Charcot and his English colleagues was further exemplified by his contribution, along with Gilles de la Tourette, of an entry on hypnotism and hysteria to the important English compendium, Hack Tuke's *Dictionary of Psychological Medicine*.

Here, however, I am concerned with the particular instance of the English translation by Thomas Savill published in 1889 by the New Sydenham Society. Savill's translation was the third in the series of Charcot's lectures. One can only guess whether this translation was commissioned as a companion piece to the others.

Savill was fairly typical of his medical generation, a man who stood at the border between a 'generalist' and a 'specialist' practice. He was from solid middle-class stock which had important ties to the medical profession; his family owned the firm that published *The Lancet*. He was educated at Stockwell Grammar School and then moved to St Thomas' with a natural science scholarship. Savill made his way to the Salpêtrière where he attended Charcot's lectures, became familiar with his teaching style, and ultimately, through the translations, gained an intimacy with the specifics of his research. He also travelled to Hamburg and Vienna, although, like many others, he failed to register and left no trace of his activities.[182]

Like many others who wanted to enhance their credentials as well as their prestige, he opted for the extra MD degree at London University. He studied abroad and, while there and back in

England, showed an abiding interest in neurology and dermatology, activities that indicated a desire for a more sophisticated clinical career. However, a complete shift to specialism was not considered entirely *bon ton* and Savill resisted the temptation to become overly involved in one area.[183] Indeed, his most noteworthy publication, *A System of Clinical Medicine*, was truly the work of a generalist and, with the help of his medical amanuensis (and later his wife) Agnes Forbes Blackadder, it went into nine editions, the last of which appeared in 1930. In sum, Savill seemed concerned to build on a reputation of gentlemanly accomplishment which included generalist public service, a strong but not exaggerated record in specialist research and a lucrative private practice.

For our purposes here, perhaps his most significant appointment was the one that he took up in 1885 when he was named medical superintendent of the Paddington Infirmary. He became expert in the workings of the Poor Law Hospitals, and urged colleagues in the profession to recognize the potential of these institutions as untilled soil for clinical research. The most significant work to emerge from this period was his *Clinical Lectures on Neurasthenia*, which appeared in 1899 and went through four editions in the next decade.

The lectures are strikingly reminiscent of Charcot's in style, plan, emphasis and approach. He speaks of the Paddington Infirmary in much the same way as Charcot spoke of the Salpêtrière, as a pathological museum rich for exploitation: 'there are close upon 600 beds available for the reception of every kind of mental and bodily ailment to which flesh is heir.'[184] Like Charcot in the *Clinical Lectures*, Savill began his own inaugural lecture to a special post-graduate clinic by describing his heroic struggle against outmoded prejudice in convincing the authorities (against, it seems, the strict letter of the law) to permit instruction using patients from the workhouses. In what could have been a paraphrase of Charcot's own remarks, he extolled the benefits of the '*anatomo-clinical method*, which consists of the careful and minute observation of cases of injury or disease of the nervous system during life, and their detailed examination, both macro- and microscopical, after death'.[185] The echoes, then, of Charcot seemed marked, although the exact nature of the Frenchman's impact is clearly impossible to determine. What is certain is that Savill held an abiding interest in neurasthenia and hysteria, continued to be *au fait* with continental scholarship, and constantly cited French authors from Briquet and Charcot to Ribot and Janet in his extensive studies.

As interesting as the translator is the society which published the work. The Sydenham Societies were devoted to providing medical men with books by way of subscription.[186] Between 1843 and 1911 they produced 230 volumes of work by important authors. The first society was founded at the high tide of the Victorian antiquarianism and aimed to offer specialized out-of-print works of historical interest. From the outset, however, the more scholarly interest of the editors clashed with the practical concerns of contemporary practitioners, who were often less than sure about the immediate utility of reprints of Greek and Arabic classics. By 1857, the membership had dwindled from 1,500 to under 700, and those who remained loyal tended to be either retired or middle-aged medical men, less likely to be interested in the most up-to-date research and clinical works. In contrast, the New Sydenham Society, founded in 1857, was notable for the young men in its ranks, and the dynamic leadership of the surgeon Jonathan Hutchinson. The new society seemed more able to satisfy its members with the production of famous and beautifully produced medical atlases and reprints of the classic works like Harvey and Hunter's folio on the gravid uterus. It also demonstrated a commitment to translating important continental research, publishing works by Koch, Charcot and Pasteur, as well as the historical works of Hecker, Hirsch and others.

The *Clinical Lectures on Diseases of the Nervous System* is worthy of this tradition. Savill's translation is of a high quality and every attempt was made to capture not only the technical meaning of Charcot's expositions, but also the unique quality of his presentations. Savill claims at the outset of the volume to have conferred with Charcot over key points. The suggestion of such a collaborative endeavour may well help to explain the exacting nature of the translation.

Notes

1. See for example the classic biography by Georges Guillain (1959) *J-M. Charcot 1825–1893, His Life – His Work*, London: Pitman Medical, trans. Pearce Bailey, pp. 133–46, 165–76.

2. Étienne Trillat (1986) *Histoire de l'Hystérie*, Paris: Seghers, p. 128.
3. See for example the revision of Charcot's notion of hysteria by one of his most famous neurological disciples: J-F-F. Babinski (1934) 'La définition de l'hystérie', *Œuvre Scientifique, Recueil des Principaux Travaux*, Paris: Masson et Cie, pp. 457–64.
4. See Elaine Showalter (1985) *The Female Malady: Women, Madness, and English Culture, 1830–1980*, New York: Pantheon, pp. 129–34 and pp. 145–64; Jacqueline Carroy-Thirard (1974) 'Figures de femmes hystériques dans la psychiatrie française du 19e siècle', *Psychanalyse à l'Université*, pp. 313–23; Martha Evans (1984) 'L'hystérie et la séduction de la théorie', *Frénésie* IV: 51–60; Gladys Swain (1983) 'L'âme, la femme, le sexe et le corps: les métamorphoses de l'hystérie à la fin du XIXe siècle', *Le Débat* 24: 107–27; Gérard Wajeman (1976) 'Psyché de la femme: note sur l'hystérique au XIXe siècle', *Romantisme* 13–14: 57–66. Mary James examines in some detail the *grandes hystériques* at the Salpêtrière from a feminist perspective in her forthcoming 'Therapeutic Practices of J-M. Charcot in their Historical and Social Context' (Ph.D. thesis, University of Essex). For an appraisal of this feminist literature as well as the other kinds of work on hysteria see Mark S. Micale (1989) 'Hysteria and its historiography – a review of past and present writings', two parts, *History of Science* 27: nos 77–8; and (1990) 'Hysteria and its historiography – the future perspective', *History of Psychiatry* 1: no. 1 (forthcoming).
5. Georges Didi-Huberman (1982) *Invention de l'Hystérie: Charcot et l'Iconographie Photographique de la Salpêtrière*. Paris: Les Éditions Macula.
6. Jan Ellen Goldstein (1982) 'The hysteria diagnosis and the politics of anti-clericalism in late nineteenth-century France', *Journal of Modern History* 54: 209–39.
7. See for example L. Chertock (1983) 'À l'occasion d'un centenaire Charcot, l'hystérie et l'hypnose', *Perspectives Psychiatriques* 2: 81–9. For Freud's own remarks concerning Charcot see Sigmund Freud (1966) *The Standard Edition of the Complete Psychological Works of Sigmund Freud*, 24 volumes, James Strachey (ed.), vol. 3, London: Hogarth Press, pp. 11–23.
8. Mark Micale (1990) 'Jean-Martin Charcot and the theory of hysteria in the male: an essay on gender, mental science, and medical diagnostics', *Medical History* 34: no. 4 (forthcoming) and 'Hysteria male/hysteria female: reflections on comparative gender construction in nineteenth-century medicine', in Marina Benjamin (1990) *Science and Sensibility: Essays on Gender and Scientific Enquiry 1780–1945*, London, Basil Blackwell.
9. J-M. Charcot (1889) *Clinical Lectures on Diseases of the Nervous System*, trans. Thomas Savill, London: New Sydenham Society. In

Lecture 15 (pp. 183–97) Charcot speaks of several kinds of nervous disorders, but comes to focus on rhythmical chorea in a young woman whose disease, he believes, has an hysterical origin; see in particular pp. 191–7.

10. Ibid., p. 9.
11. For Charcot's early years see op. cit. (note 1), G. Guillain, *J-M. Charcot*, pp. 1–15.
12. See Claire Salomon-Bayet (ed.) (1986) *Pasteur et la Révolution Pastorienne*, Paris: Payot.
13. For an overview of this history see Jacques Léonard (1981) *La Médecine Entre les Savoirs et les Pouvoirs: Histoire Intellectuelle et Politique de la Médecine Française au XIXe Siècle*, Paris: Aubier Montaigne, pp. 241–327.
14. See G. Guillain op. cit. (note 1), pp. 30–4 and G. Didi-Huberman op. cit. (note 5), pp. 21–2.
15. Léon Daudet (1956) *Les Morticoles*, Paris; Bernard Grasset. It seems likely, as Anne Harrington suggests, that the character of Foutange was a composite of Charcot and J-B. Luys, another important physician doing work on hypnosis at the Charité Hospital. See 'Hysteria, hypnosis and the lure of the invisible: the rise of neo-mesmerism in *fin-de-siècle* French psychiatry', in W. F. Bynum, Roy Porter and Michael Shepherd (eds) (1988) *The Anatomy of Madness: Essays in the History of Psychiatry* (3 vols) vol 3, London: Routledge, p. 244, n. 24. She cites the work of B. Auvrary-Escalard (1984) 'Un méconnu de l'hystérie: Jules-Bernard Luys (1828–1897)', (Université de Caen, thèse pour le doctorat de médecine), pp. 164–7.
16. Roger Martin du Gard (1983) *Le Lieutenant-Colonel de Maumort*, André Daspre (ed.) Paris: Gallimard, pp. 396–7.
17. See Maurice Agulhon (1988) *Histoire Vagabonde: Ethnologie et Politique dans la France Contemporaine*, vol. 1, Paris: Gallimard, especially pp. 101–85.
18. For the nature and importance of this patronage network see J. Goldstein (1987) *Console and Classify: The French Psychiatric Profession in the Nineteenth Century*. New York: Cambridge University Press, pp. 343–5.
19. For the story of Charcot's mentors see Bernard Brais, 'Charcot and Vulpian' (provisional title), Chapter one (forthcoming M.Phil. thesis, University of London).
20. G. Guillain, op. cit. (note 1), p. 41.
21. J-M. Charcot, op. cit. (note 9), p. 3.
22. B. Brais, op. cit. (note 9), pp. 13–14.
23. For a summary of this work see G. Guillain, op. cit. (note 1), pp. 91–132.

24. G. Didi-Huberman, op. cit. (note 5), p. 17, quoting A. Husson (1862) *Rapport sur le Service des Aliénés du Département de la Seine pour l'Année 1862*. Paris: Dupont.
25. M. S. Micale (1985) 'The Salpêtrière in the age of Charcot: an institutional perspective on medical history in the late nineteenth century', *Journal of Contemporary History* 20: 703–31.
26. É. Trillat, op. cit. (note 1), pp. 130–2. There has yet to be any indication of the way in which Charcot made this distinction. What were the symptoms which particularly distinguished the hysteric from the epileptic? As he himself acknowledged, epilepsy did not always provide evidence of organic lesion during autopsy and could, like hysteria, be described as a functional disturbance.
27. B. Brais, op. cit. (note 19), Chapter 2, pp. 17–49.
28. J. Goldstein, op. cit. (note 6).
29. For the broader context of this reformist movement, and the importance of the rhetoric of German superiority in the political struggle for improved facilities see Robert Fox and George Wiesz (eds) (1980) *The Organization of Science and Technology in France, 1808–1914*, Cambridge University Press.
30. J-M. Charcot, op. cit. (note 9), p. 6.
31. B. Brais, op. cit. (note 19), Chapter 3, pp. 78–82.
32. J-M. Charcot, op. cit. (note 9), p. 2.
33. See J-M. Charcot (1887) *Les Démoniaques dans l'Art*, Paris: Adrien Delahaye et Émile Lecrosnier; and (1889) *Les Difformes et les Malades dans l'Art*. Paris: Lecrosnier and Babé.
34. See Catherine Laurence Maire (1985) *Les Convulsionnaires de Saint-Médard: Convulsions et Prophéties à Paris au XVIII*, Paris: Gallimard; for a discussion of the ideas surrounding 'hysterical' epidemics in the first half of the nineteenth century see Jan Goldstein (1984) '"Moral contagion": a professional ideology of medicine and psychiatry in eighteenth- and nineteenth-century France', in Gerald L. Geison (ed.) *Professions and the French State, 1700–1900*, Philadelphia: University of Pennyslvania Press, pp. 181–222, and Gérard Wajeman (1982) *Le Maître et l'Hystérique*, Paris: Navarin, pp. 35–78.
35. Antoine Imbert-Goubeyre (1873) *Les Stigmatisés*, 2 vols, Paris: V. Palmé; for his fuller account of the subject see (1894) *La Stigmatisation*, 2 vols, Clermont-Ferrand: Bellet.
36. See D-M. Bourneville (1875) *Science et Miracle: Louise Lateau ou la Stigmatisée Belge*, Paris: A. Delahaye.
37. J-M. Charcot, op. cit. (note 9), p. 2.
38. M. Micale, op. cit. (note 8), 'Jean-Martin Charcot and the theory of hysteria in the male', especially Section 2.
39. A useful summary of this massive work can be found in François May

and Harold Merskey (1980) 'Briquet's *Treatise on Hysteria*', *General Archives of Psychiatry* 37: 1401–5.

40. M. Micale, op. cit. (note 8), 'Jean-Martin Charcot and the theory of hysteria in the male', pp. 11–13; page citations come from the typescript.
41. Their classic paper is J-M. Charcot and Valentin Magnan (1882) 'Inversion du sens génital et autres perversions sexuelles', *Archives de Neurologie* 7: 6–21.
42. An analysis of contemporaneous medico-legal records demonstrates that Parisian alienists looked for Charcot's hysterogenous zones and were indebted to his 'neurological' model of the disease, while at the same time applying traditional psychiatric characterizations of the hysterical personality. For more see Ruth Harris (1989) *Murders and Madness: Medicine, Law and Society in the Fin de Siècle*, Oxford: Oxford University Press, pp. 155–242.
43. For the full presentation of female hysteria see the nine lectures in (1892) *Œuvres Complètes de J-M. Charcot*, vol. 1, Paris: Bureaux du Progrès Médical, pp. 275–405 and pp. 427–57. See also D-M. Bourneville and Paul Régnard (eds) (1876–9) *Iconographie Photographique de la Salpêtrière*, 3 vols, Paris: Bureaux du Progrès Médical, and Paul Richer (1881) *Études Cliniques sur l'Hystéro-Epilepsie ou la Grande Hystérie*, Paris: A. Delahaye et E. Lecrosnier.
44. J-M. Charcot, op. cit. (note 9), p. 13.
45. M. Micale, op. cit. (note 8) 'Jean-Martin Charcot and the theory of hysteria in the male', p. 13.
46. Charcot's work on hysteria was both a part of, and a catalyst for, a wide range of new studies in the field. See Émile Batault (1885) *Contribution à l'Étude de l'Hystérie Chez l'Homme*, Doctoral Dissertation, Paris Medical Faculty; Émile Bitôt (1890) *L'Hystérie Mâle dans la Service de M. Pitres à Bordeaux*, Doctoral Dissertation, Bordeaux Medical Faculty; Léon de Casaubon (1894) *L'Hystérie Chez les Jeunes Garçons*, Doctoral Dissertation, Paris Medical Faculty; Paul Michaut (1890) *Contribution à l'Étude des Manifestations de l'Hystérie Chez l'Homme*, Doctoral Dissertation, Paris Medical Faculty.
47. J-M. Charcot, op. cit. (note 9), p. 100.
48. Ibid., p. 227.
49. Ibid., p. 237.
50. Ibid., p. 245.
51. Ibid., p. 267.
52. While hysterical men were portrayed in this instance as robustly 'masculine' in health and demeanour, homosexuals, in contrast, were depicted as 'effeminate'. See Robert Nye (1989) 'Sex difference

and male homosexuality in French medical discourse, 1830–1930', *Bulletin of the History of Medicine* 63: 32–51.

53. J-M. Charcot, op. cit. (note 9), p. 222.
54. M. Micale, op. cit. (note 8) 'Jean-Martin Charcot and the theory of hysteria in the male', pp. 21–22. It is not yet clear how neurasthenia was used in nineteenth-century France. There are indications that in the 1880s and 1890s, it was reserved for a higher social stratum. The classic French text on the subject was written by Adrien Proust and Gilbert Ballet (1897) *L'Hygiène du Neurasthénique*, Paris: Masson, and stressed the common themes associated with the illness, especially the difficulty of coping with the 'struggle for existence' in the modern world. However, in other writings, Charcot discussed male vagabonds as being afflicted by hystero-neurasthenia at a Tuesday lecture in 1889, *Leçons du Mardi*, vol. 2, p. 284, implying that their work-shy, wandering propensities demonstrated a mixed symptomatology. See J. Goldstein (1985) 'The wandering Jew and the problem of psychiatric anti-semitism in *fin-de-siècle* France', *Journal of Contemporary History* 20: 538–9. Robert Nye shows how neurasthenia was also applied, especially in the first decade of the nineteenth century, to the vagrant as a means of explaining his work-shy proclivities; see (1984) *Crime, Madness and Politics: The Medical Concept of National Decline*, Princeton: Princeton University Press, p. 176. These scattered references suggest that there may well have been a shift, or at least an enlargement, of the social classes who could be seen as suffering from neurasthenia as time wore on.
55. For a recent treatment of this subject in America, and the 'democratization' of the neurasthenic diagnosis from the professional heights to the artisanal classes, see F. G. Gosling (1987) *Before Freud: Neurasthenia and the American Medical Community, 1870–1910*, Urbana and Chicago: University of Illinois Press.
56. J-M. Charcot, op. cit. (note 9), p. 347.
57. Ibid., p. 342.
58. Ibid., p. 99.
59. A. Klein (1880) *De l'Hystérie Chez l'Homme*, Doctoral Dissertation, Paris Faculty of Medicine.
60. For the key text which enunciated the theory in full-blown form see B-A. Morel (1857) *Traité des Dégénérescences Physiques, Intellectuelles et Morales de l'Espèce Humaine et des Causes qui Produisent ces Variétés Maladives*, Paris: Ballière; for the later evaluation which summed up the theory and its implications for the study of mental pathology, see Valentin Magnan and Paul-Maurice Legrain (1895) *Les Dégénérés (État Mental et Syndromes Episodiques)*, Paris: Rueff. For the integration of the theory into the mainstream of French

psychiatry, see I. Dowbiggan (1985) 'Degeneration and hereditarianism in French mental medicine, 1840–90', in W. F. Bynum *et al.*, op. cit. (note 15), vol. 1, pp. 188–232; F. Bing (1983) 'La théorie de la dégénérescence' in J. Postel and C. Quétel (eds) *Nouvelle Histoire de la Psychiatrie*, Toulouse: Éditions Privat; for the wider cultural impact of the theory of degeneration see R. Nye, op. cit. (note 54); D. Pick (1987) 'The conception and descent of degeneration 1848–1914', Doctoral Dissertation, University of Cambridge; and J. Chamberlain and S. Gilman (eds) (1985) *Degeneration: The Dark Side of Progress*, New York: Columbia University Press.

61. For a concise rendition of the workings of morbid heredity see Charles Féré (1894) 'L'hérédité morbide', *Revue des Deux Mondes* 126: 436–52. This work is probably particularly illustrative of Charcot's own perspective, as Féré was one of Charcot's disciples.
62. J-M. Charcot, op. cit. (note 9), p. 227.
63. Ibid., p. 232.
64. Ibid., p. 237.
65. Ibid., p. 245.
66. Ibid., p. 248.
67. Ibid.
68. Ibid., p. 252–3.
69. Ibid., p. 89.
70. Ibid., p. 90.
71. Ibid., p. 101.
72. Ibid., pp. 100–1.
73. For the classic discussion about the integration of France and its effects on mentalities and daily life see Eugen Weber (1975) *Peasants into Frenchmen: The Modernization of Rural France, 1870–1914*, Palo Alto: Stanford University Press; for a more technical account see Roger Price (1981) *An Economic History of Modern France, 1730–1914*, London: Macmillan, revised edition.
74. Émile Zola (1977) *La Bête Humaine*, trans. Leonard Tancock, Harmondsworth: Penguin, pp. 365–6.
75. For a discussion of the history of trauma, especially as it relates to train crashes, see Michael R. Trimble (1981) *Post-Traumatic Neurosis: From Railway Spine to the Whiplash*, Chichester, John Wiley and Sons, pp. 5–33.
76. Ibid., p. 24.
77. Ibid., p. 45. For Charcot's own remarks on the subject, see op. cit. (note 9), pp. 224–5. For a fuller summary of the literature see Esther Fischer-Homberger (1975) *Die Traumatische Neurose: von Somatischen zum Sozialen Leiden*, Vienna: Verlag Hans Huber.
78. J-M. Charcot, op. cit. (note 9), p. 224.

79. Ibid., p. 222.
80. Ibid., p. 339.
81. See my discussion of the new legal difficulties thrown up by the problem of train crashes and accidents, especially as they related to notions of legal responsibility, Ruth Harris op. cit. (note 42), pp. 109–13.
82. Albert Blum (1893) *De l'Hystéro-Neurasthénie Traumatique* (railway spine), Paris: Asselin et Houzeay, p. 16.
83. J-M. Charcot, op. cit. (note 9), p. 227 and p. 232.
84. Ibid., p. 232.
85. Ibid., p. 237.
86. Ibid., p. 245.
87. Ibid., p. 248.
88. Ibid., p. 232.
89. For more on this point see M. Micale, op. cit. (note 8), 'Jean-Martin Charcot and the theory of hysteria in the male', pp. 38–9.
90. J-M. Charcot, op. cit. (note 9), p. 228.
91. Ibid., p. 335.
92. Ibid., p. 376.
93. For evidence of Charcot's concern with such matters see his remarks concerning Gil..'s occupation as a metal gilder and its potential dangers in ibid., p. 232: 'His occupation, in which mercury is employed, has never produced any symptoms which can be connected with mercurial poisoning. There are no signs of alcoholism.' For more background on the effects of the workplace on health in nineteenth-century France see G. Jacquemet (1977) 'Médecine et "maladies populaires" dans le Paris de la fin du XIXe siècle', *Recherches: L'Haleine des Faubourgs* 29: 349–65; V. P. Comiti (1980) 'Les maladies et le travail lors de la révolution industrielle française', *History and Philosophy of the Life Sciences* 2: 215–39; and Arlette Farge (1977) 'Les artisans malades de leur travail', *Annales, E.S.C.* 32: 993–1006.
94. J-M. Charcot, op. cit. (note 9), p. 237.
95. R. Harris, op. cit. (note 42), p. 34.
96. J-M. Charcot, op. cit. (note 9), p. 233.
97. Ibid., p. 245.
98. Ibid., p. 237.
99. Ibid., p. 405.
100. J-M. Charcot (1892) *Œuvres Complètes*, vol. 1, Paris: Babé et Lecrosnier, p. 343. See the case of Ler.., who suffered these distressing episodes in her past.
101. M. Micale, op. cit. (note 8) 'Jean-Martin Charcot and the theory of hysteria in the male', p. 35, explains that men also occasionally were

reported as having difficulties with their spouses. He cites the case of one 'Pasq' who had quarrels with his wife and episodes when he struggled with her over money for rent and their savings. Other cases involved examples of rejection by women and parental reproaches. Such instances of a male 'psychology' of domestic distress are not included in this volume of clinical lectures.

102. J-M. Charcot, op. cit. (note 9), p. 369.
103. J-M. Charcot (1887–1888) *Leçons du Mardi à la Salpêtrière, 1887–1888*, Paris: Bureaux du Progrès Médical, pp. 300–5.
104. J-M. Charcot, op. cit. (note 9), p. 250.
105. Very little work has been done on the resistance to psychodynamic interpretations in France. For an illuminating interpretive account of such issues in England see Michael Clarke (1981) 'The rejection of psychological approaches to mental disorder in late-nineteenth-century British psychiatry', in Andrew Scull (ed.) *Madhouses, Mad-Doctors, and Madmen: The Social History of Psychiatry in the Victorian Era*, Philadelphia: University of Pennsylvania Press, pp. 271–301, and Michael Clarke (1988) '"Morbid introspection", unsoundness of mind and British psychological medicine, c.1830–c.1900', in W. F. Bynum *et al.*, op. cit. (note 15), vol. 3, pp. 71–101.
106. J-M. Charcot, op. cit. (note 9), p. 247.
107. See Georges Gilles de la Tourette (1887) *L'Hypnotisme et les États Analogues au Point de Vue Médico-Légal*, Paris: Plon.
108. J-M. Charcot, op. cit. (note 9), pp. 205–6.
109. Ibid., p. 202.
110. Ibid., p. 210.
111. Ibid., p. 214.
112. J. Goldstein, op. cit. (note 54), especially pp. 534–6.
113. J-M. Charcot, op. cit. (note 9), p. 82.
114. Ibid., p. 12.
115. Ibid., p. 13.
116. Ibid., p. 373.
117. Charcot, especially in his delineation of *grand hypnotisme*, was subjected to a variety of criticisms, the most important of which came from the École de Nancy headed by Hippolyte Bernheim who in his (1891) *Hynotisme, Suggestion et Psychothérapie*, Paris: Octave Doin, pp. 167 and 169, decried the illusory nature of Charcot's work on hypnotism and hysteria. For a general introduction to debates over hypnosis in France see Dominique Barracund (1967) *Histoire de l'Hypnose en France*, Paris: Presses Universitaires de France.
118. J-M. Charcot, op. cit. (note 9), pp. 14–16.
119. Ibid., p. 40.
120. Ibid., p. 41.

121. Ibid., p. 42.
122. Ibid., p. 74.
123. Ibid., p. 75.
124. J-M. Charcot, op. cit. (note 100), pp. 320–46.
125. Ibid., p. 301; for the complete lecture see pp. 301–19.
126. For the Salpêtrière school's official statement on the matter see G. Gilles de la Tourette (1895) 'Du traitement chirurgical de l'hystérie', *Archives de Gynécologie et de Toxicologie* 22: 409–20.
127. J-M. Charcot, op. cit. (note 9). See for example in this volume the way he discusses a young woman of sixteen. He makes a point of explaining that 'she is not decked out with showy colours, like so many of these patients', an exception which proves the rule. He follows up this description by indicating that her 'moral condition' was not refined, information supplied to him by the Mother Superior in whose charge she had been. See pp. 85 and 86.
128. Ibid., p. 239.
129. Ibid., pp. 240–2 contain the pictures of the attack.
130. Ibid., p. 241.
131. Ibid., p. 242.
132. Ibid., p. 80.
133. For the full explanation of the kinds of symptoms associated with the visual field see M. Parinaud (1900) 'The ocular manifestations of hysteria', trans. Casey A. Wood, in William F. Norris and Charles A. Oliver (eds) (1900) *A System of Diseases of the Eye*, vol. 4, Philadelphia: J. B. Lippincott, pp. 727–69.
134. J-M. Charcot, op. cit. (note 9); for the maps of the visual fields in hysteria see pp. 81, 91, 104, 287, 379.
135. Ibid., p. 72.
136. Ibid., p. 74.
137. For the many body maps of this kind see ibid., pp. 268–9, 271, 285, 298–9, 300–1, 311, 327, 380–1, 392.
138. Ibid., especially pp. 261–73.
139. Ibid., pp. 264–73.
140. Ibid., p. 278.
141. Ibid., pp. 319–20.
142. See Bernard's classic (1865) *Introduction à l'Étude de la Médecine Expérimentale*, Paris: J-B. Ballière et Fils.
143. J-M. Charcot (1890) *Œuvres Complètes*, vol. 9, Paris: Bureau du Progrès Médical, pp. 213–483. These pages provide a fuller explanation of his work on metals and hypnotism.
144. For the tradition of fluidist and biomagnetic thought see Robert Darnton (1968) *Mesmerism and the End of the Enlightenment in France*, Cambridge, Mass.: Harvard University Press; Henri

Ellenberger (1970) *The Discovery of the Unconscious*, New York: Basic Books, Chapters 2 and 3; and R. Amadu (1953) 'Esquisse d'une histoire philosophique du fluide', *Revue Métaphysique* 21: 5–33.

145. For the background and importance of Burq's work see Anne Harrington (1988) 'Metals and magnets in medicine', *Psychological Medicine* 18: 21–38; and Anne Harrington, op. cit. (note 15), pp. 226–46.
146. J-M. Charcot (1882) 'Sur les divers états nerveux déterminés par l'hypnotisation chez les hystériques', *Comptes-Rendus Hebdomadaires de l'Académie des Sciences* 94: 403–5.
147. J-M. Charcot, op. cit. (note 9), p. 40.
148. Ibid., p. 70.
149. Ibid., p. 357.
150. Anne Harrington, op. cit. (note 15). Harrington, in her article in *The Anatomy of Madness*, cites the difference between Charcot's relationship to his patients and the more nuanced appreciation of their powers by those, such as Luys, who identified themselves with the neo-mesmeric tradition. See pp. 239–40.
151. J-M. Charcot, op. cit. (note 9), p. 290.
152. G. Gilles de la Tourette, op. cit. (note 107), p. 91.
153. J-M. Charcot, op. cit. (note 9), p. 293–4.
154. Ibid., pp. 258–9.
155. Ibid., p. 259.
156. For a bold discussion of these issues see L. J. Jordanova (ed.) (1986) *Languages of Nature: Critical Essays on Science and Literature*, London: Free Association Books.
157. J-M. Charcot, op. cit. (note 9), p. 121.
158. Ibid., p. 368.
159. Ibid., p. 369.
160. S. Freud, op. cit. (note 7), p. 12.
161. For more on this painting and the other artistic endeavours of the Salpêtrière see Nadine Simon-Dhouailly (1986) *La Leçon de Charcot: Voyage dans une Toile*, exhibition organized by the Musée de l'Assistance Publique de Paris, 17 September to 31 December 1986.
162. J-M. Charcot, op. cit. (note 9), p. 193.
163. Ibid., p. 87.
164. G. Didi-Huberman, op. cit. (note 5), p. 35, quoting the words of Albert Londe.
165. J-M. Charcot, op. cit. (note 9), p. 242.
166. Ibid., pp. 240–2.
167. Ibid., pp. 170, 172, 176, 177, 180, 181.
168. Ibid., p. 195.
169. For the contemporary discussion of what was owed to a patient's

privacy see the work of Charcot's colleague and friend, Paul Brouardel (1887) *Le Secret Médical*, Paris: J-B. Ballière et Fils, especially pp. 114–15, where he suggests that everything should be done to mask the identity of hospital patients. For a fuller history of the notion of medical confidence see Raymond Villey (1986) *Histoire du Secret Médical*, Paris: Seghers.

170. G. Didi-Huberman, op. cit. (note 5), pp. 241–5.
171. For an introduction to the many ambiguities in language and aim in Charcot's artistic programme, and more importantly, his collaborator Paul Richer, see the postscript by Georges Didi-Huberman (1984) in the reprinted edition of *Les Démoniaques dans l'Art*, Paris: Éditions Macula. As a physician, Richer ostensibly devoted himself to the exact reproduction, through the engraving of photographic plates, of the pathological traits he observed. As will be seen, he excelled in the representation of the grotesque and diseased, providing a portrait of illness which was both moving and hopefully instructive for the clinician. His art was indebted in theory and in practice to the contemporary naturalistic vogue prominent in the arts and literature. At the same time, Richer, as Didi-Huberman explains, was interested in a '*science du beau*' (p. 172) and, as an academician, was absorbed by notions of artistic canon and rules. For some examples of this work see pp. 172–3, especially the statue of the 'Tres in Una', which unmistakably falls into the *beaux-arts* tradition of the Academy.
172. J-M. Charcot, op. cit. (note 9), p. 324.
173. See Sander L. Gilman (1985) *Seeing the Insane*, New York: John Wiley and Sons.
174. For the drawings of hands see op. cit. (note 9), pp. 55, 56, 58, 59, 60, 61, 86, 102, 348; this last page of drawings is not attributed and may, therefore, not come from Richer's hand.
175. See M. Micale (1987) 'Diagnostic Discriminations: Jean-Martin Charcot and the Nineteenth-Century Idea of Masculine Hysterical Neurosis', Ph.D. dissertation, Yale University, pp. 125–98.
176. E. Showalter, op. cit. (note 4), pp. 167–94.
177. See Toby Gelfand (1989) 'Tuesdays at the Salpêtrière' (Essay Review), *Bulletin of the History of Medicine* 63: 133.
178. J-M. Charcot (1987) *Charcot the Clinician: The Tuesday Lessons, Excerpts from Nine Case Presentations on General Neurology Delivered at the Salpêtrière Hospital in 1887–88*, trans. and commentary by Christopher G. Goetz, New York: Raven Press, pp. xxiv.
179. Toby Gelfand (1988) '"Mon cher Docteur Freud": Charcot's unpublished correspondence to Freud, 1888–1893', *Bulletin of the History of Medicine* 62: 571.
180. J-M. Charcot (1886) *Neue Vorlesungen über die Krankheiten des*

Nervensystems insbesondere über Hysterie, trans. S. Freud, Leipzig and Vienna: Toeplitz and Deuticke.

181. See bibliography of Charcot's work in English translation at the end of this introduction.
182. I am indebted to Godileve van Heteren who has scoured her files in an attempt to find evidence of Savill's presence in Vienna.
183. I am once again indebted to Godileve van Heteren for the clarification of these points. See also Christopher Lawrence (1985) 'Incommunicable knowledge: science, technology and the clinical art in Britain, 1850–1914', *Journal of Contemporary History* 20: 503–20; and William Bynum (1985) 'The nervous patient in eighteenth- and nineteenth-century Britain: the psychiatric origins of British neurology', in W. F. Bynum *et al.*, op. cit. (note 15), vol. 1, pp. 89–102.
184. Thomas Dixon Savill (1908) *Clinical Lectures on Neurasthenia*, London: Henry J. Glaisher, 4th edition, p. 3.
185. Ibid., p. 7.
186. For the history of the societies and a bibliography of published works, see G. G. Meynell (1985) *The Two Sydenham Societies: A History and Bibliography of the Medical Classics Published by the Sydenham Society and the New Sydenham Society* (1844–1911), Acrise, Kent: Winterdown Books.

Charcot's works in English

(1872) *New Researches into the Pathology of Cerebral Haemorrhage*, no. trans., excerpt.

(1877) *Clinical Lectures on Diseases of the Nervous System*, vol. 1, trans. George Sigerson, London: New Sydenham Society.

(1878) *Lectures on Bright's Diseases of the Kidneys*, trans. by Henry B. Millard, New York: W. Wood & Co.

(1878) *Lectures on Localization in Diseases of the Brain*, D-M. Bourneville (ed.), trans. by Edward P. Fowler, New York: W. Wood & Co.

(1879) *Lectures on the Diseases of the Nervous System*, trans. George Sigerson, 2nd edn, Philadelphia, H. C. Lea.

(1881) *Clinical Lectures on Diseases of the Nervous System*, vol. 2, trans. George Sigerson, London: New Sydenham Society.

(1881) *Clinical Lectures on the Diseases of Old Age*, trans. Leigh H. Hunt with additional lectures by Alfred L. Loomis, New York: W. Wood & Co.

(1881) *Lectures on the Pathological Anatomy of the Nervous System. Diseases of the Spinal Cord*, trans. by Cornelius G. Comegys, Cincinnati: P. G. Thomson.
(1881) *Clinical Lectures on Senile and Chronic Diseases*, trans. William S. Tuke, London: New Sydenham Society.
(1883) *Lectures on the Localisation of Cerebral and Spinal Diseases*, trans. and ed. by Walter Baugh Hadden, London: New Sydenham Society.
(1888) *Clinical Lectures on Certain Diseases of the Nervous System*, trans. E. P. Hurd, Detroit, Michigan: G. S. Davis.
(1889) *Clinical Lectures on Diseases of the Nervous System*, trans. Thomas Savill, London: New Sydenham Society.
(1889) *On the Treatment by Suspension of Locomotor Ataxy and Some Other Spinal Afflictions*, trans. and ed. by A. de Watteville, London: D. Stott.
(1890) *Hypnotism and Crime*, [New York], [1890?], Excerpt, *The Forum*, April, 1890.
(1962) *Lectures on the Diseases of the Nervous System*, (facsimile of 1881 edition) New York: Hafner Publishing Co.
(1987) *Charcot the Clinician: The Tuesday Lessons. Excerpts from Nine Case Presentations on General Neurology delivered at the Salpêtrière Hospital in 1887–88*, trans. and ed. by Christopher G. Goetz, New York: Raven Press.

Reproductions of the works of J-M. Charcot in French

(1897) J-M. Charcot *La Foi Qui Quérit*, Paris, n.p.
(1969) J-M. Charcot *À Propos de Six Cas d'Hystérie chez l'Homme*, Paris, Théraplix.
(1971) J-M. Charcot *L'Hystérie*, É. Trillat (ed.), Paris, Privat.
(1972) J-M. Charcot *L'Hystérie chez l'Homme*, Paris, Théraplix.
(1974) J-M. Charcot *Leçons du Mardi à la Salpêtrière*, Paris, Retz.
(1984) J-M. Charcot *Leçons sur l'Hystérie Virile*, Michèle Oeurd (ed.), Paris, Le Sycomore.
(1984) J-M. Charcot and P. Richer *Les Démoniaques dans l'Art*, G. Didi-Huberman (postscript), Paris, Macula.
(1987) J-M. Charcot and V. Magnan *Inversion du Sens Génital et Autres Perversions Sexuelles*, in *Frénésie*, présentation Gérard Bonnet.

THE NEW SYDENHAM

SOCIETY.

INSTITUTED MDCCCLVIII.

VOLUME CXXVIII.

CLINICAL LECTURES

ON

DISEASES OF

THE NERVOUS SYSTEM

DELIVERED AT

THE INFIRMARY OF LA SALPÊTRIÈRE

BY

PROFESSOR J. M. CHARCOT,

PROFESSOR IN THE FACULTY OF MEDICINE OF PARIS; PHYSICIAN TO THE SALPÊTRIÈRE; MEMBER OF THE INSTITUTE, AND OF THE ACADEMY OF MEDICINE OF FRANCE; PRESIDENT OF THE SOCIÉTÉ ANATOMIQUE, ETC.

VOLUME III

(CONTAINING EIGHTY-SIX WOODCUTS).

TRANSLATED BY

THOMAS SAVILL, M.D.Lond., M.R.C.P.L.,

MEDICAL SUPERINTENDENT OF THE PADDINGTON INFIRMARY, LONDON; HONORARY MEMBER OF THE SOCIÉTÉ ANATOMIQUE, PARIS; FORMERLY ASSISTANT PHYSICIAN AND PATHOLOGIST TO THE WEST LONDON HOSPITAL.

LONDON:

THE NEW SYDENHAM SOCIETY.

1889.

TRANSLATOR'S NOTE.

THIS translation is from the first edition of the third volume of Professor Charcot's Clinical Lectures. Originally delivered as part of the course on Diseases of the Nervous System, these Lectures were edited by the Professor's pupils and with others were published first in the 'Progrès Médical.' Afterwards they were collected into a separate volume.

Many of these Lectures I had the pleasure of listening to, and have thus been enabled to reproduce them in the English language with greater precision of meaning than I should otherwise have done. And, it may be added, the attainment of this result has been further facilitated by the kindness with which Professor Charcot has answered questions upon points of difficulty or obscurity, where such have occurred. The French text is remarkable for its clearness and force of expression, in spite of the complexity of some of the subjects treated; and it has been my desire to preserve these qualities in the translation.

THOMAS SAVILL.

CONTENTS.

LECTURE I.

INTRODUCTORY.

LECTURE II.

ON THE MUSCULAR ATROPHY THAT FOLLOWS CERTAIN JOINT LESIONS.

LECTURE III.

I. CONTRACTURES OF TRAUMATIC ORIGIN.
II. TIC NON-DOULOUREUX OF THE FACE IN A HYSTERICAL SUBJECT.

LECTURE IV.

ON THE MUSCULAR ATROPHY WHICH FOLLOWS CHRONIC ARTICULAR RHEUMATISM.

LECTURE V.

I. REFLEX CONTRACTURE AND AMYOTROPHY OF ARTICULAR ORIGIN.
II. OPHTHALMIC MIGRAINE APPEARING IN THE EARLY STAGE OF GENERAL PARALYSIS.

LECTURE VI.

ON HYSTERIA IN BOYS.

LECTURE VII.

TWO CASES OF HYSTERICAL CONTRACTURE OF TRAUMATIC ORIGIN.

LECTURE VIII.

TWO CASES OF HYSTERICAL CONTRACTURE OF TRAUMATIC ORIGIN (*continued*).

LECTURE IX.

ON A CASE OF SPINAL AFFECTION CONSEQUENT ON A CONTUSION OF THE SCIATIC NERVE.

LECTURE X.

I. DOUBLE SCIATICA IN A WOMAN AFFLICTED WITH CANCER.

II. CERVICAL PACHYMENINGITIS.

LECTURE XI.

ON A CASE OF WORD-BLINDNESS.

LECTURE XII.

ON WORD-BLINDNESS (*continued*).

LECTURE XIII.

ON A CASE OF SUDDEN AND ISOLATED SUPPRESSION OF THE MENTAL VISION OF SIGNS AND OBJECTS (FORMS AND COLOURS).

LECTURE XIV.

NOSOGRAPHICAL REVISION OF THE AMYOTROPHIES.

LECTURE XV.

TREMORS AND CHOREÏFORM MOVEMENTS.—RHYTHMICAL CHOREA.

LECTURE XVIII.

CONCERNING SIX CASES OF HYSTERIA IN THE MALE.

LECTURE XIX.

CONCERNING SIX CASES OF HYSTERIA IN THE MALE (*continued*).

LECTURE XX.

ON TWO CASES OF HYSTERICAL BRACHIAL MONOPLEGIA IN THE MALE OF TRAUMATIC ORIGIN.—HYSTERO-TRAUMATIC MONOPLEGIA.

LECTURE XXI.

ON TWO CASES OF HYSTERICAL BRACHIAL MONOPLEGIA IN THE MALE DUE TO INJURY.—HYSTERO-TRAUMATIC MONOPLEGIA (*continued*).

LECTURE XXII.

ON TWO CASES OF HYSTERICAL BRACHIAL MONOPLEGIA IN THE MALE (*continued*).

LECTURE XXIII.

ON A CASE OF HYSTERICAL HIP DISEASE IN A MAN, RESULTING FROM INJURY.

LECTURE XXIV.

ON A CASE OF HYSTERICAL HIP DISEASE IN A MAN, RESULTING FROM INJURY (*continued*).

LECTURE XXV.

THE CASE OF SPASMODIC CONTRACTURE OF THE UPPER EXTREMITY OCCURRING IN A MAN AFTER THE APPLICATION OF A SPLINT.

LIST OF WOODCUTS.

LECTURE I.

INTRODUCTORY.

SUMMARY.—*Foundation of the clinical professorship of diseases of the nervous system.—Means of study: The Infirmary, out-patient department, laboratories.—Is it legitimate to make the teaching of neuro-pathology a special branch of medicine?—Relation of anatomical and physiological sciences to pathology.—Conditions by which those relations should be controlled.—Nosological method of study.—Anatomo-clinical method.—Functional diseases of the nervous system obey common physiological laws.—Difficulties of their study.—Simulation.*

I.

GENTLEMEN,—It is now nearly twelve years ago that in recommencing within these walls a course of instruction, which had already existed for four years, I ventured to hope that this great asylum of human miseries, where so many leaders of French medicine had achieved distinction, would become one day a properly organised centre for the teaching and investigation of diseases of the nervous system.

Where is there to be found, I asked, so much material specially adapted to this kind of study? And I pointed out that very simple modifications in the internal arrangements of the establishment would enable us to realise its value to the fullest extent.

Since then I have never ceased to enunciate these views, to establish their truth by every means in my power (both in my lectures, and by published works in which I have received the assistance of my pupils), and to declare to the world the vast material wealth that exists in this institution.

You are aware, gentlemen, that at length our wishes have been realised beyond my most sanguine expectations; and now, after seventeen years of private initiative, I recommence this course in the name of the Faculty of Medicine of Paris.

At the inauguration to-day, of the Clinical Chair of Diseases of the Nervous System, my first words, which are not without emotion I admit, must be expressive of gratitude towards those who have created it, and who have confided it to my care. Let me thank the Chamber that originated the project, the Minister of Public Instruction who promoted it, and my colleagues of the Faculty who, consulted as to the advisability of its creation, returned a favourable verdict, giving me thereby a proof of their estimation, by which I am profoundly touched.

Next, I eagerly embrace the opportunity of publicly testifying the gratitude we feel, both to the Municipal Council of the City of Paris, and also to the Administration of Public Assistance, whose prompt and liberal aid has rendered possible a scheme which without it would have encountered obstacles well-nigh insurmountable. Thanks to their help, which really took place prior to the approval of the University, we are already in possession of appliances and conveniences that form a veritable Neuro-pathological Institution.

Finally, gentlemen, it is incumbent on me to perform a duty that I find particularly pleasant, and which revives the happy friendships of days gone by. I refer to those who have done me the honour to call themselves my pupils—all of whom have now become masters, or are on the road thereto—and would offer them once more the assurance of my lively and sincere attachment, and exhort them to rejoice with us in the success of the work in which they have largely participated.

II.

I have just alluded, gentlemen, to the important modifications which, with the concurrence of the Administrator of Public Assistance, and the Municipal Council, have been gradually introduced into the department that I direct, and I will now ask your permission to enter into the question in more detail. This will give me the opportunity of indicating the benefits arising from the installation of the new professorship in the Infirmary.

This large group of buildings, as you know, contains a population of over 5000 persons, among whom are a large number that come under the denomination of incurables, and who pass the latter part of their lives here. They are subjects affected with every kind of chronic maladies, and particularly with diseases of the nervous system. Such is the quantity of material, albeit of a peculiar character, which has formed the only basis all these years of our pathological researches and our clinical teaching.

The classes which can be carried on under such conditions are surely not to be despised. The clinical types of disease which come under observation are illustrated by such numerous examples that we are enabled to take at one time a comprehensive view of an affection; and from such a vantage ground, so to speak, that the gaps made by time in this or that catagory are lost sight of. In other words, we are in possession of a sort of *living pathological museum* whose resources are almost inexhaustible.

It is true that we sometimes miss the beginnings of disease; but, on the other hand, we gain by being enabled to investigate after death the lesions which correspond to the symptoms studied minutely, and over a long period of time, during life. And who, I would ask, does not recognise the decisive influence which microscopic investigations, based on the anatomo-clinical method, have had on the progress of neuro-pathology?

The weak side of the situation which I have just indicated is too striking not to be at once apparent. In an

Infirmary, generally speaking, the well-marked cases, the so-called incurable ones, are alone admitted; the slighter and more trivial cases are not seen. And thus one is scarcely able to observe those delicate symptomatic shades, which ofttimes alone mark the onset of certain chronic diseases. And again, what hope is there of curing or alleviating our patient when the evil has, through long years, taken root in the organism, and already resisted appropriate medication?

These, then, are the chief imperfections. It was possible to remedy them by instituting, at the entrance to the Infirmary buildings, an *out-patient department,* with a dispensary attached. It was hoped that the *chronic sufferers,* who often have a difficulty in obtaining admission to the hospitals, and who even then do not invariably find the means of treatment appropriate to their state, would flock to such an institution in great numbers. In these expectations we have not been disappointed. The department has been working for two years, and cases which interest us, by reason of the special direction of our studies, have come in large numbers. I shall have many opportunities in these lectures of presenting to you those who come to the Infirmary as out-patients. These persons do not object to clinical demonstrations upon their cases; quite the contrary. They understand that the more minutely and the more thoroughly they are investigated, so much the greater is the chance of their cure or alleviation.

To make this department perfect and complete, it yet required space within the Infirmary where certain of the patients, who come to us from outside, could be temporarily admitted as in-patients. This concession we asked for many times, and at length the difficulties in the way of its achievement were surmounted. Happily for our cause it met with the support of the Director of the Public Assistance. All the obstacles were one by one removed, and now we have wards for the temporary admission of cases. They contain eighty beds—forty for women and forty for men. I know not how to thank M. Quentin for the earnestness with which he has seconded our efforts.

Thus, to the Infirmary is added an Out-patient department, and to this, hospital-wards.[1] All forms a complete whole, of which the different parts are intimately connected, and which now supplement our other means of teaching and research.

We possess a *Pathological Museum*, to which is attached a *studio for moulding and photography;* a well-fitted *Laboratory* of pathological anatomy and physiology, which is in strange contrast with the narrow, badly-lighted room, that was the only resort where I and my pupils worked, and which we dignified by the name of "laboratory," for nearly fifteen years; an *Ophthalmological room*, necessary complement to a neuro-pathological laboratory; and the *Lecture Hall*, in which I have the honour of receiving you to-day, and which is provided, as you see, with all the modern apparatus for demonstration.

We possess, moreover, a service richly endowed with all the apparatus necessary for the practice of *electro-diagnosis* and *electro-therapy;* and here numerous patients come, three times a week, to receive the treatment appropriate to their condition.

The valued assistance which my friend M. Lebas, Superintendent of the Infirmary, has rendered to us in these arrangements, is truly beyond all praise.

You see, gentlemen, the luxurious means of study that have been placed in our hands. It is for us now to turn them to account. So far as I am concerned, albeit that I have arrived at an epoch of life when the sun has passed its zenith, I hope to find enough energy still to enable me to accomplish the task.

III.

I have still, gentlemen, to make a few remarks touching the objections, the doubts, relative to questions of principle, which on the creation of the new Chair have undoubtedly presented themselves to the minds of many.

One is sure to be asked, for example, whether the official consecration of one more speciality is an event that is both

[1] Limited to the reception of diseases of the nervous system.

desirable and legitimate; and whether, if such a path were once marked out, the unity of our science might not be imperilled thereby. To this it can be briefly replied, that in the science of medicine in the present day, analysis is becoming more and more penetrating, and multiplies without ceasing the number of facts; and inasmuch as our faculties of assimilation and our power of work do not develop *pari passu;* no one could seriously pretend to embrace and to fathom the whole of the science at one time. Specialisation has therefore become an inevitable necessity. One must accept it because it cannot be averted.

Still it is important to place a limit on the indiscriminate cutting up of the science and the barren isolation of specialities, so as not to go to the other extreme, which would certainly be deplorable. I would point out that an organization having this object, already exists, so far as concerns education, in that our Faculty requires from its Fellows, from amongst whom the Professoriate is recruited, a knowledge of every branch, every department.

Moreover, the danger which would attach to a narrow specialism is scarcely to be feared in the territory of neuropathology, for that domain has to-day become, no one thinks of denying it, one of the most extensive that exist. It is one of those specialities which become enriched most rapidly; one, the cultivation of which requires from those who devote themselves to it, the widest and most general knowledge. It is then legitimate that henceforth the pathology of the nervous system should absorb all the efforts of those who would study it; and that it should claim a place among the other separate branches which, like it, by the force of circumstances, are already detached from the bosom of general medicine.

Another consideration of value in reference to the foundation of the new Professoriate, is that France has often taken the initiative in the scientific evolution which during the last thirty years has defined the limits of nerve pathology, and has thus, so to speak, rendered it a legitimate speciality. Ought she not to continue the work, or should she leave other countries to make advances in her domain?

To promote this object it was necessary to place in the

hands of a certain number of workers all the means of keeping abreast with the times. This could only be done by creating an official Chair for teaching the diseases of the nervous system; because, only an official Professoriate could worthily respond, by reason of its privileges and its duties, to the wants of education, and the exigencies of scientific progress.

IV.

It seems to me useless to enlarge on this apology for the new institution any further, or to mention any other arguments in favour of its cause. And now we must devote ourselves, as in former inaugural lectures, to initiating those who have not done us the honour of attending before, into the methods of the course, which, although of long standing, is officially confided to me for the first time to-day.

In the first place, let me again remind you that in this place we shall have to deal with clinical, or, in other words, purely practical work. That is to say, we shall always have before us a particular case, or a patient whom we wish to cure, or at any rate to alleviate. But this end, gentlemen, can only be attained by the application of information previously acquired in the different branches of medicine. True practice has nothing of autonomy in it; it lives by ideas derived from previous experience and their appropriate application. Without continual scientific renovation it would soon become a barren and stereotyped routine. It can, moreover, be affirmed, in my opinion, that apart from operations requiring dexterity, ingenuity, and other native qualities, which without doubt become perfect only by repetition, and which cannot indeed be acquired otherwise, one can affirm, I say, that the greater the pathologist the greater the physician.

This subject, therefore, before being examined practically, can be discussed, briefly at any rate, from a scientific standpoint.

In this respect, gentlemen, I must be allowed once more to declare my firm belief that the wide intervention of the anatomical and physiological sciences in the affairs of medicine is an essential condition to progress; a statement which, by frequent repetition, has verily by this time become almost a platitude.

But the point that I wish specially to insist on is this; in order that the intervention of these sciences may be legitimate, and really fruitful, it should take place under conditions which should never be forgotten. Allow me to recall to your minds the opinion which that most illustrious physiologist, Claude Bernard, thus expressed:—"*Pathology,*" said he, "*should not be subordinated to physiology. Quite the reverse. Set up first the medical problem which arises from the observation of a malady, and afterwards seek for a physiological explanation. To act otherwise would be to risk overlooking the patient, and distorting the malady.*" These are excellent words, which I have ventured to quote verbatim, because they are absolutely significant. They enable us to clearly understand that the whole domain of pathology appertains strictly to the physician, who alone can cultivate it and make it fruitful, and that it necessarily remains closed to the physiologist who, systematically confined within the precincts of his laboratory, disdains the teaching of the hospital ward.

The method most suitable to the exploration of the vast domains of pathology can be described as the *nosological.* It is, in fact, the traditional method, for it is the one which, ever since medicine has existed, has been employed to investigate morbid states, to determine their characteristics, their causation, their correlations, and the modifications which they undergo by the influence of therapeutic agents. And facts of this kind, gentlemen, I beg you to observe, necessarily constitute the very foundation of every scientific construction in pathology, and without this basis the physiology of disease would be but a vain phrase.

If it is necessary, in the category of diseases of the nervous system, to show all the power of this method, it will suffice to recall a portion of the inimitable work of that great representative of French neuro-pathology, Duchenne (of Boulogne). Without doubt his admirable study of muscular movements, made by the aid of localised electricity, could be, up to a certain point, claimed by the science of physiology. But it is not so with his grand discovery of those types of disease termed progressive muscular atrophy, infantile paralysis, pseudo-hypertrophic paralysis, glosso-laryngeal paralysis, and locomotor ataxy. These results, undoubtedly the greatest achievements of his work, because they filled spaces hitherto empty, or occupied only by confused ideas, with animated living shapes, concrete realities, recognised by all; these results, I say, were accomplished entirely by the nosological method.[1]

V.

But this method need not necessarily be restricted to the observation of the outward manifestation of disease; it can, without changing its character, be appropriately applied in exploring the domain of morbid anatomy by following the patient into the post-mortem room.

It is often said that the progress of medicine and of pathological anatomy go side by side. This is specially true in diseases of the nervous system. One example will suffice to show that the discovery of a constant lesion in maladies of this kind is the result of such a co-operation.

The description given by Duchenne (of Boulogne) of locomotor ataxy, is most striking and vivid. It rightly takes rank as a masterpiece. However, there existed for a long time a hesitation in the minds of many about accepting the disease as a real entity until the spinal lesion, which had already been described some years before by Cruveilhier, was known to be associated with this group of symptoms.

Some authors still continued to believe that the affection was functional in its origin. But all illusions of this kind vanished when it became realised that there existed, even in

[[1] The word *nosological* in English refers simply to the nomenclature and classification of disease, but it is the clinical method of investigation in its widest sense which is here implied; or that method of investigation which argues from effect to cause, commencing with a study of disease at the bedside, as distinguished from the converse method of *a priori* reasoning, with the teachings of physiology for its basis.—S.]

the earliest stages of the disease, an exact and easily recognised anatomical change, an anatomical lesion which could be detected even in the slight and aberrant forms of the disease. And it was thus, by this linking of the clinical and the anatomical features, that the different varieties came to be grouped around, and classified with, the ordinary well-marked type which alone had been indicated in Duchenne's classical description.

In this case as in very many others, it is the intervention of pathological anatomy which gives the truly practical character. It furnishes to nosography more fixed, more material characters than appertain to the symptoms alone; and thus one does not fail to grasp the nature of the connections which unite the lesions to the outward signs.

Without detracting from the importance of the results obtained in this way, it is certain that the study of morbid lesions can be utilised in another way, and from a higher standpoint; more scientific if you like. It can, when the circumstances are favourable, furnish the basis of a physiological interpretation of normal or of morbid phenomena,

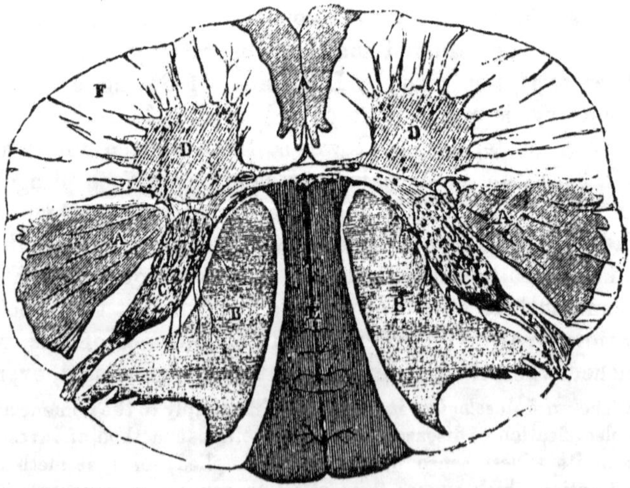

FIG. I.—A, A, lateral columns; A′, bands of Türck; B, B, posterior root zones; C, C, posterior horns; D, D, anterior horns; F, anterior root zone; E, columns of Goll.

and at the same time, as a natural consequence, give to diagnosis more penetration and exactitude.

I show you here a diagram (Fig. 1) which represents, after a fashion, the rudiments of the new spinal pathology. Here you see that the cord is divided into much more numerous regions than were formerly known by the agency of anatomy and experimental physiology alone. This is the work of the anatomo-clinical method of study. Each of these regions can be separately diseased without involvement of the neighbouring regions, and they have thus been isolated, after the manner of a successful vivisection; and to each of these circumscribed lesions there corresponds a particular symptomatology, which reveals, to a certain extent, the special functions belonging to the affected structures. Thus, we learn that the pyramidal bands are almost exclusively composed of fibres which transmit impulses from the brain directly to the cord, and by its mediation to the limbs; that the motor cells of the anterior horns hold under their control the nutrition of corresponding muscles; that the anterior horns have nothing to do with the transmission of sensitive impressions, &c. Here, then, physiology and pathology become as it were linked together.

Some analogous results have been obtained by the application of this same anatomo-clinical method to the study of localisation in the bulb, and in the cerebral hemispheres, but I will limit myself to a few remarks on this latter point.

You are aware that on the question of cerebral localisation much uncertainty exists at the present time amongst different physiologists; some deny emphatically that which others, with no less authority, affirm. We pathologists look on at these debates, not with indifference by any means, but at the same time calmly, waiting with patience until an agreement may be arrived at.

In fact, the means of research employed by us, such as I have described, have thus far put us in possession of a certain number of fundamental facts relative to man, against which the data furnished by vivisection would never prevail. Thus we know from reliable pathological observations that a destructive lesion of the pyramidal band in its progress through the capsule in front of the knee, produces ordinary permanent hemiplegia: that the destructive lesions of the posterior extremity of the internal capsule produces corresponding cerebral hemianæsthesia. As for the surface of the hemispheres one need scarcely discuss in the present day the pathological *rôle* of Broca's convolution. We know that destruction of the convolutions of the motor zone produces, if it be general, complete hemiplegia, or, on the other hand, a monoplegia only, if the lesion be circumscribed to this or that region. To the irritative lesions of these parts are attached the phenomena of partial epilepsy. Without doubt, these facts of localisation do not as yet furnish us with the elements of a fixed doctrine concerning the physiological functions of diverse cerebral regions, but, such as they are, they form most valuable landmarks for the guidance of the physician through the difficult paths of diagnosis.

VI.

From what has been said it will be understood how much importance we ought to accord in our studies to the anatomo-pathological method of research. But you are aware, gentlemen, that there still exists at the present time a great number of morbid states, evidently having their seat in the nervous system, which leave in the dead body no material trace that can be discovered. Epilepsy, hysteria, even the most inveterate cases, chorea, and many other morbid states which would take us too long to enumerate, come to us like so many Sphynx, which deny the most penetrating anatomical investigations. These symptomatic combinations deprived of anatomical substratum, do not present themselves to the mind of the physician with that appearance of solidity, of objectivity, which belong to affections connected with an appreciable organic lesion.

There are some even who see in several of these affections only an assemblage of odd incoherent phenomena inaccessible to analysis, and which had better, perhaps, be banished to the category of the unknown. It is hysteria which especially comes under this sort of proscription. But such a verdict, on no matter how great authority, would never suffice to illuminate the nosological framework. We ought rather to make the best of things as we find them, and not allow ourselves to be disheartened by the difficulties they present. Moreover, gentlemen, it is the merely superficial observation that leads men to the opinion I have just mentioned; a more attentive study makes us to see things under an altogether different aspect; and much credit is due to Briquet for having established in his excellent book, in a manner beyond dispute, that hysteria is governed, in the same way as other morbid conditions, by rules and laws, which attentive and sufficiently numerous observations always permit us to establish. Allow me to mention but one example, to recall to your minds the description of an attack of hysteria major [la grande attaque hystérique], which is reduced at the present time to a very simple formula. Four periods succeed each other in the complete attack with mechanical regularity—1st, epileptoid; 2nd, great movements (struggling, purposeless); 3rd, passionate attitudes (purposive); 4th, terminal delirium. But the attacks may be incomplete, each of the periods may appear alone, or again one or two among them will be found wanting. We understand thus how many varieties can result from these combinations; but it will always be easy to those who possess the formula to bring them under one fundamental type.

This is interesting to the physician in the highest degree, who learns thus to take his bearings in what appears to be an inextricable labyrinth. But that which I am most concerned to demonstrate here is that in the attack, and I could almost say as much of the other phases of hysteria, nothing is left to chance, everything follows definite rules,—always the same, whether the case is met with in private or hospital practice, in all countries, all times, all races, in short universally.

There is another important fact in the history of neuroses[1] in general, and of hysteria in particular, which clearly shows that these diseases do not form, in pathology, a class apart, governed by other physiological laws than the common ones.

[[1] Diseases of the nervous system apparently due to functional or dynamic causes; which are not, so far as we know, attended by any organic lesion.—S.]

It is that their symptomatology approaches, and often very exactly, to that which belongs to maladies having organic lesions ; and this resemblance is at times so striking that it renders their diagnosis extremely difficult. It is sometimes designated by the name of *neuromimesis*—this property which functional diseases have of resembling organic ones. Between the hæmianæsthesia so common in hysteria and that which arises from a central lesion, the analogy is very striking. There is the same resemblance between the spasmodic paraplegia of hysteria, and that which arises from an organic spinal lesion (rigidity, exaggeration of tendon-reflexes, loss of power without loss of muscular substance). Now this resemblance, often so disheartening to the physician, should serve as a guide to the pathologist who, besides the similarity in the group of symptoms, perceives a similarity in the anatomical seat, and *mutatis mutandis*, localises the dynamic lesion from the data furnished by an examination of the corresponding organic one.

Thus are we brought to recognise that the principles which govern pathology as a whole are applicable to neuroses, and that here also one should endeavour to complete clinical observation by anatomical and physiological investigation.

VII.

While I am speaking to you of the difficulties that the physician encounters in the study of neuroses, and of the means at his disposal for surmounting these obstacles, there is yet one point that I would wish, before finishing, to draw your special attention to. I mean *simulation*. Not that *imitation* of one malady by another, of which we spoke just now, but of intentional simulation, voluntary, in which the patient exaggerates real symptoms, or again creates all at once an imaginary group of symptoms. In fact, we all know that the desire to deceive, even without interest, by a kind of disinterested worship of art for its own sake [culte de l'art pour l'art], though sometimes with the idea of making a sensation, to excite pity, &c., is a common enough occurrence, particularly in hysteria.

Here is an element that we meet with at each step in the clinique of this neurosis, and which throws (there is no use in denying it) a certain amount of disfavour on the studies which are connected with it. But in the present day, when the history of hysteria has been so often scrutinised, ransacked so thoroughly, is it really as difficult as some appear to believe, to discern the real symptomatology from the imaginary? By no means, gentlemen, and not to deal with generalities any longer, permit me now to present to you a concrete example, chosen from many others, and calculated, if I do not mistake, to support the theory that I defend.

The example I allude to is the condition of catalepsy, produced by hypnotisation, in certain subjects of hysteria. The question is this: Can this state be simulated in such a way as to deceive the physician? It is generally believed that if,

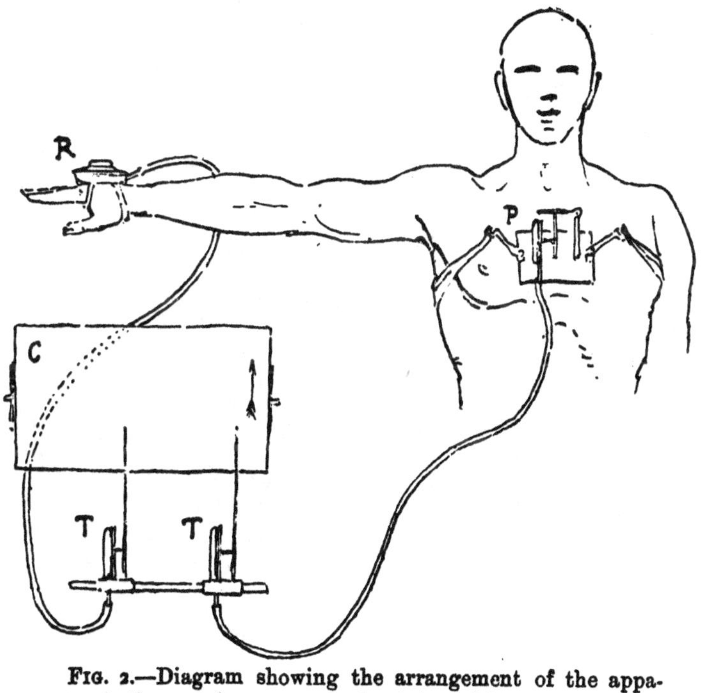

FIG. 2.—Diagram showing the arrangement of the apparatus in the experiments on cataleptic immobility. R, pressure drum of Marey; P, pneumographe; C, revolving cylinder; T, T, stylographs.

one arm of a patient in a state of catalepsy be horizontally extended, this attitude can be preserved for such a length of time that the duration alone suffices to remove all suspicion of simulation. However, our observations throw doubt on this. At the end of ten or fifteen minutes the limb begins to fall, and, at the end of twenty or twenty-five minutes at the maximum, it has fallen into the vertical position. Now these are precisely the same limits that a vigorous man, trying to keep the same position, can also reach. We must, therefore, seek some other distinguishing feature.

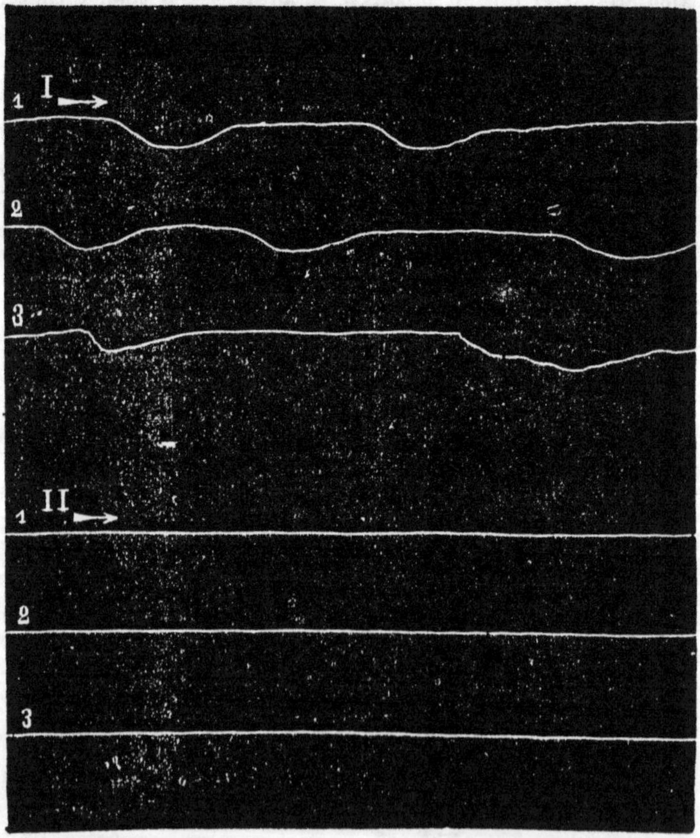

FIG. 3.—Tracings obtained from a hystero-epileptic in a state of hypnotic catalepsy. I, pneumographic tracing; II, tracing of pressure drum. Read from left to right in order 1, 2, 3.

With the healthy subject, as with the cataleptic, a pressure drum fixed at the extremity of the out-stretched limb (Fig. 2 R) will serve to register the least oscillations of the arm, meanwhile a pneumograph applied to chest (Fig. 2 P) will give the curve of the respiratory movements.

Now, I show you here, in an abridged form, what is seen in the tracings thus obtained. In the cataleptic, during the whole time of the experiment, the pen, which corresponds to the extended limb, traces a perfectly straight, regular line (Fig. 3, II).

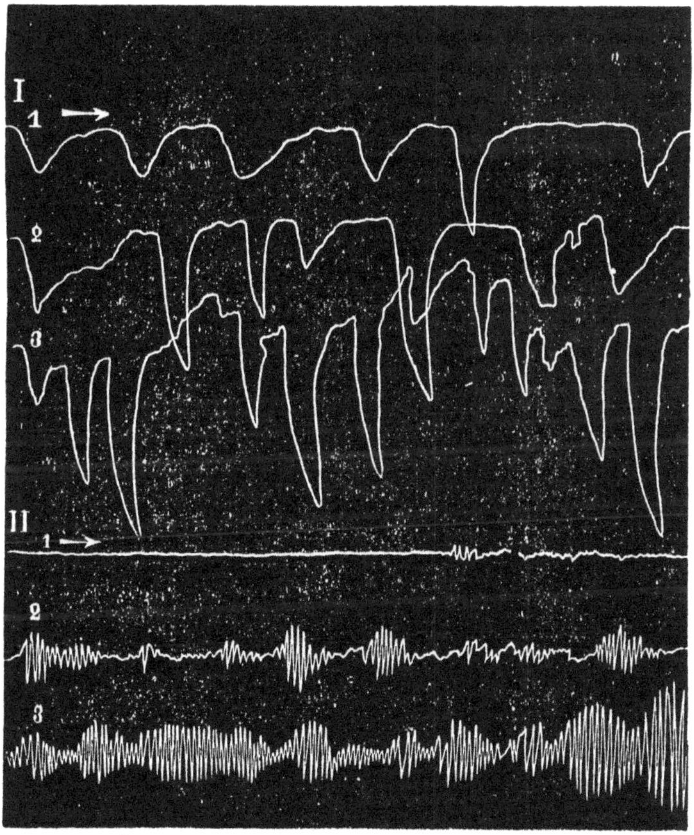

FIG. 4.—Diagram of tracings obtained from a man who attempted to maintain the cataleptic attitude. I, respiratory curve; II, tracing of the pressure drum. Read from left to right in order 1, 2, 3.

In a person who simulates, the corresponding tracing resembles at first that of the cataleptic, but at the end of a few minutes considerable differences will be seen; the straight line becomes crooked, very undulating, marked in places by large oscillations arranged in series (Fig. 4, II).

Nor are the tracings furnished by the pneumograph less significant. In the cataleptic the respiration is slow and superficial, but the end of the tracing resembles the commencement (Fig. 3, I). In the healthy person the tracing is composed of two distinct phases. At the outset, respiration is regular and normal. In the second phase there is irregularity in the rhythm, and prolongation of the respiratory movements, corresponding to the indications of muscular fatigue noted in the tracing of the limb; then deep and rapid depressions, showing the disturbance of respiration which accompanies the phenomenon of effort (Fig. 4, I).

In short you see that the *cataleptic patient* is unacquainted with fatigue; the muscles yield, but without effort, without voluntary intervention of any sort. On the other hand, the *man who simulates* succumbs under the double test, and finds himself betrayed on both sides at the same time: 1st, By the tracing given by the limb, which reveals the muscular fatigue; and 2nd, By the respiratory curve, which betrays the effort made to hide its effects.

It is useless to insist further. A hundred other examples might be invoked which would only show that the simulation, which is talked about so much when hysteria and allied affections are under consideration, is, in the actual state of our knowledge, only a bugbear, before which the fearful and novice alone are stopped. For the future it ought to be the province of the physician, well-informed in these matters, to dissipate chicanery wherever it occurs; and to sort out the symptoms which form a fundamental part of the malady, from those which are simulated, and added to it, by the artifice of the patient.

And thus do we approach, with prudence no doubt, but also with confidence, the study of these dreaded maladies, permeated, as we are, with the surety of the methods of observation we have at hand.

Time presses, and I must conclude. I shall be happy if, in to-day's sketch, I have been able to make you see the ideal towards which our efforts tend. In the solution of the problems that lie before us, all the branches and all the laws of biological science, mutually supporting and controlling each other, will be brought under contribution. But I maintain that the preponderating *rôle*, the governing and guiding principle of all, belongs to clinical observation.

In making this declaration, I am but following the precepts, and placing myself under the protection, of the classic masters of the French School; whose teachings have shed so much lustre on the Paris Faculty of Medicine, to which I count it an honour to belong.

LECTURE II.

ON THE MUSCULAR ATROPHY THAT FOLLOWS CERTAIN JOINT LESIONS.

SUMMARY.—*Traumatic joint disease, and the paralysis and muscular atrophy which follow it.—Modification in the faradic and galvanic contractility.—Contractions produced by the electric spark.—Exaggeration of tendon-reflexes.—Simple muscular atrophy.—No relation necessary between the intensity of the joint-affection and that of the paralytic and atrophic phenomena.—The extensor muscles of the articulation are most affected.—The muscular lesions are dependent on a deuteropathic spinal affection.*

GENTLEMEN,—On account of its origin, the affection from which the patient, who is about to be presented to you, is suffering would be called surgical; it was undoubtedly an injury which gave rise to it. As a matter of fact the arthritis which was the immediate consequence of the injury has ceased to exist; but the same accident gave rise also to a spinal affection of a peculiar kind which still persists, and on this account the patient claims our attention and assistance at the present time.

The man B—, aged 23 years, a telegraph clerk, has always had good health, and presents nothing of interest in his antecedents other than the fact that his maternal uncle had to be placed in an asylum on account of mental derangement. He is brought before you in bed, although he is quite able to get up and walk, because I wish in the first place to point out certain particulars which cannot well be observed unless the patient is lying down.

You will notice, firstly, that his general condition is excellent, he is healthy looking, the appetite is good, and all the organic functions act well. The only affection with which he is troubled is a disturbance in the walk, and it is, as you will see, in the right leg, or rather certain of its muscles, where the power is wanting. This difficulty of walking has existed for about one year.

A methodical examination reveals the following facts: when the patient is in bed, the right inferior extremity can execute all the natural movements excepting one, extension of the leg on the thigh. Movements of abduction and adduction of the thigh, flexion of thigh on pelvis, or leg on thigh, and all the movements of the foot on the leg, are free; but extension of the leg is wanting. Thus, when he wishes to straighten the leg after it has been previously placed in a position of semiflexion, he tries to do so by slipping the heel along the bed, or else he aids it with his hands, or the other foot. It is, you see, the extensors of the leg which are at fault, that is, the muscles which are supplied by the crural nerve, and it is especially the quadriceps extensor muscle which is affected.

The patient can oppose, although with less force than the healthy limb, passive movements of extension and flexion made at the foot or hip-joints; he can resist the strongest possible attempts made to straighten the bent knee; but he offers but feeble resistance to passive flexion of the leg on the thigh.

In the main, although there may be some relative weakness of nearly all the muscles of the lower limbs, it is chiefly the power of the quadriceps that is wanting at the present time.

This paralysis, limited to the extensors of the right knee, is shown again when the patient gets out of bed and attempts to walk.

He raises the right leg by the aid of the left foot to make up for the deficient power of extension of the right knee. He walks without support, but you notice something peculiar in his mode of progression; some of you will see also that he has much improved during the last few days; although the characters of the gait are still present, they were much more marked when he came in. Nevertheless, even now, you can see that at each step forward, although the left knee bends and straightens alternately, the right knee has hardly any such movement, all movement is in the hip; the right leg seems as if it were too long, and performs a movement of circumduction all in one piece, as if the knee-joint did not exist. Formerly, the extremity of the foot had a tendency to drop, which rendered walking still more difficult; the paresis of the muscles which bend the foot on the leg has since disappeared.

It is important to remark that there is no pain whatever on movement, such as could produce the difficulty of progression; the articulation also is perfectly free; it is in the nervous system, or in the muscles, that one must seek for the cause of this feebleness.

By a more attentive examination of the affected limb we become aware of some other important facts. In the first place you will find a diminution of volume of the entire limb, which was formerly more pronounced than it is now.

These are the measurements:

	Right.	Left.
Upper part of thigh . . .	48 cm.	52 cm.
Just above knee	37 cm.	38 cm.
Centre of calf	33 cm.	35 cm.

But, even without measurement, it is evident that the anterior surface of the right thigh is considerably flattened, it is almost hollow; the muscles of this region, moreover, are without substance and flaccid even at the moment of contraction. There is then, not only a paresis, but also an alteration of nutrition, an atrophy of the quadriceps muscle. It is possible that the right thigh and knee are relatively colder; but there is no marked alteration of the cutaneous sensibility.

To complete the description, let me add the results of electrical exploration, which reveals the state of nutrition of the muscles. At the time when he came in, eight days ago, (1) galvanic and faradic excitation of the crural nerve in the groin gave scarcely any contraction; (2) Faradisation over the points of election with completely enclosed bobbins (Du Bois-Reymond's apparatus), produced little if any reaction; the muscles might indeed have been absent. One would, after discovering this latter result, have expected to find that galvanism produced the reaction observed when the nutrition of muscles is profoundly affected, such as takes place in experimental section of the nerves, or in infantile paralysis, when there is destruction of the motor cells, or again, in severe facial paralysis. In such cases, one finds what is called in electro-diagnosis the reaction of degeneration, *i. e.* increased galvanic excitability, concurrently with a diminution or absence of faradic excitability; well, here it was not so; the galvanic current, even with fifty elements and with no matter what arrangement of poles, gave no greater contraction than the faradic current. Hence, there was a quantitative, and not a qualitative reaction; and one could conclude from this that we had before us a simple and not a degenerative atrophy.[1]

Moreover, here is a curious circumstance. This muscle which remains almost inert under the influence of the will, or under ordinary electrical excitation (whether direct or indirect, faradic or galvanic) of the nerve, contracts energetically enough when the patient, being placed on the insulated stool of a static electrical machine, is made to receive a spark either in the centre of the rectus femoris, or of the vastus internus (the vastus externus is an exception in that it has preserved a certain degree of galvanic and faradic excitability). It should be added that a sharp blow on the body of the rectus muscle produces a distinct contraction, and that percussion of the patella tendon determines very pronounced tremor, not only in the limb struck, but general, and even manifest in the two upper extremities, especially the left one. Percussion of the left patella tendon produces tremors equally intense. No trepidation can be elicited by a sudden bending of the point of the foot, either in the right or left lower extremity.

All the other muscles of the limb present normal electrical

[1] M. Rümpf has studied, under Professor Erb, the electrical reaction of muscles in cases of joint disease (of shoulder, knee, &c.). He found, and his observations were amply confirmed by those of Erb, that in these cases there is a simple diminution of electrical excitability, and never a qualitative modification, which absolutely distinguishes simple muscular atrophy from degenerative atrophy.

reactions. It was not, however, according to the patient's account, always so. Thus at one time the cheeks and the front muscles of the legs did not contract equally on the two sides, but lately he has improved. At no time has there existed any trouble of micturition or defæcation.

We must now seek for the cause and significance of all these phenomena. In summing up the whole, this patient is afflicted with paralysis, accompanied by simple atrophy, almost exclusively localised to the extensors of the thigh, and also by a profound modification, quantitative only and not qualitative, in the electric contractility.

The localisation of these troubles will help to guide us to a diagnosis. We know now, after oft-repeated observations,[1] that atrophic paralysis of the extensor muscles (or at least predominating in the extensor muscles) is a frequent complication of different idiopathic or traumatic lesions affecting the corresponding articulation: thus, one not infrequently sees atrophy of the deltoid muscle after different lesions of the scapulo-humeral articulation; or as a consequence of an arthritis, sprain, or other injury of the hip-joint, the buttock is sometimes affected in the same manner; or if it be the knee-joint which is attacked, the nutrition and mobility of the quadriceps extensor femoris is affected.

These facts, which were known to Hunter and Paget have been worked out in greater detail in later years by M. Ollivier, by M. Le Fort, and in the valuable memoir of M. Valtat, where it is shown experimentally in animals (guinea-pigs and dogs) that after inflammation of the knee-joint, artificially produced by the use of irritating injections, all the muscles of the limb are affected, but more especially

[1] J. Hunter, 'Œuvres complètes,' trad. Richelot, T. I, p. 581, Paris, 1839. A. Ollivier, 'Des atrophies musculaires,' Thèse agrég., 1869. Le Fort, 'Soc. de Chir.,' 1872. Sabourin, 'De l'atrophie musculaire rheumatismale,' Thèse de 1873. J. Paget, 'Leçons de Clinique Chirurgicale,' trad. Petit, 1877. E. Valtat, 'De l'atrophie musculaire consécutive aux maladies articulaires' (étude clinique et expérimentale), Thèse de 1877. Darde, 'Des atrophies consécutive à quelques affections articulaires,' Thèse de 1877. Guyon et Féré, "Note sur l'atrophie musculaire consécutive à quelques traumatismes de la hanche," 'Progrès Médical,' 1881, &c.

the extensors of the articulation. And that in such cases the atrophy, which presents the characters of a simple atrophy, without irritative characters, supervenes very rapidly, at the end of eight days in 20 per cent., and at the end of fifteen days in 44 per cent. of the cases.

Well, now, can this causal relationship between muscular and joint affections be applied in this case? Yes, undoubtedly; you will recognise its existence after a study of the past history of the patient, and then it will not be necessary to go far to find a cause for his condition; all his troubles date from an injury, and this injury involved the knee, solely the knee.

About a year ago, May 5th, 1881, B—, while jumping over a fallen tree, knocked his right knee; he did not fall nor did he experience much pain, still the blow was enough to tear his trousers. He could walk, and he accomplished three kilomètres without fatigue, but being obliged to descend a hill he then experienced a kind of stiffness in his knee and had to stop. It was only then that he noticed a little patch of blood on the front of his knee, but there was no swelling. When he started again he could only walk with the aid of a stick.

During the eight days which followed there was some swelling of the joint; the patient remained in bed, but there was no fever.

The doctors who saw him appeared astonished at the great contrast between the arthritis, which seemed so slight, so free from pain, and the motor weakness, which was considerable.

A silicate splint kept on for twenty-one days did not mend matters, and after taking it off there existed the same contrast, and the doctor still seemed at a loss to understand how so much loss of power could exist with such a slight and painless arthritis.

It was not till four months after the onset that the appropriate treatment was employed, faradisation, and it was only then that he began to mend and his walking to become less difficult.

In the relationship that here exists between an insignificant injury which produced so slight an arthritis, and this paralysis of one year's duration, there is nothing very astonishing if we consult the clinical history, so well known since recent investigations, of *atrophic articular paralysis* or *paralysis having an articular origin.*

If, as a matter of fact, in a large number of cases, the protopathic[1] joint affections, either spontaneous or traumatic, which determine atrophic paralyses, are painful and very severe, it is not always so, by any means. Thus a slight and easily cured sprain, a simple collection of fluid in the joint, non-inflammatory and not painful, or, like our case, a simple arthritis, can occasion the same troubles. *There is no relation necessary between the intensity of the joint affection and that of the paralytic and atrophic phenomena.*

As for the persistence of the deuteropathic[2] symptoms (paralysis and atrophy) after the cessation of the protopathic affection (arthritis), it is for the most part the rule; and that is perhaps the most interesting feature in the history of amyotrophic paralyses of articular origin, whether looked at from a pathological or clinical point of view.

The physician should certainly be aware of this important circumstance. He should not, in presence of a slight arthritis, when the weakness and atrophy are well established, risk giving a favorable prognosis, nor promise amelioration after a short while; such a prognosis would in all probability be wrong. You see, months have slipped by and the limb is still more or less useless, although the arthritis has for a long while only been evidenced by a slight thickening of the peri-articular tissues, if, indeed, there be even as much as that left.

These particulars lead us to ask what can be the physiological explanation of this singular complication of an articular affection; such knowledge might serve us as a guide in the treatment.

[1] Primary or originating (πρῶτος, first; πάθος, disease).

[2] Secondary or resulting (δεύτερος, second).

The favourite theory with most contemporaneous authors appears to be this; the articular affection reflects certain irritant impulses along the articular nerves to the spinal cord, which impulses modify the trophic centres in that organ, whence emanate the motor nerves and the nerves which regulate the nutrition of the muscles.

There exists in the spinal cord a relationship more or less direct between the cells of origin of the centripetal nerves, and the cells of origin of the motor and trophic nerves of the extensor muscles (the crural in the case with which we are concerned); hence the result produced is a constant one, and thus in the case of irritation of the nerves of the knee it is always the extensor muscles (quadriceps), or at least those principally, which atrophy. I say principally, because the irritation, once started by the articular nerves, can spread by diffusion outside the distribution of the crural nerve into the muscles of the leg or foot. In lesions of the shoulder, elbow, hip, the atrophy of the extensors always predominates, although it is possible that other muscles of the limb may also be involved.

None of the other theories that have been suggested can be accepted; thus, it has been said that the articular inflammation spreads little by little into the neighbouring muscles; but the atrophy exists equally in the entire length of the muscle, and, moreover, experiments show that the change is a simple atrophy, without a trace of inflammation, without myositis. Nor is the hypothesis of atrophy by disuse from prolonged rest admissible; the articular affection is often so slight as not to require more than a very brief rest; and, moreover, by this theory how can we explain the localisation of the atrophy almost exclusively to the extensors?

One is therefore obliged to admit that it is a deuteropathic spinal affection which gives rise to the paralysis and atrophy. But of what does the modification in the medullary centre consist? It is not a profound modification in the cellules of the anterior horns; for we know the effects of a profound alteration in these elements in infantile paralysis. Here there is the reaction of degeneration, in which we get exalted galvanic and diminished faradic excitability; except when the disease is very advanced, and the muscle is quite destroyed, and then there is abolition of both modes of excitability; in which case it is almost impossible to restore the function. In articular paralysis, on the other hand, we see that by appropriate treatment the electrical reactions are already reappearing.

It must be then only a sort of inertia, or torpor, so to speak, of the electrical elements.

Should one conclude that in a case of this kind, if we adopt an appropriate course of treatment from the very beginning, we should obtain a rapid cure? It is probable, and this leads me to speak to you of the treatment.

However, before doing so, I ought to say a word on the exaggeration of the tendon-reflexes of the lower extremities. Is it a peculiarity of the individual, or is there a morbid reflex irritability throughout the entire length of the cord, excepting that region where the motor cells are, on the contrary, in a state of torpor as we have just supposed? This latter would appear probable from an observation of other analogous facts which we are now studying, and of which I shall soon have occasion to speak to you.

But, to return to the treatment, here we have to do with a dynamic spinal lesion, without profound modification, so far as we know, and the electric treatment can certainly be adopted without fear. The results obtained up to the present time are encouraging for the future. The electric spark seems already to have played an important *rôle* in restoring the contractility of muscles where faradisation or galvanisation have produced no effect. At the present time we have ample choice; we can employ the electric spark, galvanism, or faradism. I must reserve for a future occasion the description of how this treatment should be conducted.[1]

[1] As we have just seen, in certain cases, a muscle, absolutely irresponsive to the faradic and galvanic currents, contracts very well with the electric spark. This fact, already pointed out in a lecture by M. Charcot on static electricity, shows how relative and contingent are the actual data of electro-diagnosis. It is very strange that a muscle electrically inexcitable under the usual methods (galvanisation and

In this case the spinal affection of articular origin is of a mild form, and the issue, as is usual, will doubtless be favorable. It is possible, in some cases, that both the spinal, and

faradisation) should contract normally enough from the moment that another method of electric excitation is had recourse to.

It does not, however, follow that this power of the electric spark is the invariable rule. Ofttimes the spark does not prove more efficacious than the currents in provoking contraction of the affected muscle. Indeed, we have quite recently demonstrated this state of matters in a woman the subject of incomplete atrophy of the muscles of the neck and upper extremities, with diminution (not absence) of the faradic and galvanic reactions.

But whatever practical use they may have, the facts analogous to those lately studied by M. Charcot prove the importance of static electricity in electro-diagnosis. For the future, to the faradic and galvanic reactions must be added the Franklinic (or, more euphoniously, Franklinian) reaction. Many English and American authors designate static electricity under the name of Franklinism, and its application, Franklinisation. There is at least the advantage of brevity in these denominations.

The clinical significance of this reaction remains to be determined.

Coming to the treatment of the patient, since the lecture he has been treated with static electricity (or, better, Franklinised) three times, making eight times altogether. This has produced an amelioration which contrasts strongly with his former condition, remaining stationary as he did for so many months in spite of varied treatment. His walking, &c., have improved; and moreover, strange to say, the faradic and galvanic reactions have reappeared more and more clearly. At the commencement there was no effect with the maximum faradic current, and a current of more than 20 milliampères for galvanism; but now reactions are obtained in the affected muscles with a separation of 4 or 5 centimètres between the bobbins, and 9 or 10 milliampères.

It is an important fact that these two reactions reappeared simultaneously. In both there only exists up to the present time the cathodal closing contraction. In other words, the faradic current only gives a contraction when the muscle is excited by the negative pole (in a recent article on electro-diagnosis we have insisted on the necessity of taking into consideration the direction of the current in faradism as well as galvanism); and with galvanism, also, contraction is only obtained with the negative pole, and at the moment of making the current. All which conditions, as lately explained by us, can be accurately expressed by these three letters, K, S, Z. Thus there is simply a diminution of excitability without qualitative alteration. These details confirm the opinion expressed by M. Charcot in the lecture, that we have to do with a simple atrophy.

With reference to the manner in which the electrical treatment should consequent muscular, disease may be more serious than it is here.

It is important to bear in mind that the paresis and the atrophy are not the only deuteropathic trouble that can result from an articular lesion. This group of facts is somewhat complicated. Thus arthritis, or traumatic joint mischief,

be conducted, we have, as the Professor says, the choice between faradisation, galvanisation, and Franklinisation. In the actual state of matters it would be difficult to assign a reason for giving a preference to one or the other of these means. The most simple course would be to continue the static electrisation. Its good effects have been evident up to the present time, it is a convenient application, and we are not thereby prevented from having recourse to the exploration of the ordinary reactions.

It remains to indicate precisely how the treatment should be carried out. We know by experience that the electric spark acts in a most efficacious manner on the nutrition of muscles, and in this way we have successfully treated a long-standing facial paralysis of peripheric origin, in which the ordinary electrical reactions were quite abolished.

But the point on which we insist is that to obtain therapeutic results, strong sparks administered from a metal point or ball are not indispensable. With this patient these have simply been used for purposes of exploration; for the treatment it is sufficient to produce a much weaker discharge from a brush, *one incapable of giving rise to any contraction.*

By this proceeding we have succeeded in a case of considerable atrophy of rheumatic origin. M. le Professeur Agrégé Regimbeau (de Montpellier) has also established, quite independently, analogous facts (oral communication).

Practically this is valuable information, for it is not always convenient to produce a violent contraction in the affected muscle.

Theoretically, it is well to note that the most evident trophic effect is produced by an electric discharge, the *quantity* of which, compared with ordinary galvanic currents (in electrotherapy), might almost be overlooked. Hence it is expedient to accept with reserve the views of authors who take their stand on the physiological properties of the current, attributing the trophic effects to the quantity, no doubt by analogy, with the chemical effects. It is very probable that the question is not so simple as thus stated.

Upon the whole, the patient who forms the subject of M. Charcot's lecture, gives us ample justification for bringing static electricity more and more into use at the Salpêtrière.

In the present stage of electrotherapy it is inexpedient to lose sight of any material contribution. It is from experience alone that one must draw arguments for or against static electricity.—ROMAIN VIGOUROUX.

may produce, by reflex action, a contracture limited, to the muscles of the joint, or involving the whole limb. These cases are not infrequent, and it is known, that under these conditions the joints assume a flexed position, the flexors overpowering the extensors. In other cases the atrophy and contracture combine.

These varieties of spinal disease, produced by the influence of a cause always the same in appearance, are particularly interesting to us, and we shall have occasion to return to them when speaking of several patients which are now in the wards.

LECTURE III.

I. CONTRACTURES OF TRAUMATIC ORIGIN.
II. TIC NON-DOULOUREUX OF THE FACE IN A HYSTERICAL SUBJECT.

SUMMARY.—I. *The influence of traumatism in determining the seat of certain diathetic manifestations.—Contracture of traumatic origin in subjects who present spasmodic rigidity in a latent state.—Exaggeration of tendon-reflexes in hysterical patients.*—II. *Typical case of tic-non-douloureux of the face.—Contracture of the muscles of the face in a hysterical patient.—Simulation.*

GENTLEMEN,—At the present moment our wards contain a large number of cases of very great interest, many of which are well worthy of being presented to you. Now some of these can well be postponed for a future occasion, but there are others in whom the symptoms that I want to show you are of an evanescent character, and may even disappear all in a moment in a most unexpected way; so I believe it will be prudent to seize the opportunity of showing you some of these latter cases to-day.

I.

In the first patient that I am going to show you, you will recognise the influence which the most common traumatic lesions have on the local development of the phenomena of hysteria, and on development of contracture in particular.

We have known for a long time that certain diseases, which are pathologically dependent on a diathesis, are sometimes developed at the instance of a traumatic lesion. It is usual for these diseases to localise themselves at first in parts where the wound, the contusion, or the sprain is produced. It is so in articular rheumatism for example, and in gout; and, as I long ago remarked, nothing is more common in a gouty subject than to see, in addition to the regular spring or autumn attacks, a supplementary attack, following a fall for instance. And the peculiarity is that whereas the spontaneous attacks become localised in the usual place, the supplementary attack will be situated in the shoulder or the knee, or some other joint which has been the seat of a contusion or the sprain. This is the commonly accepted opinion in the present day, and during the last few years Professor Verneuil and his students have realised the full value of the importance which attaches itself to the study of facts of this kind, from a surgical point of view.

But what is less known perhaps is that certain local phenomena of hysteria, and in particular the contracture of a limb, manifest themselves sometimes in the same way and under the same influences.

I will commence at once the narration of the case, and as we proceed I will point out the lessons to be drawn from it.

This stout woman, aged 34, is one of our oldest inmates in the division for common epilepsy; she has been here in fact for more than twelve years. She belongs to the class of cases that comes under the denomination of *hystero-epilepsy with distinct crises.*

I ought perhaps to give you a short explanation of the meaning of this phrase. It means that this woman is the subject of two diseases of which the outbreaks appear separately; at one time the hysterical crises are present (the *attacks*, as we say here), at another time the epileptic seizures (the *fits*). On the other hand, the phrase *hystero-epilepsy with mixed crises* is meant to include those cases where hysteria alone exists, but in which also the malady is characterised, in its complete outbreaks, by four periods, one of which, the first (epileptoid or hystero-epileptiform phase), bears the likeness of epilepsy. We have proposed for this form the term *hysteria major* [*la grande hystérie*] so as to replace the long phrase "hystero-epilepsy with mixed crises," which sometimes leads to confusion.

This patient is, at the present time, suffering from Hysteria Major and from true Epilepsy also, of which she has attacks during the night, accompanied by biting of the tongue, involuntary emissions of urine, &c. Formerly, that is prior to five years ago, the hysteria predominated over the epilepsy; thus in 1874, 244 attacks (of hysteria) were counted, and 62 fits (of epilepsy); but since 1876 the *attacks* have shown a tendency to disappear, and the *fits*, although they also have been less frequent and occurred mostly at the catamenial periods, have decidedly held the chief place.

It was one of the peculiarities of the hysterical attacks in B—, when they used to occur side by side with the epileptic fits, that they were frequently followed by contractures of the right lower extremity, lasting fifteen days, a month, or more. Hemianæsthesia and ovarian tenderness [ovarie][1] existed at that time on the right side; it was on the right side also that the symptoms premonitory of an attack occurred (buzzing in the ear, beating of the temple, &c.).

The hysterical phenomena have almost completely disappeared of late years, and the patient has been considered by us during the last five or six years no longer as an hysterical one, but rather an epileptic, whose seizures were generally diminishing, if not in intensity, at least in number.

Now, on May 16th, that is a fortnight ago, a symptom appeared which shows that hysteria is by no means extinct in this woman, and that the diathesis persists up to the present time, albeit in a latent condition. B— went as usual to her work, there having been nothing particular in her behaviour during the few preceding days, when suddenly and purely by accident, and without having experienced any giddiness or vertigo—she is very explicit on this point—she took a false step on the top of the staircase, fell heavily on her left side, and slipped like an inert mass down a flight of a dozen steps. Two of her companions

1 "Ovarie" is a term used in France for a series of phenomena (sighing, laughter, crying, sometimes convulsions, &c.) produced by pressure on the inguinal region.—T. D. S.

lifted her up directly; she was not much hurt, and the only trace of the injury at the present time is a bruise over the left external malleolus. But, immediately after the fall, her walking became very difficult, and the reason of this difficulty was a rigidity of the joints (hip, knee, ankle) of the left inferior extremity, the one that had been injured.

We saw the patient on the morning of the next day and found her in the same condition as she is to-day, and which I will now demonstrate to you.

The patient is lying on the right side. The left lower extremity is rigid from end to end. Voluntary extension and flexion are both impossible, attempts at passive movement are equally useless, in whatever direction the force be applied. The flexor and extensor muscles are both in action, as you see, only, the extensors, as is usual in this kind of contracture, predominate; the thigh and leg are straight out; the foot is in a state of plantar flexion, as a consequence of the predominating action of the calf-muscles; in other words, the three segments of the limb are in a straight line, the foot being in a position of talipes equinus.

I should add that the limb, which is like a rigid bar, is also adducted; if one succeeds in bending the limb away from the middle line it springs back to its original position. Moreover, this limb has undergone rotation inwards at the hip-joint, so that the knee-cap and the point of the foot look almost directly inwards. For the rest, there is no articular pain or swelling, no vestige of the fall, if we except the bruise in the neighbourhood of the external malleolus above mentioned.

I should like you to observe that this strained position of the limb came on almost suddenly. This, as I have already pointed out, is one of the characteristics of the hysterical spasmodic contracture in distinction to contractures of organic origin. Thus, in the spasmodic paraplegia of transverse myelitis, of disseminated sclerosis, &c., this condition is not arrived at all of a sudden. In the first period there is paralysis with flaccidity of the limbs, though there is exaggeration of the tendon-reflexes; in the second stage spasmodic attacks of rigidity occur; in the third, there is a condition of rigidity, either in a position of extension or semiflexion; and lastly in the fourth stage, which is very rarely, if ever, seen, there is an invincible rigidity, which may be compared to an iron bar.

One of the most interesting characters of hysterical contracture is, you see, that it can reach its maximum all in a moment.

The occurrence of contracture under the circumstances just narrated in a subject known to have been affected with hysteria in a marked degree, and to have been formerly attacked with contracture, would naturally make us suspect that a *hysterical storm* was imminent. We ought therefore to inquire whether other hysterical *stigmata* were not developed in her after the fall, at the same time as the contracture. Now, as a matter of fact, it is so; hemianæsthesia, which was formerly on the right side, but which had disappeared for some years, has reappeared, though it is on the left side now, the side on which she fell, and on which there exists the contracture.

The anæsthesia occupies the whole of the left side, the limbs, trunk, and the face, excepting the parts immediately round the organs of sense, an exemption which sometimes happens. There is no ovarian phenomena [ovarie].[1]

Besides these symptoms there is nothing worthy of your attention, except perhaps insomnia, which she has had for the last five days, and the fact that the catamenial period commenced at its natural time two days ago. Now, it is at the menstrual period that she is usually attacked with the epileptic fits, and it was then that she was formerly attacked with the hysterical seizures. It is very probable that she will have a manifestation of this kind in a few days; after which the contracture may disappear in the same manner as it came, that is to say, suddenly, or very nearly so. It is on that account that I was so anxious to present this patient to you to-day, for it is possible that we might not have another opportunity of showing you a case of hysterical contracture of traumatic origin for a very long time.

But, you will ask me, are you quite convinced that the

[1] *Vide* note, p. 34.

injury has had the influence which you suppose on the development of the spasmodic rigidity of limb? May it not be simply a fortuitous coincidence? The reasons in support of the theory I hold are not wanting.

1. Let us first take the arguments which are independent of hysteria. I have already had occasion to point out the analogies that exist between the spasmodic paralysis of hysterical patients, or such as are not due to any organic spinal affection, and the spasmodic paralyses, hemi- or paraplegic, due to organic lesions of the brain or cord.

Thus, in hemiplegia consequent on a lesion of the brain occupying the internal capsule in the course of the pyramidal band, the limbs may remain flaccid. But the contracture exists there, in a latent state as it were, as is shown by the exaggeration of the tendon-reflexes (foot- or knee-jerks); and, sometimes by perseverance, by repeated blows on the patellar tendon, a temporary contracture lasting several minutes can be produced.

Well, under these circumstances, there is an imminence of contracture which can be brought on by the occurrence of a traumatism, and it will manifest itself in the part which is the seat of the contusion, sprain, &c. In this manner a contracture was produced and persisted for several months in the case of a woman recorded by M. Terrier. Sufficiently numerous examples of this kind could be quoted, relative not only to hemiplegia but also to paraplegia, which take on a spasmodic character under the influence of an injury.

Moreover, to determine a contracture in a limb which is paralysed and flaccid, the injury need not necessarily be violent; an ill-timed faradisation, the application of a blister or an antimonial plaister, can produce the same effects as a blow.

The theory which best enables us to fix these facts in the mind is the following. There exists in cases of paralysis due to a material lesion a hyper-excitability of the grey substance, and particularly of the motor cells of the anterior horns, a special state which I propose, for want of a better term, to describe by the name of *strychnism*. Then, cutaneous irritations, irritations of the centripetal nerves in general, augment the already excited condition of the motor cells; the measure overflows, and the centrifugal nerve transmits the irritation to the muscles which it supplies.

2. Now, to return to hysteria. In many hysterical patients, chiefly on the anæsthetic side, but sometimes everywhere a little, there exists an exaggerated reflex excitability. And one finds also a paresis, a well-marked dynamometric weakness. Hence it is not astonishing to find that an excitation of the centripetal nerves, whether of the tendons or of other parts, produces the same effects as in cases where there exists a lesion of the nervous centres. Under these conditions, paralysis of the limbs without rigidity becomes transformed into a paralysis with contracture.

I could mention numerous cases of this kind, and some of them are reported in the appendix to the first volume of my lectures delivered at the Salpêtrière. In one case a contracture of the wrist followed a blow on the back of the hand and lasted for several months. Or again, I have seen the same symptoms after crushing the hand in the machinery of an engine; another hysterical patient, whose foot had been violently pressed against the bar of a chair, was attacked with a contracture of the foot; and so on. Brodie, who was well aware of these facts, and who, indeed, was the first to publish them in 1837 in his work *on certain local nervous affections*, mentions contracture of the upper extremity following pricks of the fingers.

These facts are all the more interesting since a contracture determined by an injury is often the first manifestation of the hysterical diathesis. For example, an ordinary injury is followed by a contracture in a young person who till then is not known to have any nervous symptoms; examine the case very thoroughly, and in all probability you will find some accompaniment that will demonstrate the presence of hysteria; it will be very surprising if you do not find some hyperæsthesia, anæsthesia, ovarian pain, or some indication of that kind.

3. I can give you further evidence of this tendency to contracture which exists often in a very marked degree in cer-

tain hysterical subjects—not always subjects of Hysteria Major, but of the affection in its commoner form.

I can show you now, in passing, two young persons who are the victims of this affection, whose flippant air and taste for finery, rendered manifest by the ribbons and flowers with which they are adorned, offer a marked contrast to the aspect of our first patient, whose oft-repeated epileptic seizures have left traces of a profoundly affected intellect on her physiognomy.

One of them has disseminated patches of anæsthesia and left ovarian phenomena [ovarie], and she has spontaneous contractures after her attacks; the other patient is anæsthetic on the left side, her right side is analgesic, and she has ovarian phenomena on both sides. Now you see that by repeated percussion of the patellar tendon, or the tendo Achillis, the leg of either assumes a position of extension, and the foot is bent into a position of talipes equinus. This attitude is fixed, the rigidity of the limb is absolute, it is impossible to either flex or extend it; in short, it is a very characteristic contraction, which will probably last for several hours unless we can undo it by the same proceedings which were employed to provoke it. That which has just been done on the inferior extremity can be repeated on the superior. If we take a pleximeter and with repeated small blows strike the flexors of the finger at the level of the wrist, you see that the fingers assume a position of exaggerated flexion, and remain fixed in a state of contraction.

I think that enough has been said to demonstrate the influence of traumatic causes on the development of contracture in hysterical patients; and also in those who are predisposed thereto by certain organic lesions quite apart from hysteria. We shall have many occasions, in the course of our studies, to apply this interesting idea to the explanation of certain phenomena otherwise inexplicable.

But, returning to the contracture of B—, what can be done for it? In the first place, we must wait and see whether, as is usual, the disease will of itself come to an end. But if it persist? Since the disease is unilateral we have some hold on it; we may be able by the aid of a magnet or of agents of the same kind to bring about a transference of the contracture to the opposite side, and it is possible that at the end of a large number of such transfers, the contracture may disappear altogether.

II.

At the present time there is a little patient attending the out-patient department whose history is made up almost entirely of hysterical phenomena, if indeed there be aught else. She is a young Jewess from St. Petersburg, fifteen years old; she has never menstruated; she has been attending the Clinique for about six weeks. She comes to Paris in the hope of being cured, having been unable to obtain relief elsewhere. I know not if we can give her what she seeks, or rather what her father asks for her. You will understand soon why I make this reservation.

The case seems to be one of *facial tic non-douloureux*, but the affection in this girl appears to have special characteristics which show considerable departure from the normal type.

Now here, gentlemen, is a woman whom I shall have occasion to show you for another purpose, and who is afflicted with facial tic non-douloureux in the form generally seen. She is an "hysteric" of many years' standing, and indeed she is one still, albeit that she is fifty years of age, and has not had hystero-epileptic attacks for a long time. But she has hemianæsthesia of the left side, and on the same side she has had facial tic for four or five years. This tic appears in spontaneous paroxysms which are repeated with greater or less frequency during the day, and which consist of blinking of the eyelids, and a very rapid quivering, some 200 times per minute, of the left lateral commissure; the platysma participates in the convulsion in some degree. That is the ordinary type.

Now examine our little patient; here the spasm is produced only when we wish. You see that with a little pad on the right eyelid nothing particular occurs in the face. But, we are about to raise the pad; if we raise it slightly, without uncovering the globe of the eye, which is permanently protected by the contracted eyelids, a contraction of the muscles of the right side of the face is at once produced. If we uncover the eye, the spasm occurs more energetically still, and results in a frightful distortion and fixed expression of countenance. The same result is always obtained; repose when the pad is there, contracture as soon as it is removed.

Thus there is a remarkable difference between this case and the preceding. So much so that we are obliged to ask ourselves whether it is not one of those singular instances of simulation with which the history of hysteria teems.

It should be stated at once that the affection we now see was preceded a year ago by a spasm of the right orbicular muscle which came on without known cause, and without pain. A little while after this, nervous paroxysms came on, which were accompanied by laughing, crying and shouting. In August last, the spasm of the face as we see it now supervened after a local electrisation.

Let us examine matters more closely. The existence of a blepharospasm in nervous or hysterical subjects is not a rare occurrence, and would surprise no one. That the spasm should spread to the face is not strange. It is seen in numbers of cases, and nothing is more natural than that this spasm should be held in check by pressure directed to certain points. De Grœfe some while ago called attention to the existence of these points of stoppage which the physician should seek for, and which the patients themselves often find out quite empirically. In the case before us the stoppage point would be the eyelid itself, or the supra-orbital arch.

But here is where the strange part of the case commences. The pressure exercised by this little pad is such a small matter; and moreover it is not a question of the pressure alone, which ought to be efficacious whether applied by us and tightening it up with a bandage, or done by the patient herself. It is not so here, and thus there is a personal influence in the matter which gives us material for much thought. I will even go further and say that in my mind there is not only a suspicion, but a conviction. Yes, this young woman simulates, or at least exaggerates. I willingly admit the reality of the blepharospasm; but, as for the spasm of the muscles of the lower part of the face and the platysma I believe it to be superadded, invented, simulated.

It is probable that the same opinion entered into the minds of the physicians who saw the young girl at St. Petersburg, at any rate an operation for section of the nerve-trunk was prepared, the patient was chloroformed, but they went no further. Nevertheless, the spasm has persisted in the same condition as you see it to-day.

But, you will ask me, what possible motive could this young girl have for simulation? I have already had occasion to point out to you [p. 14] that hysterical people often simulate without any very distinct end in view, by the worship of art for its own sake. But is not the love of notoriety motive sufficient? To deceive, or think she deceives, the physicians of St. Petersburg, then those of Paris, next the Faculty of Vienna, and thus to make a tour through the whole of Europe, is not this sufficient motive?

I should add that when the patient was placed on the stool of an electric machine, with the eyelids uncovered, she soon displayed evident signs of fatigue; after a quarter of an hour she became quite breathless, a cold sweat covered the body, and a more or less genuine nervous storm seemed imminent. We did not care to push the experiment further.

Under these circumstances what is to be done? We do not wish just yet to make known our opinion either to the father or the child; we are following an expectant treatment. I hope that the little patient will remain with us some time yet, and that I shall have another opportunity of showing her to you.[1]

[1] Since the lecture, Madlle. A— has been isolated from her family. She came into the Infirmary on May 27th, and the only treatment employed has been the application at a distance of magnets to the same side as the spasm, and a few applications of static electricity. On the 1st of April [? June], under the influence of electrisation, the spasm diminished momentarily and the sensibility was increased. Nothing particular occurred until June 18th, but on that day she had an acute attack, with loud cries and some contortions, predominating on the right side—that of the spasm. These attacks have been repeated

several times since. During the month of July use had been made almost daily of the magnet at a distance. The contracture of the lower part of the face insensibly disappeared; and on July 26th nothing but the blepharospasm remained. Next day, after being vexed, she had rather a violent attack, and since then the eye has remained open quite normally, but the attacks have recurred several times.—CH. F.

LECTURE IV.

ON THE MUSCULAR ATROPHY WHICH FOLLOWS CHRONIC ARTICULAR RHEUMATISM.

SUMMARY.—*Muscular atrophy in acute, subacute, or chronic joint disease.—Relation between the localisation of the atrophy and the seat of the joint disease.—Types of primary chronic articular rheumatism :* i. *Generalised or progressive primary chronic articular rheumatism.* ii. *Fixed or partial chronic articular rheumatism.* iii. *Heberden's nodes. — Generalised chronic rheumatism determines amyotrophies which predominate in the extensor muscles of the affected joints.—Exaggeration of the tendon-reflexes.—With the amyotrophy there exists a contracture in a latent state.—Spasmodic contracture of a reflex articular origin.*

GENTLEMEN,—I am about to present to you a patient who will bring back to your minds the subject of amyotrophic paralyses[1] which recently occupied our attention.

You will doubtless remember the young telegraph clerk who, after receiving a blow on the right knee that lighted up transient arthritis in the joint, suffered for nearly a year from atrophic paralysis, chiefly of the right quadriceps extensor, which rendered his power of walking very imperfect during all that time.

Traumatic lesions are not by any means the only causes which can give rise to such a condition. It is well known that the most diverse lesions can lead to the same result. The fact is established beyond doubt as regards acute articular rheumatism, acute gout (Bouchard, Debove), and

[1] Paralyses due to muscular atrophy (*α*, neg., *μῦς*, a muscle, *τροφη* nutrition).

gonorrhœal rheumatism. And what has been said of acute and subacute arthropathies can now be affirmed of chronic articular rheumatism. In all these joint affections, acute and chronic, the muscular atrophy occurs according to the law already pointed out [p. 24], that is to say, the atrophy always predominates in the extensors of the affected joint. Thus in arthritis of the hip the muscles of the buttock are chiefly involved, if the knee is attacked it is the quadriceps extensor femoris, if it is the elbow, then the triceps brachialis is the seat of the atrophy, and so on.

This relationship between the seat of the articular affection and the localisation of the muscular atrophy is sufficiently constant to be of service in cases which present difficulties of diagnosis. For example, in diseases of the hip, in certain cases of *morbus coxæ senilis* in an early stage, when the physical signs are scarcely appreciable on account of the depth of the articulation, a marked flattening of the buttock of the corresponding side, due to atrophy of the lower fibres of the gluteus maximus, can be regarded as a very significant symptom.

Long enough before joint disease was recognised as a cause of muscular atrophy, Adams[1] called attention to this flattening of the buttock in certain chronic affections of the hip-joint.

The case which I am about to bring before you belongs to the category of chronic articular rheumatism. It may be within your recollection that I have proposed to collect the many various forms under which this affection appears into three fundamental groups :[2]

1. *Generalised or progressive primary chronic articular rheumatism.*—This is the nodular rheumatism of some authors ; it follows a chronic course from the commencement, and presents an invariable tendency to become generalised. It is the small joints of the extremities, especially those of the hands, and most often the metacarpo-phalangeal joints which are involved in the first instance, and they are

[1] Adams, 'A Treatise on Rheumatic Gout,' &c., London, 1857.

[2] Charcot, 'Traité de la goutte de Garrod,' note, p. 602 ; 'Maladies des vieillards,' 2e Ed., 1874, p. 197, et suiv. ['Syd. Soc. Transl.,' p. 180.]

generally attacked symmetrically. Then in due course the other articulations are almost invariably involved. During the tedious progress of the malady the patient has severe attacks of pain, from time to time, which are frequently accompanied by febrile symptoms.

2. *Fixed or partial chronic articular rheumatism.*—This disease, which presents the same characteristic of chronicity from the outset as the preceding, generally remains localised to one or two of the large joints in which it produces profound alterations. It is well known to the surgeon under the name of dry arthritis, or of morbus coxæ senilis when it is the hip that is affected. The pains that accompany it are less intense, and fever is wanting.

3. *Heberden's nodes.*—This is the affection described by Heberden under the name of *digitorum nodi.* Very generally, but incorrectly, this is confused with gout. It is found almost exclusively in the articulations of distal phalanges; while the metacarpo-phalangeal joints, which are specially prone to be involved in the first variety, are free.

I need scarcely say that dry arthritis forms the anatomical substratum of all these clinical varieties, although a slight modification in the anatomo-pathological type is found in each. These three forms, in fact, are not absolutely separate; one passes into the other by insensible grades. There are undoubtedly cases which occupy an intermediate position, and the one we are about to study partakes of the characters both of partial and also of generalised chronic articular rheumatism; it is a partial chronic rheumatism which has a tendency to spread to a great many joints.

The man named L—, 51 years of age, and by occupation a hair-dresser, enjoyed good health till he was forty-four years old. For the last nine years he has occupied a dark, damp room on the ground floor behind his shop, where he often suffered from the cold at night. The influence of a damp habitation is often mentioned, and correctly so, as one of the principal determining causes of chronic rheumatism; and it is very remarkable that the articular pains frequently do not appear until some years after the evil influence has commenced; there is as it were a sort of incubation period. Thus was it in our patient, and it was not till after five years' residence in this unhealthy room that the first symptoms of joint mischief appeared. The joints were affected in the following order : the wrists first, next the shoulders, then the ankles, knees, hips, elbows, and last of all the fingers, and the cervical articulations to a slight degree. This gradual invasion was spread over a period of four years. The pains were slight and the swelling ill-marked; he has never had either rigors or fever; he has never been obliged to take to bed; he gradually became aware of a stiffness in certain movements of his wrist incidental to his occupation, then a rapid loss of flesh and great weakness came on, making it difficult for him to walk, and soon he was obliged to give up his occupation.

At the present time it is easy to recognise the affected joints, the alterations that have taken place in them being so well marked. Many of the joints are the seat of crackling, the left shoulder and the knees being the worst. They contain a small quantity of fluid, and the soft parts around are evidently swollen. Crackling is to be detected pretty equally in the wrists, the elbows, and some of the finger-joints in both hands. In a word, without going more into detail, we find in a large number of joints the classic signs of a dry arthritis.

But the point which should most occupy our attention is the loss of substance in the muscular parts. It is not a general emaciation in the strict acceptation of those words, but a localised muscular atrophy which affects certain muscles or groups of muscles; and we shall find that it predominates in the extensors, a point worthy of our special attention. Thus, on the shoulders the deltoids are flattened, in the arms the triceps muscles are wasted, while the biceps still preserve considerable substance. The buttocks also are considerably flattened, corresponding to the affection of the coxo-femoral articulations. In the thigh the quadriceps is much more atrophied than the flexor muscles, and the same rule obtains for all the diseased joints.

The modifications in the electrical reaction of the muscles is here again simply a quantitative and not a qualitative one.

Only one muscle forms an exception to this statement; the vastus externus of the right side, which gives the reaction of degeneration, in that the faradic excitability is weaker and the galvanic is stronger than normal. This is the only exception; everywhere else the electrical reactions indicate a simple atrophy without marked alteration in the nutrition. Some of the atrophied muscles are the seat of very manifest fibrillar contractions, the deltoid, for example, the quadriceps femoris, and the buttocks. And some of these muscles are easily excited to contraction by direct percussion, as you can see in the left deltoid particularly.

Side by side with these trophic changes in the muscles is a motor weakness, more accentuated in proportion as the muscular atrophy is more advanced. The patient finds walking very difficult, more on account of the amyotrophic paresis than the pain in the joints. The dynamometric force of the hands is considerably limited; it is represented by 10 for the right and 12 for the left hand, the average normal strength being represented by about 80.

By a more detailed investigation one recognises that in the upper extremities it is the extensors that have lost most power; thus, while it is easy enough to prevent extension of the elbow, the arm when placed in a position of flexion can effectually resist efforts to straighten it. The same condition, *mutatis mutandis*, can be made out at the wrist-joint, and also at the knee.

You see then that the essential features of this case are in entire accord with those we have seen in the young telegraph clerk whose atrophic paralysis appeared as a consequence of an injury to the knee. Hence, we may infer that the joint lesions of generalised chronic articular rheumatism determine, in the same way as traumatic arthritis, a reflex irritation of the spinal centres, which produces in like manner an amyotrophic paralysis, predominating in the extensors.[1]

[1] M. Debove ('Progrès Médical,' 1880, p. 1011) has had the opportunity of studying under the microscope the atrophied muscles in a case of chronic rheumatism, and has observed certain characters which enable us to class these amyotrophies among myopathies of nervous origin, *i.e.* there is an irregularity in the atrophy, which attacks not

But, between the two cases, there is a very marked similitude on another point also.

As an interesting feature in the case of the telegraph clerk, I referred to the exaggeration of the tendon-reflexes, which was present not only in the affected limb, but also in the healthy one; and we concluded therefore that the spinal affection, developed in consequence of the arthritis, whatever it might be, was much more extensive than might at first have been supposed. Well, this same exaggeration of reflex excitability is to be found in the patient whom I show you to-day, and in a still more pronounced degree. Jerking upwards the point of the foot produces a very manifest trepidation, which is increased if the patient endeavours to resist the movement. In order that you may fully realise the exaggeration of the patellar reflexes, I will cause the patient to sit on the edge of a chair. You see that the effect of striking the patellar tendon, either on the right or left side, is to produce at every stroke a movement in the shoulders, and particularly in the left one. Every time that the patellar tendon is struck, no matter of which leg, there is a contraction of the deltoid, trapezius, and pectoralis major; the shoulder is perceptibly elevated, and drags along with it the whole of the upper extremity.

Thus we find in this case the essential elements of a spasmodic paralysis at a stage when the permanent contracture, although not actually developed, is nevertheless imminent. And these phenomena are sometimes so pronounced that physicians of considerable experience have been led to think that the spinal lesion is the primary one, the joint disease and muscular atrophy being secondary. But the evolution of the phenomena is against such a view. The arthropathies are in reality the primary facts, the spinal affection which produces the amyotrophy is only secondary.

It is important to add that, apart from this increased reflex excitability as evidenced by exaggerated tendon-reflexes both of the upper and lower limbs, no other

only the fibres of the same muscle in different degrees, but even the fibrils of the same fibre; and the sclerosis of the interstitial connective tissue has a like irregularity.

symptom can be discovered which could be connected with a spinal lesion. No abnormality of cutaneous sensibility, no girdle pains, no urinary trouble, &c.

From what has just been said, you will be led to infer that in cases where amyotrophic paresis is a leading feature, contracture exists, so to speak, in a potential or latent condition. I may here point out to you that if in certain arthropathies, such as the preceding case, the amyotrophic paralysis forms the predominating feature, it is not the same in other joint affections where, on the contrary, spasmodic contracture holds the chief place.

It is well known to surgeons that, in certain joint diseases, in the painful forms especially, the affected joints become rigid. They become fixed ordinarily in a state of flexion; in hip disease, for example, the thigh becomes flexed on the pelvis; in pulpy degeneration of the knee-joint, the leg becomes flexed on the thigh, and so on.

There have been many discussions on the cause of this rigidity of the joint, and the consequent deformity. You are aware that in the school of Bonnet, of Lyons, great stress was laid on the instinct of the patient, who endeavours, so they say, to adjust the joint in that position which gives him the least possible pain. Others have attributed influence to the weight of parts, the fluid in the joint, &c.; always relegating the involuntary spasmodic contraction to quite a secondary position. In the present day, however, it is this reflex spasmodic contracture, of an involuntary kind, to which most surgeons attach their faith, and in this way they have come back to Hunter's doctrine. In a book but little known in France,[1] the late Mr. Hilton, Surgeon to Guy's Hospital, has very clearly expressed what may be regarded as the prevailing opinion on this point. "When," said he, "the joint cavity is inflamed or irritated in any way, the influence of this condition is transported to the spinal cord, and thence reflected by the mediation of the corresponding motor nerves to the muscles which move the joint." M. le Professeur Duplay in several passages of his book, and Pitha also, support this theory.

[1] 'Rest and Pain,' &c., 2nd edition, London, 1877.

Now, in this instance we have a spasmodic contraction of both the flexors and extensors at the same time, though it is the former which determine the character of the deformity. It does not seem in such cases to be an intentional, or instinctive contraction, the object of which is to lessen the pain; for in many cases of joint disease, and especially disease of the hip-joint, one knows that it is often necessary by applying extension to oppose this very contracture in order to ease the patient's pain. Furthermore, M. Masse[1] has made the interesting observation that whereas these contractures are often enormously increased during sleep, they become much less during the waking state, when the patient is in a condition to oppose them.

Without denying accessory causes, one is bound to admit, under the circumstances, that reflex spasmodic contracture is the principal agent in producing the joint deformity. Such an opinion finds, I believe, full confirmation in the study of those remarkable deformities which are so frequently met with in generalised or progressive chronic articular rheumatism (knotty rheumatism).

This was the conclusion that was forced upon me in my inaugural dissertation thirty years ago, and to which, with your permission, I will refer. Yet, the exposition of all the facts relative to this question will demand more time than is left at our disposal to-day, and I must therefore resume this subject in the next lecture.

Moreover, it will not be without interest to indicate more clearly that side by side with amyotrophic paralyses, there exist spasmodic contractures which are also connected with alterations in the joints; that these contractures, like the amyotrophies, are due to a spinal affection developed along a reflex path; and lastly, to bring into view the relationship that exists between these two series of phenomena apparently so different from each other.

[1] 'Influence de l'attitude des membres sur leurs articulations,' Montpellier, 1878, p. 104.

LECTURE V.

I. REFLEX CONTRACTURE AND AMYOTROPHY OF ARTICULAR ORIGIN.

II. OPHTHALMIC MIGRAINE APPEARING IN THE EARLY STAGE OF GENERAL PARALYSIS.

SUMMARY.—I. *Chronic articular rheumatism.—Reflex contracture of articular origin.—Deformities in chronic articular rheumatism : 1. Type of extension ; 2. Type of flexion.—The hand of athetosis ; hand of paralysis agitans.—Articular deformities of chronic rheumatism are due to a spinal affection produced by the same mechanism as reflex acts.*

II. *Progressive general paralysis.—Ophthalmic migraine at the outset.—Scintillating scotoma.—Hemianopsia.*

GENTLEMEN,—The first patient to whom I wish to direct your attention to-day presents an illustration of dry arthritis of the hip, and you will recognise in her the flattening of the buttock, due to atrophy of the gluteal muscles, which is capable, as I pointed out in the last lecture, of assisting us in the diagnosis of difficult cases.

The patient is a woman, sixty-two years of age. She has not, so far as we can discover, been exposed to the ordinary causes of chronic articular rheumatism, at any rate she has not lived in a damp place. She has worked a sewing machine for several years, and it is this, she thinks, which has produced the disease of the right hip. All the other articulations are sound. The malady started about a year ago with stiffness in the joint ; then she had attacks of pain, worse at night, starting at the lower border of the buttock, shooting down the thigh and inner side of the knee. At one time there was crackling in the joint, but there is none now. At the present time she has scarcely any spontaneous pain, and there is no tenderness on striking the great trochanter; there is no marked shortening of the limb, but it has a considerable tendency to assume a position of rotation outwards, as those of you even at a distance can detect by the direction of the foot. The patient can walk fairly well, and after she has made the first few steps, she scarcely limps at all; but when she is seated it is impossible for her to cross the right leg over the left, although she can cross the left one over the right. The physical signs and the loss of function render it impossible to doubt the existence of an articular lesion, but even if these were less marked our attention would be directed to the joint by the flattening of the right buttock, which is very distinct. And not only does the buttock appear very wasted, but on palpation it feels softer and more flaccid than normal. On the right side the fingers can easily touch the ischium, but on the left it is not so; and you can see, moreover, that the great trochanter seems much more prominent on the right side, indicating some atrophy of the gluteus minimus.

I was anxious to show you this patient because the case ought to be classed in the same group as the amyotrophies of articular origin which we are at present studying.

I must now add some further details to the facts I have already laid before you relative to the spasmodic contractures that follow joint lesions, and are sometimes accompanied by muscular atrophy. I attempted, following the doctrine of Hunter, to prove that these contractures are produced by a reflex mechanism started in the diseased joint. The excitation of the articular nerves reacts on the spinal centres, which in their turn reflect this excitation along the path of the motor nerves to the muscles, both flexors and extensors, of the joint.

The spasmodic contracture is generally limited to the flexors and extensors of the affected joints. But, in some cases, as a consequence of the diffusion of the spinal lesion, the muscular spasm becomes more generalised, and may even extend to all the muscles of a limb. I have already drawn attention to cases of this kind connected with hysteria, but, judging by recorded cases, such contractures involving a whole limb, consequent on a lesion limited to a single joint, may be observed quite independent of hysteria.

The cases reported by Duchenne (of Boulogne), and described by him under the name of *reflex contractures of articular origin*, may be mentioned in support of this statement, and there is another by M. Dubrueil (of Montpellier).[1] M. Dubrueil's case was that of a young man, 16 years of age, who fell from the top of a ladder and sprained his left ankle; three days later contracture appeared not only in the muscles of the foot, which was flexed and in a state of adduction, but in those also which act on the knee and the hip. The subjects in whom contractures of arthritic origin tend thus to become generalised are evidently predisposed thereto, and in this respect the cases may be said to be akin to the hysterical neurosis.

In order to finish this subject it remains for me to show, as I promised, that the deformities of progressive chronic articular rheumatism (nodular rheumatism) are due, in like manner, to a spasmodic contracture of the muscles, developed by reflex action secondary to the joint lesions.

I endeavoured some years back to show[2] that the deformities observed in such cases, so far as the upper extremities are concerned, can all be brought, no matter how different they may seem, under two fundamental types, to which all accessory forms may also be referred.

The symptoms common to both types are these: the hands are generally in a state of pronation and slightly flexed; the deformities are usually symmetrical; there is ordinarily a deviation of all the fingers towards the ulnar border of the hand (Fig. 4).

Now, the characters distinctive of the two fundamental types are:

[1] Dubrueil, 'Leçons de clinique chirurgicale,' Montpellier, 1880, p. 5.

[2] Charcot, 'Etudes pour servir à l'histoire de l'affection décrite sous les noms de goutte asthénique primitive, nodosités des jointures, rheumatisme articulaire chronique (forme primitive),'' 'Thèse de Paris,' 1853.

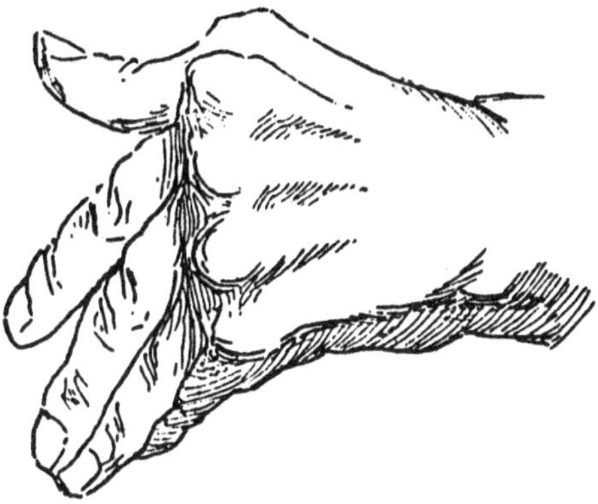

FIG. 4.—Representing the deviation of all the fingers towards the ulnar side of the hand in chronic rheumatism. (Drawn by M. P. Richer.)

First type, or type of extension.—Beginning at the free extremities of the fingers, you will notice (*a*) flexion of the ungual phalanges, (*b*) hyper-extension of the second phalanges, (*c*) flexion of the proximal phalanges. The woman named D—, who is brought before you, presents this deformity in a very characteristic manner. She is now forty-nine years old, and the malady commenced when she was twenty, after three years' residence in a damp house. She has most of the other joints also affected (Fig. 5).

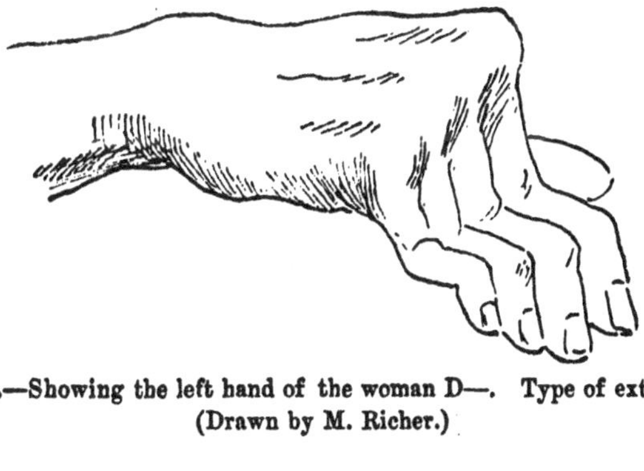

FIG. 5.—Showing the left hand of the woman D—. Type of extension. (Drawn by M. Richer.)

You will find the same deformity in the hands of the woman M—, who has had the disease since the menopause (Fig. 6).

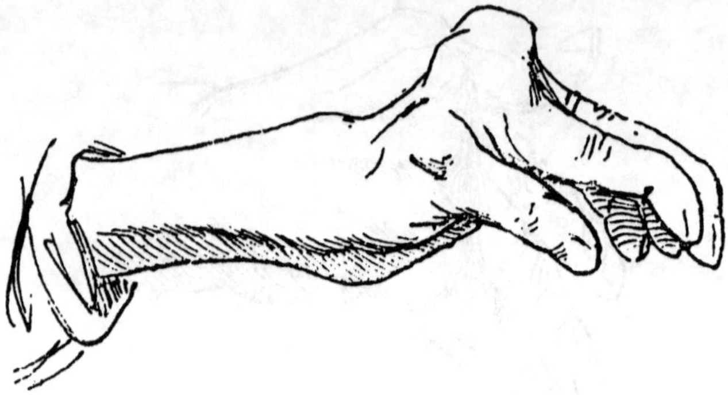

FIG. 6.—Showing the left hand of the woman M—. Type of extension. (Drawn by M. Richer.)

Second type, type of flexion.—Here we have a hyper-extension of the ungual phalanges, and a flexion of the second phalanges, as you see in this patient (Fig. 7).

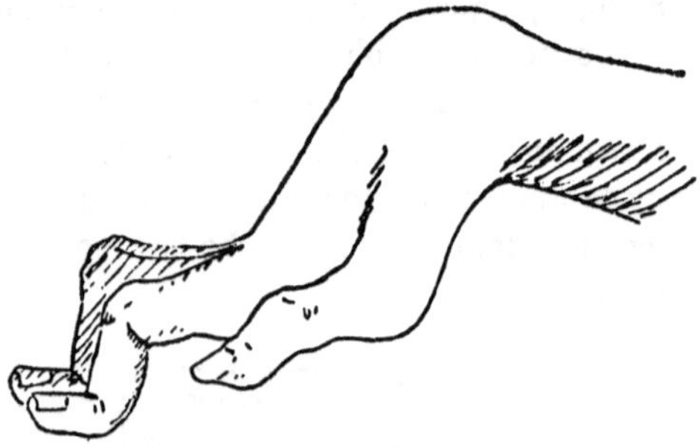

FIG. 7.—Right hand of the woman X—. Type of flexion. (Drawn by M. Peugniez.)

Such are the deformities which are due, quite as much as those occurring in the other joints of the same patients (knees, elbows, &c.), to a spasmodic contraction of the muscles.

You will remark that the spasmodic contraction has long since ceased in both of these patients; but the resulting deformities persist nevertheless in consequence of the thickening of the periarticular tissues, the subluxations, the shortening of the ligaments which have existed all this long while, wherever the joints have been maintained in a faulty position by the spasmodic muscular contracture.

What are the arguments that can be advanced in favour of the theory I hold?

1. It seems impossible to admit that these strained unnatural positions can be the attitudes instinctively assumed by the patients themselves, in order to avoid pain as much as possible, while maintaining the articulation in a fixed position. In examining such patients during an acute exacerbation of the affection one recognises that, far from endeavouring to bring about these forced attitudes, they strive against these spasmodic contractures, these cramps as they call them, to which they are subject.

2. The accumulation of fluid within the synovial cavities gives greater mobility to the joints, and favours the action of the contracted muscles; but this element cannot be invoked as a predominating cause of the deformity. Moreover, all the joints which in the hand undergo deviation have not been attacked with hydrarthosis, or even inflammation.

One can add also, without fear of contradiction, that the weight of the parts plays but a very ineffectual part in the production of such deformities.

Therefore, by a process of exclusion, we can affirm that muscular contraction is the only influence which is worthy of our support.

I should add that there are other powerful, though indirect, arguments which can be produced in favour of this theory. I can show you that these same deformities of the hands, these same articular deviations, which are seen in nodular rheumatism, are also found, with so many of the same characteristics that they may be mistaken the one for the other, in cases where there exists no joint affection at all, and where rigidity of muscles is the only disease present. Thus, for example, in spasmodic infantile hemiplegia, from which the patient before you now is suffering, there is a spasmodic contracture of all the muscles of the upper and lower extremities of the left side. It dates from infancy, and the patient is an epileptic, though it is an epilepsy of a special kind. Never has there been a trace of arthritis, certainly not in the hands. Now, in this hand, which shows the involuntary movements of athetosis, and in which consequently there is an increased articular mobility in certain movements when the patient stretches out the hand, one sees a deformity resembling our first type, the type of extension (Fig. 8).

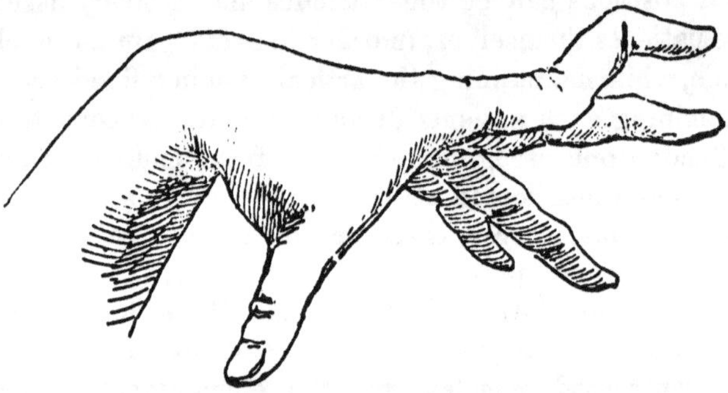

FIG. 8.—The hand of athetosis, resembling the deformity in the type of extension. (Drawn by M. P. Richer.)

The same remarks will be found to apply to Parkinson's disease. A long while ago I pointed out these deformities, which can only be explained by prolonged contracture of antagonistic muscles. It is well known that in paralysis agitans the muscles of the limbs and trunk are in a state of permanent tension, and thus determine a rigidity of the parts as firmly as if they were welded together. The most common deformity in the hand reminds us of a hand which has the attitude of holding a pen in the act of writing. It is the contracture of the interossei which produces it. But in certain cases one meets with a deviation of the hand wholly comparable with that which is seen when the joints are affected with nodular rheumatism. In the case before you you will recognise the type of flexion (Fig. 9). Under these circumstances again, the deviation is produced solely by muscular action, the joints are in no wise affected.

Such then, gentlemen, are the different arguments which appear to me to show that in chronic articular rheumatism the distortion of the joints is due to a spinal affection developed after the mechanism of a reflex act.

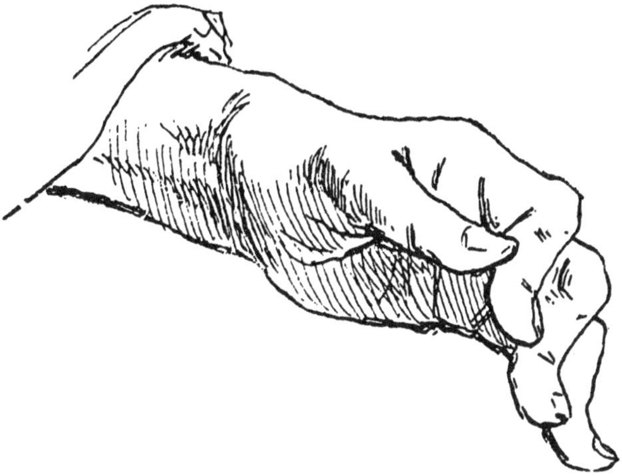

FIG. 9.—Hand of paralysis agitans, resembling the deformity of the flexion type. (Drawn by M. P. Richer.)

And this brings us again to the statement that joint affections, when they reflect back their pathogenic influence on the spinal centres, sometimes determine an exaltation of the functions of the nerve-cells, whence is derived the contracture of muscles; but sometimes, on the other hand, they lead to a depression of these same functions, which results in amyotrophic paralysis.

It should be added that these two kinds of spinal affection are sometimes found combined in the same subject. Thus, in nodular rheumatism, for example, at the very same time when contracture occurs in the muscles, one sees many of them, and especially the extensors, undergoing a more or less marked atrophy. Depression and exaltation of the functions of the ganglionic elements represent, under these circumstances, the two successive stages of the same morbid process. But, it is in such cases that the functional depression of the nerve-cell seems to be developed primarily, at the very outset; as indeed appeared to be the order of events in the cases of amyotrophy which I showed you when we commenced this subject. But you have doubtless not forgotten that, even in those very cases, the conditions which prepare the way for muscular contracture and predispose to it, namely, the exaggerated reflexes, are found combined, as it were, with the muscular atrophy.

There is not then, as one would at first imagine, an opposition or contradiction between these two kinds of phenomena. Whether it be contracture or amyotrophy which follows a joint lesion, the spinal lesion is fundamentally the same. These two kinds of phenomena represent, as it were, two extreme phases of the same morbid process.

In conclusion, I should like to point out to you that this same combination, this same succession of amyotrophy and contracture, is not by any means a unique occurrence in the clinical history of spinal affections. It is found very well marked in amyotrophic lateral sclerosis, of which I recently showed you a case.[1]

---

[1] Since this lecture M. Charcot has received from M. Dreschfeld, Professor of Pathology at Manchester, the photograph of the hand

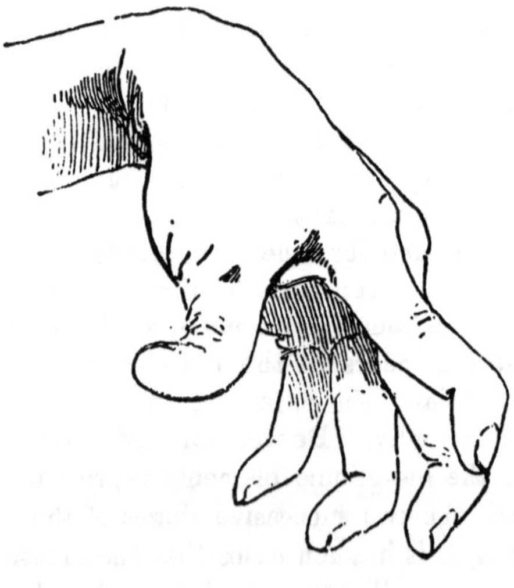

FIG. 10.—Voluntary deformity resembling the extension type of chronic rheumatism. (Drawn by M. P. Richer.)

of a student at the College who could, by stretching out the second phalanx and flexing the first and third, produce at will a deformity

II.

Enough has been said concerning spasmodic contractures and amyotrophies of articular origin. Now I want to show you a patient whose disease is of quite a different kind. He is the subject of progressive general paralysis, and, if we consider his present condition alone, we shall see that the case is quite an ordinary one, and the diagnosis of it is easy enough to establish.

Mr. L—, a Professor of History, came to France to study law; he is now 35 years of age. He has the following symptoms:—characteristic embarrassment of speech (which is almost unintelligible), fibrillar trembling of the tongue, characteristic tremors of the hands, a collection of intellectual and moral phenomena, which are grouped under the term *paralytic dementia.*

Nothing could be more typical than this case for it is well known, in the present day, that there exists a form of general paralysis, which is unattended by "grandiose delirium"

---

analogous to that of chronic rheumatism (Fig. 10). A pupil studying at the Salpêtrière can in like manner produce the same distortion at

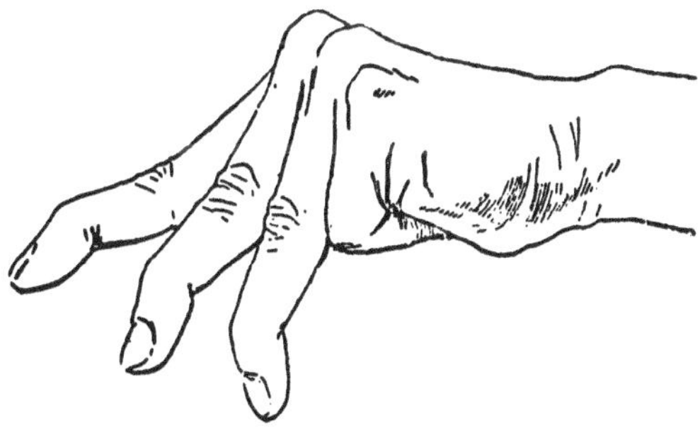

FIG. 11.—Voluntary deformity resembling the extensor type of chronic rheumatism. (Drawn by M. Richer.)

will (Fig. 11). These facts show clearly that the deformity is produced exclusively under the influence of muscular action.—Ch. F.

[délire ambitieux], and recognised as the paralytic variety, or general paralysis without madness.

But what constitutes the interesting part of the case is the narration of the symptoms with which it commenced, given in a most intelligent manner by the young wife of the patient.

I would remind you that, according to M. Jules Falret,[1] general paralysis, although it assumes an almost uniform symptomatology when it has reached its full development, appears under many different aspects at its commencement, and that these can all be classed under four types or varieties.

1. *The expansive variety*, with delirium of greatness, satisfaction with oneself, and one's surroundings, &c. These patients are worth millions of money, or may have pretensions to poetry, &c. This grandiose delirium [délire ambitieux] generally partakes, at the outset, of the characters of dementia (Falret). Their ideas are changeable, contradictory, absurd; very different from those of ambitious monomaniacs, who are logical. These mental troubles are accompanied by a certain difficulty in the articulation of sounds, inequality of pupils, tremors, and uncertainty of movements.

2. *The melancholic variety* contrasts strongly with the preceding.

(*a*) Melancholic delirium, the patients believe they are ruined, dishonoured, &c.

(*b*) Sometimes there is an association of hypochondriac ideas, fear of death; they imagine that they have maladies which do not in reality exist, say that they cannot swallow or micturate, that their passages are blocked, &c. These troubles may be very marked at the outset, but they are soon followed by embarrassment of speech, inequality of pupils, &c.

3. *Paralytic variety*, characterised by the absence of maniacal ideas, only there are profound modifications in

[1] J. Falret, "Recherches sur la folie paralytique," 'Thèse de Paris,' 1853.

character, outbursts of passion and emotion without motive, impairment of memory. In this form motor troubles predominate, embarrassment of speech, fibrillar tremors of the hands and tongue, uncertainty of the walk, staggering. This is general paralysis without insanity. These patients are conscious of their decadence, they are able, up to a certain point, to fulfil their social duties, in spite of their enfeeblement of intelligence.

4. *Congestive variety.*—In this form a series of so-called congestive attacks occur, separated by comparatively healthy intervals, and being repeated a variable number of times before the characters of general paralysis become permanently established.

These so-called congestive attacks take different forms; thus at one time it is an apoplectiform attack followed by a temporary hemiplegia, at another it is an epileptiform seizure; or again a condition frequently seen is one where, without loss of consciousness, there is a numbness of one hand, or the lips, a temporary embarrassment of the speech and ideas, a transitory aphasia, &c.

It is this congestive variety in an early stage which occurred in our patient, and in him the different kinds of attack seemed to succeed each other.

But the point to which I wish especially to draw your attention is that most of his attacks were preceded by a collection of symptoms usually known under the name of *ophthalmic migraine.*

The phenomenon presented, in the early attacks, certain characters from which one would have thought, considering the state by itself, that it was connected with a mild affection, although in reality, as the sequel showed, we had to do with the commencement of a grave, incurable disease.

I shall not enter now on the history of ophthalmic migraine; it is a subject that will occupy our attention on some future occasion. I will simply remind you that in an ordinary attack of ophthalmic migraine of the typical kind, a luminous figure appears in the visual field which is at first circular, then semicircular, of a zigzag shape like the drawing of a fortification, agitated with a very rapid vibratory movement; the image is sometimes white and phosphorescent, and sometimes it presents more or less marked tints of yellow, red, or blue. That is what is known as scintillating scotoma (Fig. 12).

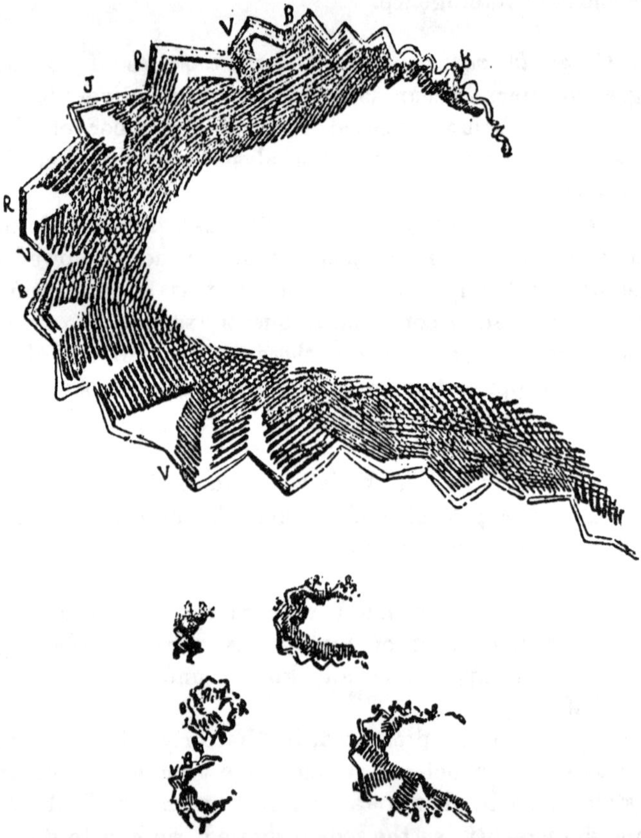

FIG. 12.—Different phases of the scintillating scotoma, after Hubert Airy (the letters indicate the different colourations: R = red, J = yellow, B = blue, V = green), 'Philosophical Transactions,' 1870.

The scotoma is often replaced by a temporary hemianopsia of the field of vision sc that the patient sees only half the object.

An examination of the field of vision, which is very important in such cases, reveals a hemianopsia, generally homonymous and lateral, but not usually extending quite up to the fixation point (Fig. 13).

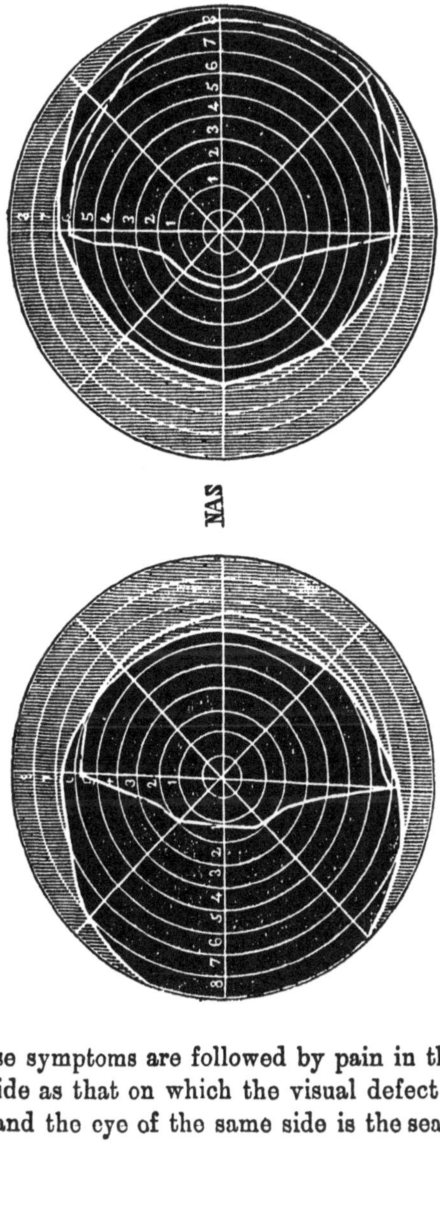

FIG. 13.—Representing homonymous retraction of the visual field in a case of ophthalmic migraine. (From the thesis of M. Féré, 'Des troubles functionels de la vision par lésions cérébrales,' 1882, p. 109.)

These symptoms are followed by pain in the temple on the same side as that on which the visual defect or the spectra occur, and the eye of the same side is the seat of a tense pain not unlike that experienced in acute glaucoma.[1] Vomiting terminates the attack, and the patient gets well again.

Such is the ordinary course of events in simple cases of ophthalmic migraine. In other cases of migraine, various other troubles are superadded, to which Piorry was the first to call attention.[2] There may be, for example, a numbness of the hand, or of the side of the tongue, an aphasia, or temporary derangement of speech, epileptiform attacks, &c.[3]

Now, migraine, even in its graver forms, and with frequent recurrence, may appear in the course of a disease, or rather of an habitual indisposition; yet it is not followed perhaps after ten, twelve, fifteen, years' duration by any serious consequence.

But do not, with the knowledge of these facts, which are doubtless those most usually met with, always give a favorable prognosis; hesitate to commit yourself, investigate matters more closely, and reserve your decision.

Several events may happen; thus as I have pointed out, there are scarcely any of the usually transitory phenomena of ophthalmic migraine which may not become permanently established; and thus, aphasia, hemiopia, paralysis of a limb, after having come and gone in a transitory way several times, may persist indefinitely after a fresh attack.

Lastly, a combination not often met with is that in which these very symptoms of migraine figure amongst the early symptoms of the congestive form of progressive general paralysis. This combination is undoubtedly rare, and has not been noted, I believe, by authors; however, I have met with it on three or four occasions.

This is briefly M. L—'s history. Ever since he was two years old he has been of an irritable and fussy disposition. However, he successfully passed his law examination before the Faculty of Paris last July. The first symptoms which attracted attention occurred in September, 1881. Then he

[1] Dianoux, "Scotome scintillant ou amaurose partielle temporaire," 'Thèse de Paris,' 1875.

[2] Priory, 'Traité de médecine pratique,' p. 75.

[3] Ch. Féré, "Contribution à l'étude de la migraine ophthalmique" ('Revue de Médecine,' 1881).

had the *first attack*, which consisted of ophthalmic migraine with scintillating scotoma, and weakness of vision on the right side, accompanied by embarrassment of speech, paralysis and numbness of the right arm. This lasted for eight days, and then he was quite well again. Eight days later he had a *second attack*, without loss of consciousness, but with difficulty of speech. The intelligence was obscured for twenty-four hours, and then, to all appearance, he recovered completely; but he was still nervous and irritable, though he was able to resume work.

In the month of February, 1882, he had a *third attack* with the same symptoms of migraine, only this time there were, at the commencement, convulsive fits of an epileptiform character with loss of consciousness. This condition continued for two hours, during which he seems to have had a series of convulsions which presented the peculiarity of predominating on the right side. After this seizure the difficulty of speech persisted.

Eight days later he had a *fourth attack* of the same nature, with a relapse of the difficulty of speech and weakness of right arm. Lastly, on May 5th, he had a *fifth attack*, with paralysis of the right arm, followed on the morrow by paralysis of the right lower extremity. During the ensuing five or six days he could say nothing but the words "à cause que." The right arm remained paralysed for a month. It was from this time that his intellectual troubles really began; and he became childish. He is docile, but very changeable, crying or laughing on the slightest pretext. He can scarcely write spontaneously, but he has managed to copy a page with a trembling handwriting. The memory is as feeble as the judgment and will. From time to time he experiences the scintillating scotoma. He advances, as you see, with a staggering gait; his hands tremble and his tongue also; his speech is scarcely intelligible; his physiognomy is characteristic, look vacant, eyelids drooping, &c. The right pupil is more dilated than the left; they act feebly to light but better for accommodation.

The lesson, gentlemen, to be learned from all this, is that one must not allow one's judgment to be led away, because, in the immense majority of cases, scintillating scotoma, together with the other phenomena which accompany it, are things of but little importance.

Beneath a benign exterior it is possible that there may lie the commencement of a grave disorder, such as should not be overlooked.[1]

[1] Since this lecture was delivered and published in the 'Progrès Médical' M. Parinaud has published a case of a similar kind ('Archives de Neurologie,' T. V, p. 57).—CH. F.

LECTURE VI.

ON HYSTERIA IN BOYS.

SUMMARY.—*Hysterical contracture.—Amblyopia.—Hysterogenic zones.—Phases of the hystero-epileptic attack.—Hysteria in boys; the attack; permanent symptoms.—Importance of isolation in the treatment.*

GENTLEMEN,—I propose in to-day's lecture to bring before you a youth who has been attending here for several weeks, and who presents a series of interesting nervous symptoms. All these symptoms, as you will see, can be attributed to hysteria, and the case will enable me to show you briefly the leading features of this malady as it occurs in the male sex, and especially in early life.

But, in the first place, I think it will serve as contrast, and to bring out the features of this particular case if I recall to your minds some of the chief phases of hysteria in women, as it occurs in the classical type of hystero-epilepsy with mixed crises, *la grande hystérie,* such as we so frequently see in many of the patients in our wards. I will show you again two of the hysterical patients whom I have already shown you several times. One is a woman named B—, 34 years of age, who presented, as you will remember, a good example of hysterical contracture developed under the influence of an injury.[1] During five days the contracture existed in all the articulations of the left lower extremity; and in addition to that we discovered that there was an absolutely complete hemianæsthesia on the same side, complete at least so far as

[1] See p. 33, *et seq.*

general sensibility was concerned. A certain degree of hemianæsthesia still persists, but the contracture has disappeared.

What else has happened since the last time we saw the patient together? The catamenia have appeared, but the hysterical seizures, on which we counted to put an end to the contracture, have not occurred. The only fits that she has had, which were three in number, presented all the characters of epilepsy; they took place in the night without premonitory symptoms, the loss of consciousness was complete, there was biting of the tongue, &c. They had no influence on the rigidity of the limbs, and we decided therefore to try the application of a magnet to the neighbourhood of the contracted limb. Several incidents occurred, and finally the contracture yielded. Now you see the left leg is almost completely flaccid.

I should add that the tendency to contracture in this patient does not seem to exist now, for they tell me that the application of the magnet to the neighbourhood of the limb no longer produces rigidity.[1] The same can be said of faradization, which is productive of no result.

One more fact to note: Faradization with Du Bois Raymond's apparatus even at its *maximum* has not produced hitherto, any sensation. However, yesterday we found, after a little perseverance, that the sensibility had slightly reappeared all down the left side. This circumstance makes one think that in this patient the hysterical tendency, which has so lately reappeared, is about to cease, and that soon everything will revert to its former state. Probably the sensibility will become re-established on the left side, and the hysterical manifestations will not return, at any rate for a time, although the patient will remain liable as heretofore to epileptic seizures.

Matters have not quite reached this point with the young Jewess whom you saw about three weeks ago. You will remember that she had had contracture of all four extremities for six months. Whether under the influence of static

[1] It may be pointed out that the same agent which causes a disappearance of stigmata in hysterical subjects is frequently capable of causing their reappearance when they are not present.—T. D. S.

electricity or whether spontaneously we are not sure, but her condition has improved. The contracture has disappeared, first from the upper extremities, then the left lower extremity, remaining, however, in the right; and the anæsthesia, which during the contracture was present in all four limbs, only persists in the right side now. After a certain number of modifications, obtained by the prolonged application of a magnet, the right lower limb has regained its normal mobility, but the hemianæsthesia still persists.

You see that the patient does not feel pricking or even prolonged and severe faradization. Another fact should be mentioned, namely, that faradization, acting on the muscles and on the nerve-trunks, produces muscular contractions which do not cease after the current is withdrawn, but which pass into a state of permanent contracture. Here, for example, is the ulnar deformity of hand [*griffe cubitale*] determined by excitation of the nerve behind the elbow; here is club-foot produced by faradization of the calf-muscles. You see thus that the contracture exists all the while in a latent state, and that the slightest excitation is sufficient to reproduce it for a long time, perhaps as a permanency.

I have pointed out in these two patients the existence of hemianæsthesia. It is a phenomenon which occupies an important place in the clinical history of hysteria, and is very frequently met with, in some degree at any rate. Allow me to dwell for a moment on this trouble of sensibility.

The young girl Bl— presents the hemianæsthesia of hysteria in a form that is altogether characteristic, and suitable to study. On the left side there is insensibility to pricking, cold, and all forms of stimuli. This loss of general sensibility is found in the upper extremity, the lower extremity, half of the trunk and the head. You see that this girl bears the most intense faradization without suffering the slightest inconvenience, and that the anæsthesia occupies not only the skin but even the deeper parts, the muscles and nerve-trunks; for one is able, by exciting the nerves and muscles, to determine, without producing pain to the patient, a pronounced and more or less durable contraction.

It is rare if the general sensibility alone is affected. The sensorial organs of the same side of the body as the anæsthesia are usually attacked also. In general there is a diminution of taste, hearing, and of smell. But I want specially to call your attention to the visual troubles, so interesting from a diagnostic point of view. In most cases, when there is insensibility of one side of the body and of the face, a more or less pronounced disturbance of vision is also manifested in the corresponding eye, a sort of amblyopia which rarely amounts to amaurosis. A methodical study of this modification of vision shows the following:

1. Retraction, often very marked, of the field of vision. Sometimes, when the anæsthesia is double, or when there is an analgesia of one side and anæsthesia of the other, there exists a retraction of the visual field of both sides, but much more marked on the side where the troubles of general sensibility are more pronounced. This retraction of the visual field is most interesting to the physician. The patient can neither simulate nor exaggerate it, and not uncommonly it is very accentuated, although the troubles of general sensibility may be but little marked.

2. Another phenomenon which generally accompanies this limitation of the visual field, consists of a diminution of the acuteness of vision. There often exists a disturbance in the perception of forms, and sometimes there is a cloudiness of luminous perceptions.

3. But a fact which ought particularly to attract our attention in hysterical amblyopia, is the presence of dyschromatopsia, and, to a degree even more pronounced, of achromatopsia, that is to say, a diminution or an absolute loss of the notion of colours. One knows that, in a normal state, all parts of the retina are not equally apt in the perception of colours; thus under physiological conditions the visual field for *blue* is wider than that for *yellow*, and that for *yellow* than that for *red;* and then after red, *green*, and *violet*, which is only perceived by the most central parts of the retina. In hysterical amblyopia the characters of the normal state are modified in such a way that the circles representing the limits of the visual fields for all colours are concentrically retracted. The violet circle may be so retracted as to become lost; and then the patient, placed in

front of the colour, will be unable to name it; the same phenomenon repeats itself with the green, red, &c. The yellow and the blue may perhaps be the only colours the perception of which remains. But even they may disappear, and then we have total achromatopsia, the patient only recognising the forms of objects, which appear grey, like an uncoloured photograph seen through the stereoscope.

There is, however, in many hysterical patients a not infrequent exception to the rule which I have just mentioned, namely, that the notion of the two colours, blue and yellow, remain, although the others have disappeared in the achromatopsia. I must point out this anomaly, although I am not now making a complete study of hysterical achromatopsia, because it is met with not only in most of the hysterical women under our observation, but also in the cases of male hysteria of which we are about to speak. The exception consists of the fact that the extent of the visual field for red remains larger than that for blue; so that, although the patients may have lost the power of perceiving violet, green, blue, and yellow, the perception of red remains. Here is a case that has been studied by Dr. Parinaud, which clearly demonstrates the phenomenon in question.

In the young girl N—, the right eye is affected to a certain degree with a retraction of the visual field for all colours, which remain, however, in their natural order. In the left eye there is manifest retraction of the visual field for white light, the different colour fields are narrowed and in a more marked degree than the opposite side. But, besides that, and this is what constitutes the anomaly, the field for *red* has remained more extended than that for yellow or for blue; this last is next to the green, and has become substituted for the red. If this retraction progresses, it may happen that the perception of all colours will disappear, excepting that of red. I dwell on these anomalies because we shall find them in a certain degree in the hysterical boy whom you will see to-day.

I will not discuss the nature of these visual troubles in hysteria. I will only remind you, in passing, that these phenomena are unaccompanied by any modification appreciable to the ophthalmoscope. There are modifications neither of the refractive media, nor of the back of the eye, there are not even vascular changes; they are exclusively dynamic troubles, as they are called. I ought, moreover, to remark that these phenomena are not altogether peculiar to hysteria, excepting perhaps that which relates to the field of vision for red; for, with the exception of this last peculiarity, they may be met with in central lesions of the brain occupying the internal capsule.

We ought to refer to another symptom in the patient now under examination. There exist, on the anæsthetic side, two *points*, or rather two *areæ*, where sensation is exaggerated. One of these points corresponds to the ovarian region, the other to the lumbar region right and left of the spinous processes. These are the *hysterogenic points* or *areæ*, which are frequently found in hysterical patients, and which sometimes occupy other positions than those now indicated.

Thus, H—, whose anæsthesia is general, but more pronounced on the left, presents three hysterogenic zones: the ovarian, the left lumbar, and the bregmatic.

What are these *hysterogenic zones?* They are more or less circumscribed regions of the body, pressure on which, or simple rubbing, produces the symptoms of an aura, which may be followed, if you persist, by an hysterical attack. These points, or rather patches, are, moreover, possessed of a permanent hyper-sensibility, and before an attack are the seat of a spontaneous painful sensation which consequently forms part of the *aura*. Sometimes this latter consists of palpitations, sometimes of a burning sensation. An attack, once started, may often be arrested by energetic pressure on these same points. It is an interesting fact and worthy of notice, that these points are not met with on the limbs,[1] but they are to be found on

[1] Since the delivery of this lecture M. Gaube has published some interesting observations on hysterogenic zones. According to these investigations, which were conducted under the direction of Professor Pitres, of Bordeaux, hysterogenic zones have been found to exist on the superior or inferior extremities, and these zones were found to have the same properties as those met with on the trunk or head (Gaube, "Recherches sur les zones hystérogènes," 'Thèse de Bordeaux,' 1882).—CH. F.

the anterior surface of the trunk in the middle line (base of the sternum, xyphoid appendix), just below the clavicle (Fig. 14), below the breasts and in the ovarian regions of women, in the inguinal region of men; on the posterior

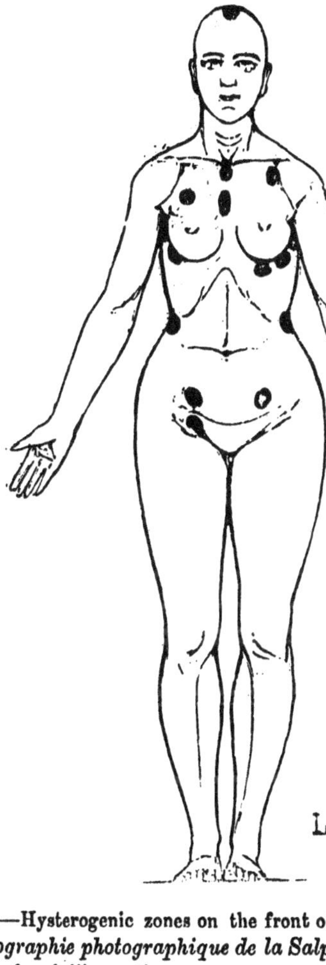

FIG. 14.—Hysterogenic zones on the front of the body (taken from the '*Iconographie photographique de la Salpêtrière*,' by Bourneville and Regnard, vol. iii, p. 48).

surface (Fig. 15), between the shoulders, sometimes at the angle of the scapula, in the lumbar region to right or left of the middle line, or over the coccyx. In men it is not uncommon to find that the testicle, especially if it presents an abnormality of position or development, is the seat of a partial hysterogenic zone; or perhaps the prepuce is exceedingly sensitive, and exhibits the same peculiarity. In the

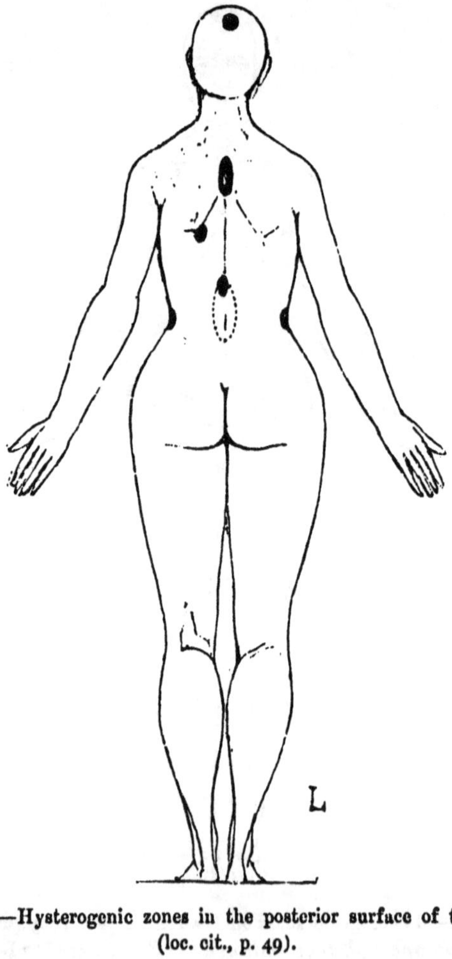

FIG. 15.—Hysterogenic zones in the posterior surface of the body (loc. cit., p. 49).

head these patches are sometimes to be found about the level of the bregma, on one side or the other.

The extent of these zones is very variable; they are not often larger than a five-franc piece.

In order to complete these preliminaries upon which I have been dwelling so long, it would be necessary for me to recall the general characters of the severer form of hystero-epilepsy (la grande attaque hystéro-épileptique), but I think it will suffice if I refer you to former lectures.

Such are the phenomena which are met with in the more pronounced form of hysteria in women, and on which I wish at the outset to fix your attention. Well, the greater number of these characters are to be found in the hysteria of men.

But does hysteria exist in men?

To this question, whether hysteria also attacks individuals of the male sex, we can undoubtedly reply in the affirmative; and we can add moreover that it is by no means rare.

In a recent thesis, M. Klein,[1] a pupil of M. Ollivier, has collected not less than seventy-seven cases of hysteria in men. The proportion, according to M. Briquet, is one man to twenty women. This figure is undoubtedly a slight exaggeration. Nevertheless, my experience enables me to affirm that hysteria is met with frequently enough in men; and that it is attended with all the characters ordinarily seen in the female sex.

I will only mention one case by way of illustration.

A youth of 17 years, S—, from Moscow, came to consult me for the first time last year. He is a tall thin lad, amongst whose antecedents there is an uncle the subject of melancholia. The patient himself is imaginative, writes poetry, is fond of music, reads novels with avidity. He has no malformation of the genital organs. For several months he has been subject to attacks coming on nearly every day about five o'clock in the evening. In the way of permanent symptoms, he has left hemianæsthesia, and on the same side, a costo-sternal hysterogenic point. Brisk friction on this point induces an attack. The spontaneous attacks are preceded by melancholy, beating of the temples, and the sensation of a ball which spreads from the precordial region upwards to the larynx. Whether spontaneous or provoked, the attacks consist of an epileptoid stage, more marked in one half of the body, tonic and clonic spasms which predominate on the

[1] Klein, "*De l'hystérie chez l'homme,*" 'Thèse de Paris,' 1880.

left side; he loses consciousness, but does not bite his tongue. After which his body assumes the arc of a circle with an abdominal convexity. In the third stage, he gets up and walks with his eyes wide open, and utters a cry of terror (seeing his dead mother.) At the conclusion of an attack, laughter, tears, and yawnings occur; he asks for something to drink, trembles, says he is cold, &c. By way of summing up,—the hemianæsthesia, the existence of a hysterogenic zone, and the character of the attacks which have just been described, amply suffice to establish the diagnosis; it is not epilepsy certainly, it is hysteria. A tonic treatment, the employment of hydrotherapeutic methods, and certain alterations in the intellectual hygiene, will tend to promote recovery.

But well-marked cases of hysteria are met with not only in manhood and adolescence, but are seen even in childhood before puberty. This is proved by well-authenticated observations. It would seem, according to M. Klein, that hysteria in the male is most frequently seen about twenty-four years of age; but I think this statement needs confirmation.

According to my own observations, hysteria is more common than is generally believed in boys about twelve or thirteen years of age. It is met with, as you know, in the other sex very frequently at the age of ten or twelve years. Moreover, cases having all the characters of *hysteria major* do occur in children both male and female. As an example of this last kind, I may mention the case of a little boy of 13 years old, whom I saw in consultation with a very distinguished physician, who displayed the greatest scepticism about hysteria in general, and particularly about hysteria in childhood. In presence of the epileptiform attacks, it was asked whether it was not true epilepsy, or perhaps a consequence of some serious encephalic lesion, a cerebral tumour for example. The epileptiform seizures existed without doubt, but they were only part of a series of other manifestations; they were followed by the great movements, during which the child threw himself into the arc of a circle, &c. I was a witness of one of these seizures. I sought for a hysterogenic point, and it was found in the left flank; I pressed upon it and the convulsive movements ceased, although consciousness did not return. In the intervals of the attacks there existed a left hemi-hyperæsthesia; besides which this boy had an effeminate air, and was surrounded by the playthings of a little girl.

I prescribed tonics; isolation, so as to withdraw him from the influence of his parents, who petted him too much; and hydrotherapy. A cure was effected in less than three months. Unhappily, this child succumbed three years afterwards to a pericarditis consequent on scarlatina; but the nervous symptoms had never again appeared.

Among all the published cases of hysteria in boys, that of MM. Bourneville and d'Olier[1] is perhaps the most remarkable, both on account of the care with which the details of the case were studied, and the accentuated character of the symptoms. It is an illustration of hystero-epilepsy, of *hysteria major* [la grande hystérie] in the strictest sense of the term. The child was 13 years old, born of a family which numbered amongst its members several epileptic idiots, and one child with depraved instincts. The child in question, however, was good-tempered and intelligent. In the intervals of the attacks, left hemianæsthesia and amblyopia were found to exist, and three hysterogenic zones (bregma, left iliac fossa, and lumbar region). The bregmatic point was the most sensitive.

The least shock, the least friction, applied to this point produced an attack; and even the comrades of the patient, having learned the secret, gave themselves the wicked pleasure of initiating the convulsive seizures by these simple means. Strong pressure arrested an attack with the same facility. The fits were always the same; epileptoid period, period of great movements, with the attitude of an arc of a circle, then passionate attitudes with violent cries. He had, between November, 1879, and December, 1880, not less than 582 such seizures. He had no true epileptic fits, and there was no permanent impairment of intellect, in spite of the frequent repetition of the seizures.

[1] Bourneville et d'Olier, 'Recherches cliniques et thérapeutiques sur l'épilepsie, l'hystérie et l'idiotie,' 1881, p. 30.

The case of the child whom I am about to show you is less complete, less precise; and less rich, if I may say so, in the very accentuated phenomena. It is a case of *minor* rather than *major* hysteria, although I do not think it is the less interesting, if only on account of the surrounding circumstances.

He is a young Jew of 13 years of age, a native of Southern Russia. Both his parents are in good health; the father is very impressionable and nervous, but without anything very characteristic. You see the child is clothed in the uniform of a Gymnasium at . . . . . (Southern Russia), which he has attended for the last three years. He has worked hard; he has a bright, intelligent look, but he is small and pale. He has complained for rather more than a year of pains in his head, but it is only during the past five months (in January) that the headache has become intense, returning every evening about five o'clock, and followed shortly afterwards by convulsive attacks.

The original diagnosis seems to have been somewhat uncertain; an organic lesion was mentioned, and the prognosis given was very unfavorable. The father, who loves his son to distraction, undertook the voyage, came to Paris, and brought him to us fifteen days ago, imploring us to give him the means of cure, which he had been unable to obtain in his own country. From the very first interview we were able to give him hope. The affection is not so serious; not only will the child live, but we can affirm without hesitation that the child will make a complete recovery.

If we bear in mind, apart from the other circumstances of the case, that this young person is the subject of a persistent cephalalgia, with a point of exaggerated sensibility on the vertex, and that for five months the attack has occurred every day at the same time, we should have a strong presumption of *hysteria*, which a more careful investigation tends only to confirm. In the periods between the fits we have ascertained that there is a loss of sensation to pricking, to cold, and to faradization on the right side; the taste, smell, and hearing are also weak on the same side. He complains that he cannot see clearly with the right eye, and a methodical examination of the visual field shows a retraction more marked on the right side (Fig. 16), and with that eye he can only identify red. Besides these symptoms there are patches of hyperæsthesia on the cranium,

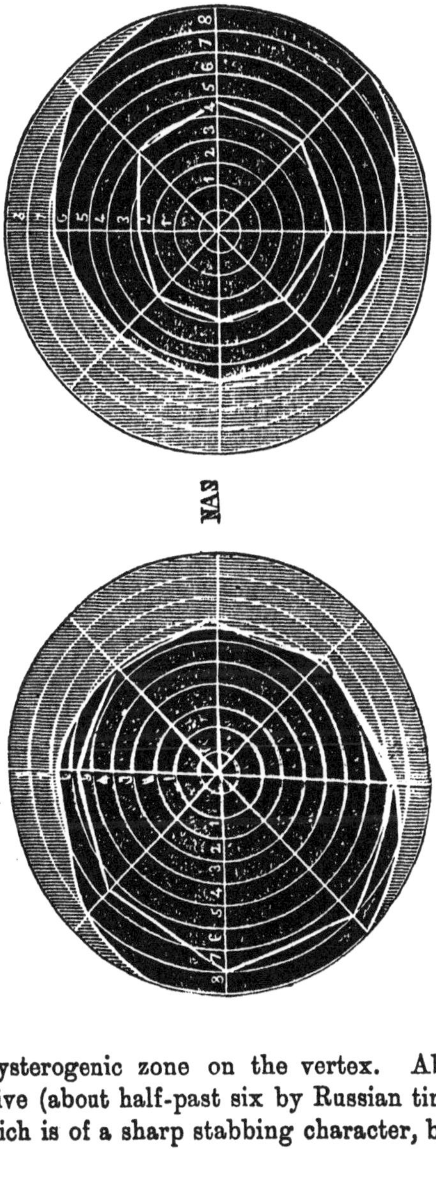

FIG. 16.—Retraction of the field of vision predominating on the right side in the case of the child B—.

and a hysterogenic zone on the vertex. About half-past four or five (about half-past six by Russian time), the headache, which is of a sharp stabbing character, becomes worse, and is followed by tinkling in the ears. He has not the sensation of a ball, but a sort of thoracic constriction.

The attack may generally be cut short by chloroformization. Left to himself he lies down on his left side, with his head on a little cushion that he always has with him, sobs, and doubles himself up. The upper and lower extremities are bent, he hides his head in his hands, and assumes somewhat the position of emprosthotonos ; he can be roused quite easily. This lasts three or four minutes, then the limbs unbend, the eyes fill with tears, and all is finished; no laughter, no crying, no delirium.

It is interesting to notice the deportment of the father at the expected time of attack. He takes out his watch, which is set to the time of his country; about six o'clock he questions his son, and asks him if he is suffering. If the reply is "Yes," he displays an amount of solicitude which is respectable no doubt, but which certainly tends to foster the patient's condition and to maintain the regularity of the symptoms.

It is not necessary after the preceding account to discuss the differential diagnosis.

It would be superfluous to compare this case with those other more classical ones which I have described to you at the commencement of the lecture, and to point out the analogies which prove that they all belong to the same family. We have here to do with hysteria, nothing but hysteria; the idea of any intracranial organic lesion may be dismissed at once.

Hence the prognosis, which is in general relatively favorable, is absolutely so in this case. There is no doubt about the result, because, hysteria occurring in boys is not so rebellious, according to my experience at any rate, as when it occurs in little girls.

I shall prescribe: 1, isolation, so as to withdraw him from the paternal solicitude, which serves only to perpetuate the excitable nervous condition; or at least I shall enjoin a firmer and less sympathetic behaviour on the part of the father; 2, the employment of tonics; 3, static electricity and hydrotherapy. These, I believe, will effect marvels. I hope that the father will not refuse to consent to the employment of these methods, and that he will be able in a few months' time to take back his son to the Gymnasium of . . . . completely cured.[1]

[1] At first the patient underwent treatment by static electricity every other day, and bath-treatment daily, at the same time as a restorative regimen was pursued. But the father would not consent to be separated from the child, and every day at the same hour he was in waiting for the attack, which in fact did not fail to produce it in the same manner as it had done before the treatment was commenced. At the end of a month's unsuccessful attempt, he decided to place his child in a sanitorium; but during the greater part of the day he roved continually around the establishment, questioning those who came out as to the condition of his son, who knew what was going on and did not feel completely abandoned. Several weeks passed thus, and nothing occurred; the distressed father wished to give up the treatment. It was only after much trouble he was made to understand that until then only a fictitious isolation had been adopted; that, in consequence, the treatment had been altogether incomplete; and that it was necessary for him to absent himself altogether, so that his son should have no doubt he was alone, quite alone, and would only be liberated when cured.

This was done, and what took place subsequently proved the therapeutic value of complete isolation in cases of this kind. At the end of four or five days the attacks became modified, less regular and less severe. Fifteen days later and the attacks no longer occurred; then the bregmatic hysterogenic zone disappeared; and when the patient departed, about one month after the commencement of effectual treatment, traces of amblyopia were all that was left of the former symptoms. (Ch. F.)

LECTURE VII.

TWO CASES OF HYSTERICAL CONTRACTURE OF TRAUMATIC ORIGIN.

SUMMARY.—*Latent hysteria without convulsive attacks.—Permanent spasmodic contracture of traumatic origin.—Two cases compared, one in a woman, the other in a man.—Heredity.—Ulnar deformity of hand; experimental study of the deformity by electricity, and by putting in action the phenomenon of neuro-muscular hyperexcitability.*

GENTLEMEN,—In the lecture to-day, which inaugurates the new academical year, I shall call your attention to two cases that have recently come under our observation, and which several among you have already had the opportunity of examining. These two cases seem to me to be quite worthy of occupying our attention for a while, for they present some striking analogies; so much so that they seem to be cast as it were in the same mould, and for several reasons merit careful comparison.

They both, in fact, offer an illustration of hysteria, anomalous by the absence of convulsive seizures. They have besides this, another trait in common, to wit, the existence of a spasmodic contracture limited to one of the hands, and developed, as it would seem, under the influence of an external stimulus.

If one of these cases occurs in the female sex, as is the rule; the other, on the contrary, attacks the male; and this is a circumstance which should undoubtedly excite your interest.

Briefly put: 1. Hysteria, latent and wanting in that pathognomonic feature of the disease, the convulsive attack; 2. Permanent spasmodic contracture developed under the influence of an injury. These are the two points which I wish especially to emphasise in our study of these two cases; which are of different sex truly, but between which there is, as I shall attempt to show, a marked degree of similitude.

I. After these preliminary remarks, I will commence at once with an account of the first case.

The patient is a girl of about 16 years old, and as you see, of delicate appearance. Her physiognomy is calm enough, and presents nothing very peculiar. She is not decked out with showy colours, like so many of these patients; she does not belong to the buoyant, expansive variety of the disease. But, it may be noted in passing, these placid hysterical subjects are not always the easiest to manage.

A few facts in her antecedent history should be mentioned. After the death of her mother from pulmonary phthisis, she was placed, at the age of 11, in a home under the direction of a religious sisterhood. We learn, and this is a point of interest, that her father died in the Orleans Lunatic Asylum, where he had lived for three years before his death. The disease for which he was admitted into the asylum seems to have been progressive general paralysis, if one may judge by the fact that he had several convulsive attacks, after which he remained paralysed. One of her brothers, 13 years old, who is kept in a charitable institution, is almost an idiot.

These facts deserve some attention because, as you know, neuropathic heredity figures conspicuously in the etiology of hysteria. This cause can be invoked in 30 instances out of every 100 according to Briquet. In conformity with the nomenclature proposed by M. Prosper Lucas there are two kinds of heredity, *homonymous heredity* or the *heredity of similitude*, where hysterical parents beget hysterical offspring; and the *heredity by transformation*, the parents having been affected with some other affection of the nervous system, such as insanity, epilepsy, &c.

There is scarcely anything worth noting in the previous history of the patient herself besides a severe bronchitis, which lasted three months. There is a complete absence, whether in the past or the present, of any of the phenomena of convulsive hysteria. Our patient seems to be absolutely unacquainted with hysterical globus, spasms, or convulsions.

As regards her moral condition, the information furnished by the Superior of the Sisterhood where she lived is not very explicit: "She has an extreme fondness for liberty; her conversation and her mind are not refined." What is there behind this monastic reticence? At present we know of nothing; but perhaps we shall know by-and-by.

Now I come to the principal fact, the deformity of the left hand, which represents as you see a veritable club-hand [main-bot], and which I designate hysterical (Fig. 17).

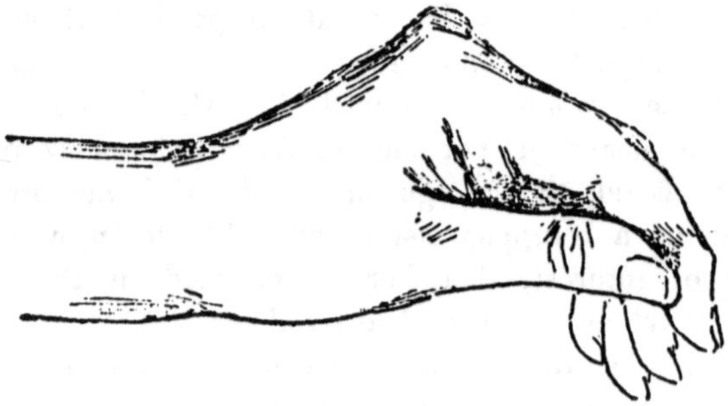

FIG. 17.—Hysterical contracture of the left hand. Drawn by M. P. Richer.

I shall tell you presently what are the circumstances under which this deformity was developed; at present I will only mention the fact that it has lasted for one year. During all that time the deformity has been permanent; there has been no cessation, no alteration, except during a period of two months, when it was modified under the influence of treatment.

The wrist is free, so also are the other joints of the upper extremity. The deformity is therefore limited to the hand. The first phalanges are flexed on the metacarpus, the other phalanges only present a slight degree of flexion. The fingers, thus flexed as a whole, are squeezed one on the other, forming a sort of cone, of which the summit corresponds to the extremities of the terminal phalanges. The thumb, in a state of adduction, is itself strongly pressed against the index finger.

It is easy to satisfy oneself that the muscular rigidity is the sole cause of the deformity, and that the joints and the ligaments are not affected. The attempts at reduction sufficiently demonstrate this. Chloroformization would be able to give us instantaneous proof; but we feared a perturbation which would have prevented you from studying this deformity *de visu*.

Furthermore, we find here the characters of a spasmodic contracture. If, in fact, the flexors are especially affected, and determine the kind of deformity, the extensors are also undoubtedly attacked; for it is as difficult to exaggerate the flexion as to produce extension. This simultaneous action of antagonistic muscles is one of the characters of spasmodic contracture, to which I shall return.

In passing, there are some other particulars worth mentioning. The deformed hand is colder than the other, and has a bluish tint, denoting a manifest trouble of the vaso-motor nerves. There exists an atrophy, or rather a slight emaciation, not only of the hand, but also of the other segments of the limb. The forearm and the arm are about one centimetre smaller than those of the opposite side; it is not a true muscular atrophy, but rather a wasting from prolonged repose. We find, moreover, a diminution of general and special sensation over all the half of the body on the same side as the deformity.

We have here, note it well, a permanent contracture in the true acceptation of the term. It is to be found morning and evening, it persists also during sleep. Of this we can easily satisfy ourselves, thanks to the circumstance that the patient is devoid of sensation on this side, and the exploration can be made without waking her. Hence, any suspicion of trickery can be entirely dismissed from the mind.

Perhaps, before going further, it may be interesting to enter into some detail relative to the physiology of this contracture.

What are the muscles which specially act to determine this defective attitude? In the first place it is the interossei; for, as Duchenne (of Boulogne) has shown, these muscles serve the purpose of flexing the first phalanx, in addition to which, the palmar interossei have the action of drawing the fingers towards an imaginary line passing through the longitudinal axis of the middle finger, and consequently of drawing them all together. But the interossei are not alone affected, for the two distal phalanges are also flexed, and this attitude is due to the action of the superficial and deep flexors.

Therefore one must recognise the action not only of the ulnar nerve, which supplies the interossei, but also of the median, under the influence of which the flexors contract. But, besides this, the participation of the median nerve is also shown by the attitude of the thumb. You will notice in fact that the thumb is not only in a state of adduction, but also at the same time in opposition; for, not only is it carried inwards, but the nail faces, not directly outwards, as in simple adduction, but somewhat forwards. Simple adduction of the thumb is determined by the adductor, *i. e.* the true interosseous of the first space, which is supplied by the ulnar nerve; but the other movement is produced by the opponens, which is supplied by the median.

Moreover, we need not confine ourselves to simple assertions relative to the mechanism of this deformity of hand. We are prepared to demonstrate the condition which has just been described by means of localised electricity, after the method of Duchenne (of Boulogne). This kind of experimentation is rather difficult on normal subjects, because of the pain produced by faradization; but that difficulty does not exist in anæsthetic hysterical subjects, who lend themselves, as it were, to the investigation by not experiencing any pain.

I bring before you again the woman B—, a hystero-epileptic with left hemianæsthesia. A black point has been marked just within the tendon of the flexor carpi ulnaris; it is the point of election for faradization of the ulnar nerve at the level of the wrist. You see that faradization produces a *partial ulnar deformity of hand* [*griffe cubitale partielle*], which recalls that of our patient, and in which the interossei and adductor of the thumb are alone in action. If, again, we excite the ulnar nerve at the level of the bend of the elbow we determine a *total ulnar deformity of hand* [*griffe cubitale totale*] with flexion of the last two fingers; this latter movement being due to the action of the ulnar segment of the deep flexor.

These same facts are even more easily studied in subjects who can be plunged into a state of hypnotic lethargy. We can in fact profit by the *neuro-muscular hyperexcitability* with which these subjects are affected, and produce the same movements by irritating the nerve with some hard body, simply with a stick, without faradization. The advantage of this mode of experimentation is that the attitudes which result are enduring, as you observe in this patient, in whom you see me produce, by simple pressure on the ulnar nerve at the wrist, the interosseous deformity of hand [*la griffe interosseuse*]; or, if you like to press on the nerve at the bend of the elbow, the complete ulnar deformity of hand [*griffe cubitale totale*]. After having brought back the hand to the interosseous deformity, you see I can reproduce exactly the deformity of our first patient by exciting the opponens muscle in the palm of the hand. I should like you to observe that in this hyperexcitable subject the hand, contracted in a state of flexion, presents all the characters of spasmodic contracture; the attitude is fixed, and the flexors and extensors are both contracting. It is therefore evidently an influence of the cord. But that is a point to which we shall return.

After this digression, it is time to come back to our patient. It has just been shown that the case before us is one of spasmodic contracture, but now it remains to be seen that it merits the term hysterical, and that the relatively favorable prognosis applicable to this class of case can be given here; or, in other words, one can hope that in spite of its long duration and tenacity it will yield to appropriate treatment.

This diagnosis can be based, firstly, on the very *intensity* of the contracture, which rarely presents itself to such a degree when it is due to an organic lesion, a lateral sclerosis of the cord. Secondly, on its *permanence*, always in the same degree, night and day. In hemiplegic patients the contracture generally relaxes under the influence of sleep.

Thirdly, the circumstances under which the defective position was produced are of great importance. More than a year ago, 2nd November, 1881, the patient, in breaking a pane of glass, produced an insignificant wound on the back of the hand, over the position of the second metacarpal bone, which healed in four or five days. It was this slight injury that determined the contracture: this is a feature of great importance. Besides this, the onset was sudden and without pain. Finally, the deformity persists long after the wound is healed. Without doubt, among the subjects of organic lesions (cerebral, or spinal, descending sclerosis) one may see the same condition arise in consequence of an injury. But under these circumstances, generally speaking, the onset is not so sudden, and there is not the same disproportion between the triviality of the injury and the intensity of the contracture; and, moreover, it has not the same persistence after the cure of the peripheral irritation.

This tendency to contracture in hysterical patients, this *contracture diathesis*, which can be lighted up by a trivial injury, is very pronounced in some people. I observed a long time ago that certain hysterical subjects, after a sudden movement, in throwing a stone for example, remained with the arm in a state of contracture. We can reproduce the same phenomenon in the woman M—, whom I show you. You see that I can, by suddenly bending the foot, determine a talipes equinus, which will only yield to prolonged massage. You notice that this contracture is produced in the waking state, and that it has the same intensity as that which we produced just now, by means of the neuro-muscular hyper-excitability in hypnotic sleep.

Applied to the case of our patient, you perceive that this series of considerations enables us to presume that the affection is of an hysterical nature. But this presumption, already a strong one, becomes changed to certainty when a more attentive study has enabled us to reveal characteristics which establish more and more clearly the fundamental nature of the case.

Although the convulsive attacks are wanting in this patient, she nevertheless presents a number of nervous troubles, which constitute quite as much the characteristic stigmata of hysteria.

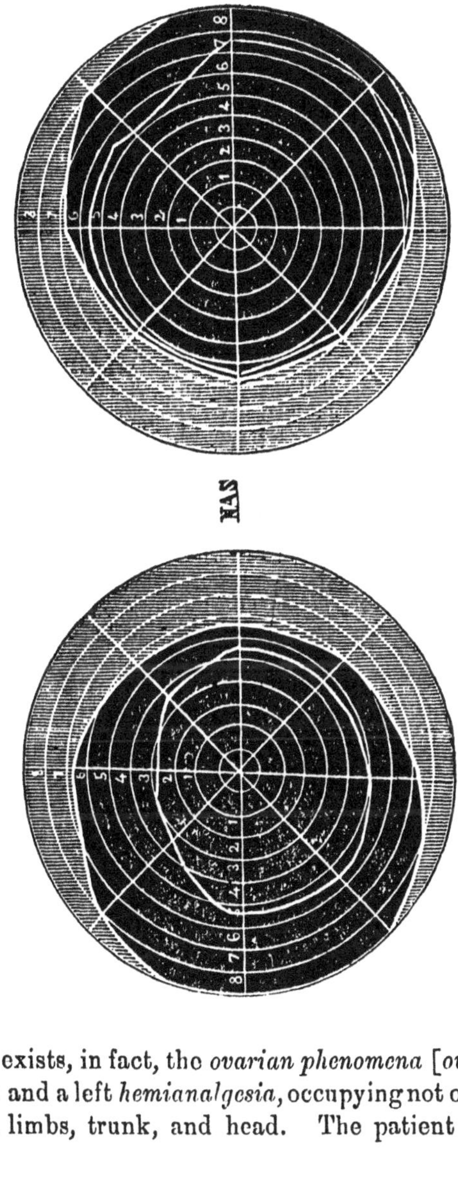

FIG. 18.—Retraction of the visual field.

There exists, in fact, the *ovarian phenomena* [*ovaric*] on the left side; and a left *hemianalgesia*, occupying not only the hand but both limbs, trunk, and head. The patient is quite unaffected by faradization of the skin. There is, moreover, a *sensorial hemianæsthesia.* The organs of sense are affected in the same manner as the integuments which protect them. This point belongs to a question which we have already had occasion to study in the clinique in a general manner;[1] and in this particular case a deficiency has been demonstrated to exist in the sense of hearing by a physician, M. Walton,[2] now visiting our wards. Smell and taste are also affected. It is the same with vision; there exists a retraction of the visual field (Fig. 18) for the perception of light, and for the perception of colours, with a transposition of the red circle to the exterior. There is a diminution of the acuteness of vision, which is represented by a sixth of the normal.

We find then in our patient all the characteristics of an hysterical hemianæsthesia, with ovarian phenomena. These troubles of sensation could only be determined by a central cerebral lesion placed within the sensitive crossway, by alcoholism, or by lead poisoning. But since we find no other sign of these affections in this patient, we are obliged to conclude that all the pathological phenomena are of a purely hysterical nature. And in short you see that all the phenomena, which at first sight seemed so irregular, so strange, is fully explained.

Gentlemen, the hour is already late, we must postpone the continuation of this investigation till the next lecture.

[1] Ch. Féré—"Sur quelques phénomènes observés du côté de l'œil chez les hystéro-épileptiques, soit en dehors de l'attaque soit pendant l'attaque" ('Soc. de Biologie,' 1881, et 'Arch. de Neurologie," 1882, T. iii, p. 281).

[2] G. L. Walton—"Deafness in Hysterical Hemianæsthesia" ('Brain,' part xx, 1883).

LECTURE VIII.

TWO CASES OF HYSTERICAL CONTRACTURE OF TRAUMATIC ORIGIN (*continued*).

SUMMARY.—*Investigations into simulation, catalepsy, and contracture.—Hysteria in the male, frequency, heredity, adult age.—Masked forms.—Contracture of traumatic origin.*

GENTLEMEN,—You have not forgotten that in the last lecture I proposed to draw a comparison between two cases which came under notice here about the same time; in both of which there exists a contracture of an hysterical nature, supervening after an injury; a wound through the breaking of a pane of glass in one case, a superficial burn in the other. These two cases, I pointed out, are drawn together by the most striking analogies, although the one is a young girl of 16 years old, while in the other we have a vigorous man, a blacksmith of 35 years of age, married, and the father of several children.

The young girl has already been the subject of most attentive study. But the male subject, which we were not able to bring before you the other day, has now been confided to our care by M. Debove, in whose wards he was, at Bicêtre. I will gladly take the opportunity thus afforded to me of submitting this man to a very thorough examination before your eyes. I do it the more willingly because it is undoubtedly a rare case, instructive in the highest degree, and consequently well worthy of absorbing your attention for a time.

But before coming to this case, it will be convenient I

think to complete a few details about the young patient with whom we were occupied in the last lecture.

You are well aware, gentlemen, that when we are treating of hysteria, the physician should always have present in his mind the possibility of simulation, under which the patients either exaggerate real symptoms, or sometimes even create an entirely imaginary symptomatology. Everyone knows that the desire to lie, to deceive, sometimes even without motive, by a disinterested cultivation of art for art's sake, sometimes with the view of making a sensation, of exciting pity, &c., is a characteristic common enough in hysteria. It is an element that is met with at each step in the history of this neurosis, and which throws a certain amount of disfavour on the study of it.

But in the present day, gentlemen, since the clinical history of hysteria has been ransacked so many times and so thoroughly, is it truly so difficult as some would have us believe, to discern the real from the false symptomatology, *i. e.* from that which is imaginary, simulated? No, gentlemen, it is not; and not to remain among vague generalities in regard to this matter any longer, allow me to recall to your minds a concrete example, chosen amongst many others, and upon which I dwelt last year.

I refer to the catalepsy induced in hysterical subjects. The question is this: Can this state be simulated so as to deceive a physician experienced in these matters?

It is generally believed that if a cataleptic subject is placed with the arm horizontally extended, this attitude will be preserved so long that the duration alone is sufficient to do away with all suspicion of simulation. This statement is not quite accurate according to our observations. At the end of ten or fifteen minutes the cataleptic arm begins to descend, and at the end of twenty to twenty-five minutes it resumes a vertical position according to the law of gravity. Now, a vigorous man attempting to preserve the same position is able to attain the same limit. One must, therefore, seek some other distinctive character.

Let us apply both to the healthy person who simulates and to the cataleptic patient,—1, a reaction drum to the extended arm, so as to register the least oscillation of the limb; 2, a pneumograph to the chest, so as to obtain the respiratory movements. These are the results which are obtained: *a*. In the cataleptic patient the pen, which corresponds to the reaction drum connected with the arm, traces on the registering roller a straight, perfectly regular line; in the healthy subject, on the contrary, the straight line at first oscillates, then becomes broken, and finally presents great oscillations arranged in series. *b*. The signs afforded by the pneumograph are even more significant. In the cataleptic patient the respiration remains slow, superficial, regular up to the end: whereas, in the person who simulates the tracing presents two distinct parts; at first the respiration is regular, and normal; then, corresponding to the oscillations of the limb, which indicate muscular fatigue, one observes an irregularity in the rhythm and extent of the respiratory movements,—the rapid and deep respiratory depressions which accompany the phenomena of effort.[1]

To recapitulate: 1. The cataleptic patient is unacquainted with fatigue, the muscle yields without effort, without voluntary intervention. 2. The person who simulates, when put to the test, is betrayed both by the tracing of the limb which indicates muscular fatigue, and by the respiratory tracing, which shows the effort destined to mark the effects of fatigue.

We have within the last few days made a somewhat analogous arrangement to put the contracture of our young patient to the test. The forearm was laid on a table to which the back of the hand was solidly fixed by the aid of a bandage. A little sling containing the thumb was fixed by a cord passing over two pulleys and supporting a balance plate in which was placed a weight of one kilogramme (Fig. 19). The experiment lasted about half an hour, during which time the thumb was gradually raised, and became more and more detached from the index finger. After the experiment the thumb immediately returned to its first position without any appearance of fatigue, and quite as firmly as before.

During all the time the pneumograph applied to the front of the chest registered every respiratory movement, and this was what the tracing revealed. The respiration was

[1] See p. 14, *et seq.*

regular, not too deep, equal from the commencement to the end, quite normal; there was nothing, therefore, absolutely nothing which recalled the respiratory trouble that characterises the phenomenon of effort (Fig. 20, A, B).

For the purpose of comparison, a vigorous young man, one of our clinical clerks, was placed exactly under the same

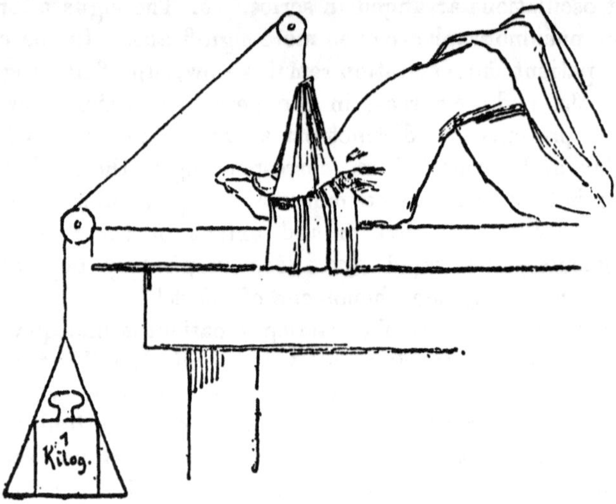

FIG. 19.—Experiment intended to verify the reality of the contracture of the hand.

conditions. He voluntarily placed his hand in the peculiar attitude presented by the contracted hand of our young patient. The thumb was applied tightly against the index finger at the outset of the experiment, it was submitted to the same continuous traction during the same space of time, that is to say, half an hour. It yielded little by little, and became separated by degrees from the index finger against the will of the experimentalist, who resisted all the while. There was nothing up to that time to distinguish the simulator from the patient, but it is in the respiratory tracing where the contrast becomes manifest. At first, that is for the first few minutes, the respiration was equal and regular, but it soon became disordered, the respirations became prolonged, marked by deep depressions, and separated by large flat-topped curves. It was then that the phenomena of effort became evident. (Fig. 20, C, D.)

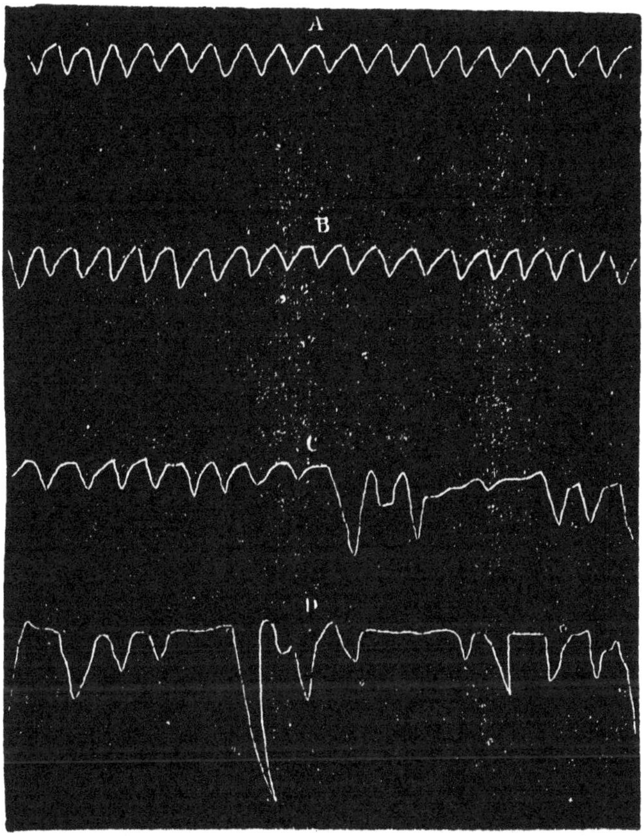

FIG. 20.—The lines A and B represent the respiratory movements of the patient; the lines C and D those of a simulator. Read from left to right.

Thus you see, by an experiment of this kind, that fraud, if it was a fraud, would have been easily recognised, since we have in the study of the respiratory curve the means of discovering it.

Evidently it is not possible to surround oneself with too many guarantees, in clinical studies of hysteria. But please to notice, gentlemen, that this test, to which we have put the little girl, is a sort of crucial experiment; we have already collected numerous and sufficient proofs of the legitimacy of the affection.

I think that I have sufficiently insisted, and that it is well established in your minds, that the phenomena which we have studied together in the preceding lecture are perfectly legitimate pathological phenomena, in which the will of the patient counts for nothing, absolutely nothing. And now I hope to enable you to recognise in a minute that what has just been said concerning the little girl, can be equally applied, step by step, to the case of the male subject whom we are now going to consider more particularly.[1]

At the commencement, it will not be out of place to say a few words relative to the hysterical neurosis, in so far as it affects the male sex.

And firstly, does hysteria occur in the male sex? Yes, undoubtedly, and it is met with much more frequently than would at first be supposed. This subject, male hysteria, is one of those which have been specially investigated by physicians of late years. Thus, one is able to count not less than five inaugural dissertations on this special subject presented to the Faculty of Paris between 1875 and 1880. Briquet in his excellent work has stated that for every twenty hysterical women, one man is met with, at least in Paris, affected with the same malady. This figure I confess appears to me to be a trifle too large. M. Klein,[2] the author of one of the theses, to which I have already alluded, and which was written under the supervision of M. Ollier, has been able to collect from different authors seventy-seven cases of male hysteria, to which he has added three other personal observations, bringing the number up to the respectable total of eighty cases. Hence one is bound at least to conclude that hysteria in men is not such a very rare affection as is generally supposed.

[1] The patient was subjected to the repeated application of a magnet, and the contracture finally disappeared. In the lecture of January 12th, 1883, M. Charcot was able to show the patient completely cured of her deformity; but still preserving the permanent stigmata of hysteria as described above. —CH. F.

[2] P. 77.

Another fact is shown in the same work; namely, that when it occurs in men, hysteria is very often hereditary. This circumstance occurred twenty-three times out of thirty. It is generally maternal heredity, and *similar*[1] heredity; thus it frequently happens that hysteria in the mother begets hysteria in the son.

Another general rule derived from a perusal of these various contributions, is that the hysterical symptoms in the male appear most frequently, at an adult age, after fourteen years at any rate, and according to the opinion of M. Reynolds, who has studied this question in London, between twenty and thirty years of age, or it may be later. Without doubt, hysteria in the male may begin in the child before puberty, from five to fourteen years; but hysteria is more common in the male adult. And here is another point worthy of mention; those adult men who are a prey to the hysterical neurosis do not always present, far from it, feminine characteristics; they are, at least in a great number of cases, robust men presenting all the attributes of the male sex; they may be soldiers or artisans, married and the fathers of families; men in whom one would be very astonished, unless forewarned, to meet with an affection considered by most as an exclusively feminine disease.

Lastly, I should add that in man, as in woman, the neurosis may manifest itself in a masked or latent form. It is perfectly well established, on the other hand, that it can appear in man, endowed with all the attributes belonging to the type of hystero-epilepsy, *hysteria major*, great hysteria [la grande hystérie]. Last year I cited several cases which were very appropriate illustrations of these points. Time does not permit me to say anything just now touching the analogous mental modifications in the two sexes. I must confine myself to a statement of the following facts.

1. Sensorial and sensitive hemianæsthesia—that stigma which almost surely characterises the hysterical condition, after one has carefully excluded certain affections which occasionally produce it (focal capsular lesions, plumbism,

[1] *Vide* p. 84.

alcoholism)—in a word, hysterical hemianæsthesia, are met with in man just as well as woman. Though it does not, perhaps, amount to a retraction of the visual field for luminous perception, or to the transposition of the limits of the visual field for colours. These are not met with in like frequency.

2. The ovarian phenomenon [ovarie], one of the most frequent symptoms of feminine hysteria, is usually wanting in the male; but in them, in some cases at any rate, pressure on the testicle, when it is retained in the canal, provokes or arrests an attack.

3. Instead of the *ovarie,* we find in men hysterogenic points, having the same characters as in women; but in him the points of election are chiefly in the bregmatic region, or on one of the sides of the chest or abdomen, and a very favourite place is in the left flank.

4. The series of phases of the severe attacks of hystero-epilepsy [hysteria major] are found equally in man and in woman. (See amongst others the cases of MM. Bourneville and d'Olier, of M. Fabre (of Marseille), without counting the four or five cases of the same kind that I have personally observed.)

5. Paraplegic or hemiplegic paralysis, with exaltation or diminution of the tendon-reflexes, is a phenomenon which is occasionally seen; much more frequently, it may be said, than contracture, which seems to have been rarely met with.

But you ought not to expect to find all this assembly of phenomena united in one male subject. The hysterical neurosis can be present, and undoubtedly does very often appear in the male without its great classical attributes, that is to say, in a masked form, just as it does in the patient who is about to occupy our attention. I hope, however, to be able to convince you that, in spite of the absence of its chief attributes, it is nevertheless with hysteria that we are dealing, nothing but hysteria.

The patient is a man 34 years old, a blacksmith, father of four children, robust enough, and without any sign of effeminacy. I may tell you at once that we have not been able to find in him any antecedent taint of a neuropathic order, neither hereditary nor personal; no moral emotion can be ascertained as the actual cause of the complaint, and, indeed, no other cause of any sort excepting the burn. On June 26th last a bar of iron heated to a white heat touched his forearm and left hand. The burn, though slight, took six weeks to heal, and at the present time there remains a violet-red patch of 3 or 4 centimetres [1¼ inches] broad, and 10 or 12 long [4 or 5 inches], occupying the lower part of the forearm and the back of the hand. The accident does not seem to have caused much emotion, and the contracture does not seem to have followed the injury immediately; strange to say it became developed gradually. In the history of hysterical contracture due to a traumatic cause this is an exceptional circumstance. A few days after the accident, says he, his arm felt heavy, it became difficult to bend his fingers, feeling as though they were benumbed; but as for the contracture, it came on without the intervention of a fresh cause seven weeks later.

It was on August 15th that he felt pain in the arm, and he could not sleep; and the next day his hand presented the characteristic interosseous deformity, although the thumb was unaffected. Then, the following day, flexion of the fingers came on, and finally the thumb became firmly applied to the fingers. Since then we have seen flexion of the wrist, and then pronation of the forearm, successively occur.

Let us study this singular deformity of hand a little more closely. It consists you see of a permanent contracture of certain muscles, a contracture so pronounced that it resists every attempt at reduction, and which for three months has not ceased to exist, not only during the day, but also, and on this point I lay much stress, during the night. The shoulder and the upper arm are free, the forearm is in a state of pronation. The hand is flexed on the forearm; the four fingers are flexed to such an extent that the nails dig into the palm of the hand. The fingers are strongly pressed against each other, and the thumb is strongly pressed against the posterior surface of the second phalanx of the index finger (Fig. 21).

Here, the most simple physiological analysis shows that

it is chiefly by the action of the median nerve, which supplies the superficial and deep flexors of the wrist, that this attitude is produced. But the ulnar nerve also plays a part, for the adduction of the fingers is due to the action of the interossei. It may be added that there is also contracture of the extensors, as in all spasmodic contractures.

Observe this attitude of a closed, energetically closed, fist, complicated with a flexion of the hand, which is also very forcible. It is, you will notice, an exceedingly forced attitude, an attitude difficult to preserve even for a short time (Fig. 21).

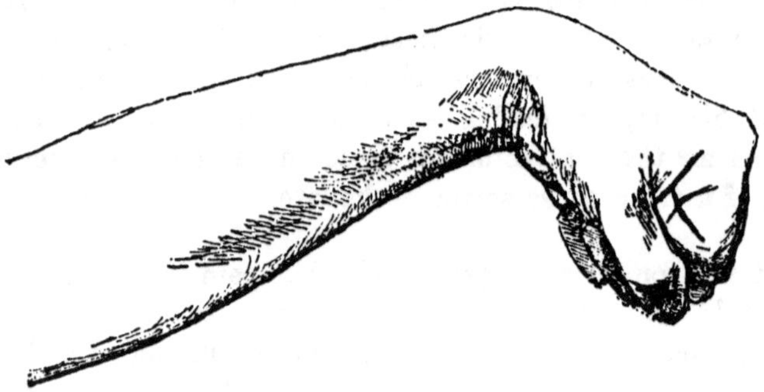

FIG. 21.—Contracture of the left hand. (Drawing by M. P. Richer.)

This is a favorable opportunity to remind you of an ingenuous observation of Duchenne. You know that the extensors of the fingers and those of the entire hand are in a sort of antagonism. If you bend back your closed hand as much as possible, and if you then endeavour to extend the fingers, the hand becomes slightly flexed. It is because the effect of extending the hand is to shorten the extensors of the fingers, and consequently to place them in a situation less favorable for their action; whereas on the contrary, when the hand is extended the conditions are more favorable for the flexors to act. For an analogous reason, if you flex the entire hand, the fingers can more easily be brought into a condition of complete extension.

Let us now consider the combined action of the flexors of the hand and those of the fingers; here, also, there is a sort of antagonism. Thus, in order to strongly flex the fingers and clench the fist, as in pugilism, the hand itself must be extended, and thus the action of the extensors favours that of the flexors. If, on the contrary, the fist being closed, you strongly flex the wrist, then you will notice that the flexion of the fingers relaxes, and that the fingers have a very marked tendency to become unbent. You can only maintain the hand flexed in this position by the help of very strong effort. This, gentlemen, is a fact of a sort which dispels the idea of simulation. It is very much to be doubted whether any resolute person could maintain, without hesitation or intermission, for several hours, and still less for several days, the truly pathological attitude of this patient. It is certain, at any rate, that one cannot imagine a man capable of maintaining it during profound sleep. In this patient the attitude is preserved during sleep; M. Debove has assured himself of it, and we have assured ourselves of it on several occasions. We propose, moreover, to submit the patient to the pneumographic test; and I doubt not but that we shall obtain the same results as in the case of the young girl whom you have already seen.[1]

You will acknowledge, I think, that we have to do with a perfectly legitimate pathological deformity, and not a simulated one; a true symptom, and not an imaginary one artificially produced by the voluntary intervention of the patient. It remains for me to show that, as in the case of the girl, it is hysteria with which we have to deal.

I have already said that it is a masked form of the neurosis; the patient has had no attacks, there are neither antecedent circumstances, nor any psychic modifications to note. But if we refer to the observation which was made by M. Debove on October 1st, and also that which was made by us a week later we find the following symptoms:—1. A left hemianalgesia; pricking produces no pain but a simple sensation of contact; cold is less well perceived over the whole of the left side of the body. 2. A very distinct lessening of the taste, hearing, and smell, on the left side. We have taken regular

[1] The experiment was made under the same conditions and with the same result as in the young girl. It may be added, that under chloroform only incomplete resolution of the contracture was obtained, though a complete resolution had been formerly obtained by M. Debove at the Bicêtre Hospital.

measurements of the visual field. On both sides there is retraction, but more on the left; the visual field for colours is proportionately smaller, but the concentric circles which

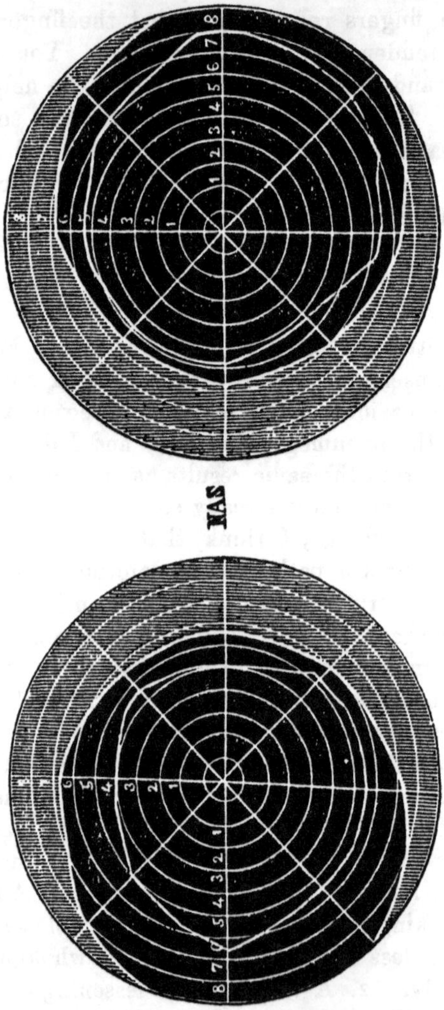

Fig. 22

represent the field for each colour have preserved their relations and their reciprocal proportions; there is no transposition; no achromatopsia; no dyschromatopsia (Fig. 22). 3. All traces of a hysterogenic zone are wanting.

What else could it be but hysteria, in the absence of any circumstance capable of being connected with a focal capsular lesion, with plumbism, or with alcoholism? And in presence of a contracture, a deformity of the hand, which considered by itself carries with it the indisputable mark of a hysterical origin, surely we are justified in concluding that in this patient all the phenomena which have come under our notice belong to hysteria, nothing but hysteria. They present a truly striking analogy to those we have just met with in the girl whom we have been studying.

Such was the condition of the patient on October 7th. Since then, under the influence of treatment, the symptoms have been slightly modified. A magnet was applied to the side of the contracture, and then the sensation returned, without transfer, to the left upper extremity, to the trunk, the head, the arm, but not to the hand or the wrist. In the midst of this treatment the patient went out, fearing, for special reasons, lest he should be cured too quickly. But he came back again a few days ago, and a fresh application of the magnet was made, which has this time caused the insensibility of the hand to disappear, and has produced a numbness and commencing rigidity in the opposite side. M. Debove was not far wrong in the fear which he expressed of modifying too profoundly a situation which he knew that I desired you to witness.

At the present time the contracture alone exists in this man; the hemianæsthesia has completely disappeared, though there exists a painful feeling of cramp in the contracted part, which sometimes troubles his sleep. It is therefore now essentially a latent case, but a case, nevertheless, of whose hysterical nature, if I succeed in my hopes, you will by-and-by have not a shadow of doubt.[1]

[1] The repeated application of the magnet had no other result than bringing back the sensibility to the contracted member. After that the patient was a martyr to some very acute sufferings in the forearm and hand, due partly to the penetration of the nails into the flesh, and also in a certain measure to the contracture itself, for the flexor muscles especially were very sensitive (these spontaneous pains had already been noted, although they were less intense, when the patient was anæsthetic). As he persistently asked for some surgical interference, preferring to submit to amputation

rather than undergo such pain any longer, M. Charcot decided to have recourse to stretching of the nerve which was the main element in the production of the deformity, the median. This operation, which had already been suggested by M. Gillette, surgeon at the Bicêtre, was performed on December 26th, 1882, by M. Terrillon, surgeon at the Salpêtrière. The operation was performed in the upper part of the arm, and the median nerve was twice raised on a director to the height of about 8 centimetres [three and a quarter inches] from its natural position. After recovering from the chloroform the patient experienced tingling, accompanied by pains in the forearm and hand, but the contracture seemed to persist. After a sleep of three or four hours he awoke without pain in the forearm and hand; the contracture had almost completely disappeared, although the fingers could not be quite extended. Since then the situation has further improved although the extension of the first phalanges is still incomplete, due, as it would seem, to a retraction of the fibrous tissues; and, moreover, the contracture is replaced by a paresis of the muscles at first attacked. When showing the patient cured in the lecture of January 12th, 1882, M. Charcot made the observation that, besides this retraction of the fibrous tissues which may be seen sometimes after hysterical contractures of long duration, there exists a peculiar glossy condition of the skin at the extremities of the fingers, and particularly of the index finger, which seems to taper off like a spindle.

LECTURE IX.

A CASE OF SPINAL AFFECTION CONSEQUENT ON A CONTUSION OF THE SCIATIC NERVE.

SUMMARY.—*Contusion of the left buttock.—Continuous pains, intermittent pains.—Early muscular weakness.—Muscular atrophy.—Troubles of micturition, of defæcation, and of the genital functions.—Persistent atrophy of the muscles supplied by the lesser sciatic nerve of the left side.—Electrical exploration.—Paresis and atrophy of the gluteal muscles of the right side.*

GENTLEMEN,—The patient who is about to be brought before you, and who forms the object of our lecture to-day, offers in my opinion a very singular example of an organic spinal affection developed after an injury, not of the cord itself, but of a peripheral nerve.

I am well aware that there already exists among the records of our science a certain number of facts tending to show that certain lesions of the extremities, or of the nerve-trunks, can be reflected back to the spinal centre, and there determine alterations more or less profound; but I doubt if any of these facts present, in the same degree as this case, the conditions of clearness and simplicity so necessary to ensure conviction. This will become evident, I think, from the account of the case, upon which I will enter at once.

The patient is a man, 40 years of age, vigorous, and of good constitution, as you see. He is the father of two children.

A. I ought to mention, in the first place, that in his history prior to the actual complaint, there is no circumstance which can be said to have contributed to the development of the spinal affection with which he is now afflicted, nor of the sciatic pain from which he has suffered. This man has confessed that from 27 to 36 years of age, when he was occupied as a brewer's drayman, he indulged in numerous alcoholic debauches; he has had delirium tremens, and has evinced for some time the characteristic tremor of hands. But for the last four years he has much improved in this respect, and since he has followed the occupation of a carpenter, he has lived a sober life. It would appear that he has not had syphilis; he has certainly not had gonorrhœa; he has not lived in a damp room; he has never been particularly exposed to cold, nor has he suffered from rheumatic pains.

B. The circumstances under which the pathological conditions we are about to investigate came to be developed are as follows. On December 28th, 1881, in the carpenter's shop where this man works, a joist of 3 metres 30 long, [11 feet] terminating in a square surface whose side measured about 10 centimetres [4 inches], which was being moved rapidly in its long axis on a bench by another workman, struck him violently on the left buttock. He thinks he can indicate precisely the exact spot where he was struck; and he points to a place midway between the ischial tuberosity and the great trochanter, a few centimetres below the lower border of the gluteus maximus muscle. Even now, when he presses on the spot the patient experiences a painful sensation. I should like you to remark, as a fact somewhat strange, that no ecchymosis nor tumefaction appeared at the seat of injury either on the same or succeeding days.

If you will be good enough to look at this anatomical diagram, you will at once perceive that the place where the patient was struck corresponds precisely to the course of the greater and lesser sciatic nerves, just after they have passed through the great sciatic foramen. These two nerve-trunks therefore were capable of being, they must have been, affected by the blow.

Although injury to the gluteal region is not rare, far from it;[1] yet it should be remembered that contusion of the sciatic nerve is not a very frequent occurrence.

For such an injury to take place, certain very special conditions are necessary. It may take place when the blow

[1] Concerning this subject, see an interesting article by M. le Dr. Bouilly, 'Arch. gén. de médecine,' 1880, T. II, p. 655.

is produced by the extremity of a beam or shaft, by the butt-end of a gun, or the corner of a piece of marble; then the nerve is squeezed as it were between the external object and the bony surface, from which it is only separated by the gemelli and the quadratus femoris. But otherwise, and this is most frequent, when the buttock is struck by a more or less flat surface, the nerve-trunk is protected. You see that the conditions of a contusion strictly limited to the sciatic nerve existed in the injury; and there is nothing to make us suppose that the coxo-femoral articulation has ever been involved in any way whatever.

Next it is important for you to understand what were the earlier symptoms in this case. These pointed to an affection exclusively limited to the sciatic nerve. The symptoms did not differ at the commencement, which was marked by a sudden onset, from those which belong to ordinary sciatica, *ischias nervosa*, Cotugno's disease. This will appear from the following.

The blow was violent enough to throw the patient to the ground. But he soon got up again, and at the same moment he was seized with pain along the course of the sciatic nerve and its branches. The pain which he experienced from that moment, and during a period of about three months, consisted of two elements:

(*a*) *Continuous pain*, localised along the course of the nerve-trunk, particularly in certain places where it was exacerbated by pressure. We have discovered the existence of certain tender spots: 1, a *superior femoral point*, seated at the lower border of the gluteus maximus muscle between the ischial tuberosity and the great trochanter; 2, a *peroneal point*, corresponding to the place where the nerve goes round the head of the fibula; 3, an *external malleolar point*; 4, a *dorsal point on the foot*. On two of these points, blisters have been applied, of which you can still see traces. These pains were also accompanied by a permanent and very painful sensation of tingling in the foot and the leg.

(*b*) Besides the constant pain there existed *intermittent pains*, coming in twinges, severe, sudden, shooting, and uniting, as it were, one fixed painful spot with another. These painful twinges were accompanied by very evident clonic spasm, in which the leg would be suddenly flexed on the thigh. The patient's pains, both fixed and intermittent, the tinglings and the spasms were especially bad at night, increased by the heat of the bed, to such a degree that he acquired the habit of passing his nights seated in a chair.

So far, we have drawn a clinical picture which could be applied perfectly well to a case of idiopathic spontaneous sciatica, of rheumatic or any other nature.

Even in the first few weeks which followed the accident, a certain degree of muscular weakness was manifest in the left lower limb, considerably impeding the walking and even standing powers, which could not be entirely connected with the fear which the patient evinced of increasing the pain, for this functional impotence persisted even at a time when the pain was becoming less. About three months after the accident the pain had almost completely ceased, but the muscular weakness had very greatly increased; for during the ensuing month it was impossible for him to stand upright and preserve his equilibrium without the support of objects around him. At the end of another month, the fifth after the accident, he was scarcely able to walk a few steps in his bedroom, by pushing a chair before him; and it was only at the end of six months that he was able to walk with the aid of a stick, or without support for a quarter or half an hour, and then not always without fatigue, such as he can do to-day.

This muscular weakness of a limb after sciatica is not a rare occurrence, as you know, when the neuralgic affection has been severe. It is accompanied in such cases, as MM. Bonnefin and Landouzy have remarked, by a more or less pronounced atrophy of the muscular substance of the limb. An atrophy of this sort certainly existed at that time in our patient, although he did not notice it. You will see directly what are the facts on which this assertion is founded.

Functional weakness and concomitant muscular atrophy, in common sciatica, cannot, you are aware, be attributed to prolonged repose. In fact, according to the observations of M. Landouzy, it appears quite early in the disease (at the end of fourteen days), after the onset of the first pains, and even in those cases where the limb has not been placed at rest. The theory generally accepted in order to explain this muscular dystrophy in ordinary sciatica is, as you doubtless know, the following. It is admitted that the irritation, with which the centripetal nerve-tubes are affected, mounts as it were towards the spinal centre, by way of the posterior roots, and extends to the cellules of the corresponding anterior horns, which are consequently affected. The lesion, slight or serious, dynamic or organic, of which they are the seat, has the effect of suppressing, for a shorter or longer time, their trophic action. Consequently, the muscles which are supplied by the centrifugal nerve-tubes, arising in these ganglionic elements, become in their turn the seat of a more or less transitory or permanent dystrophic lesion. One of the proofs which are advanced, and it is not the least powerful, in favour of the intervention of the spinal centre in this mechanism is that the atrophy often attacks muscles which do not come within the distribution of the nerve which is affected by the neuralgia. Thus, for example, in cases where the pain has occupied exclusively the trunk of the great sciatic, the atrophy may be found not only in the muscles supplied by this nerve, but also in the gluteus minimus and medius, which are supplied by the superior gluteal coming directly from the first sacral pair.

However, contemporary observations tend to show that in common idiopathic sciatica, functional weakness, and the muscular atrophy which accompanies it, do not last very long after the pain has disappeared. But it is not altogether thus in traumatic sciatica, at least if one can judge from a case which M. Seeligmüller has published of sciatica coming on after a difficult confinement which necessitated the use of the forceps. In that instance the neuralgia was followed by a paralytic atrophy affecting the calf-muscles, which resisted every measure employed for its relief. We shall see that dystrophic lesions, quite as grave and involving a large number of muscles, have occurred in our case.

But I wish now to dwell for a minute on a series of facts which occurred about three months after the injury, which form a fundamental part of all the mischief, and prove unmistakably, in this patient, the participation of the spinal centre.

Well, about May 15th, at a time when the pains were becoming less, though the muscular weakness was increasing, the patient experienced a painful feeling as of a bar across the lumbar region, extending to both sides, and lasting for several days. Two or three days afterwards he became unable to micturate. The next day he urinated drop by drop, involuntarily, and without knowing it. Then he went to the Necker Hospital, where he was seen by M. Guyon, and a catheter was passed. It was proved there that he had no urethral retraction, no enlargement of the prostate gland—facts which later explorations have confirmed. Since that time the patient has continued to pass a catheter two or three times a day; when he neglects to do it, the urine runs away drop by drop. At the present time the condition in this respect is somewhat ameliorated; he sometimes urinates voluntarily, though not without effort. But most frequently he is obliged, as formerly, to use the catheter regularly.

You will not fail to perceive that this persistent incontinence of urine necessarily implies an involvement of the spinal cord. It is almost possible even to localise the lesion within a very little. The region referred to is the one where experimentation (Goltz, Budge) has placed the centre of the vesical reflexes; it occupies the inferior extremity of the lumbar enlargement, and corresponds to the point of emergence of the four last sacral nerves.

You doubtless know that the experiments to which I allude localise the centre for the muscles of the rectum, and those also for erection and ejaculation, in the same region. Well, the clinical facts show that in this patient these two centres are also affected. In fact, the same day when the incontinence of urine commenced, he had also incontinence of fæces, and it still exists to a certain degree. It should also be added that erections were absent about the same time, and are still wanting.

Here is a series of symptoms which, I repeat, demonstrate beyond doubt the existence of a spinal lesion; and this lesion, it may be affirmed, is not purely dynamic. We have to do with a material lesion, anatomical, probably of an inflammatory nature; in short, a myelitis.

A thorough examination of the patient's lower limbs will furnish us, moreover, with additional and weighty arguments in support of this statement.

The patient was admitted into the Salpêtrière on November 8th last, in the same state as you see him now. He habitually walks with the aid of a stick, which he holds in his right hand. But it is possible for him to walk without support for about half an hour; then he suffers extreme fatigue, especially in the left leg, and he is absolutely obliged to stop. It is curious that the left limb only should be complained of by the patient. Nevertheless the right inferior extremity is also seriously involved, as we shall see directly.

An examination of the left inferior extremity reveals the following. The limb, compared with the right, is somewhat wasted in every part; according to the measurements, there is a difference of several centimetres in favour of the corresponding parts of the right side.

The leg and the foot are cold and mottled with red spots, besides which the foot is slightly tumefied. This condition reminds us of what is seen in certain cases of long-standing infantile paralysis. The sensibility, especially the electric sensibility, is lost over nearly the entire surface of the left limb. The cutaneous reflexes are normal on both sides.

The patella-reflex is exaggerated on the right side, normal on the left. When you strike the left patella tendon, the patient being seated, it produces a curious phenomenon which probably also indicates spinal intervention; at each stroke the right thigh is seen to go towards the median line with a distinct movement of adduction.

Now let us proceed to an examination of the movements of the left leg. First of all as to the muscles supplied by the lumbar plexus, which have preserved their normal power. (*a*) In the muscles supplied by the crural nerve, the movement of flexion of thigh on pelvis, performed by the psoas and iliacus, is preserved and is forcible; movement of extension of leg on thigh are also normal. (*b*) Movements of adduction are also normal.

It is easy to see, on the other hand, that the muscles supplied by the greater and lesser sciatic nerves, the two nerve-trunks simultaneously contused, are, for the most part, profoundly affected. (*a*) The gluteus maximus is soft and flaccid. You are aware that, according to Duchenne, these two muscles are not of much use in standing, but come into play in movements requiring energetic muscular action, such as in the act of mounting a chair. You see that our patient is unable to perform this feat without help, and even then he prefers to do it with his left leg. (*b*) The posterior muscles of the thigh, flexors of the leg. (*c*) The muscles which produce plantar flexion, and dorsal flexion of the foot are also profoundly affected. It is impossible, for instance, for the patient to support himself on tip-toe.

Thus all the muscles supplied by the great or lesser sciatic nerves, or almost all, are seriously involved. Such a muscular weakness might doubtless be explained, by itself, by supposing the existence of a lesion of the motor nerve-tubes, developed in consequence of the contusion below the point struck. But this explanation is insufficient when it is borne in mind that the gluteus medius and minimus of this same left side also participate in the alteration, and that these muscles are supplied by the superior gluteal nerve, which is derived directly from the upper branches of the sacral plexus.

It is known, chiefly by means of Duchenne's researches, that these muscles have the action, both in standing and walking, of fixing the pelvis in such a manner as to prevent its inclination to the right or the left, according as the muscles of the left or right side respectively are in action.

If you observe the patient in a standing position, you will at once perceive that the iliac crest of the right side is on a lower level than the iliac crest of the left. The pelvis is therefore inclined towards the right. This right-sided inclination corresponds also to the relative lowering of the right great trochanter, and the lowering of the corresponding gluteal fold. It should be added that the right shoulder is lower than the left, and that the spinal axis is rightly inclined towards the right. This inclination of the pelvis towards the right side, of itself enables us to suspect a weakness of the left gluteus medius and minimus muscles, whose function it is to lower the left iliac crest so as to place it on the same level as that of the right side.

This weakness is even more obvious if the patient raises his right foot from the ground, as in taking the second step in marching; you see then that the pelvis and the great trochanter of the right side become lowered, even more than it was just now. Under normal conditions, at the moment when the right foot starts for the second step in marching, the pelvis, owing to the action of the left gluteus medius, ought to undergo a slight movement of lowering on the left side, and elevation on the right; but this is not the case here, quite the contrary.

When the patient walks, this failing of the gluteus medius is brought out very clearly at each step by a very pronounced lowering of the iliac spine and trochanter of the right side; and as a result the pelvis undergoes a series of large oscillations, quite obvious and significant.

The gluteus minimus and medius muscles are therefore affected, and profoundly affected. Now, these muscles are innervated by the superior gluteal nerve, which in its origin has nothing in common with the great and lesser sciatic nerves. This participation of the gluteal nerve can scarcely be explained except by the existence of a spinal lesion.

The existence of this spinal lesion, already evidenced by the paralysis of the vesical and anal sphincters, and by weakness of the genital reflexes, is still further shown when we carefully examine the *right* lower extremity, in which there is a marked weakness of the gluteal muscles and most of the muscles of the leg.

This paresis of muscles of the right side is accompanied, as on the left, by an atrophy, an easily appreciable diminution of volume, though it is not so striking as on the left side.

It is expedient that we should consider for a moment this atrophy of six months' duration. The question to settle, and we shall see how interesting a one it is, not only from a theoretical but a practical point of view, is this, is the atrophy that we have here a simple one, unattended by alteration of the fibres ; or is it a degenerative atrophy, one which is attended by a profound modification, a degeneration, of the muscular elements ? You know that the prognosis depends, in a measure, to the solution of this question. Simple atrophy usually yields under the employment of appropriate means, whereas in the degenerative atrophy treatment is powerless.

Are we in possession of the means of clinically making this distinction ? Yes, certainly; the means consist in a methodical electrical exploration, which to be complete should be made successively by the aid of both kinds of current, faradic and galvanic.

In the galvanic exploration (constant current) I may remind you that one of the poles, the indifferent one, is applied to the chest, and the other is applied to the nerve or muscle which it is wished to examine. The latter can be made to become at will either the positive pole (An. *Anode*), or the negative pole (Ka. *Kathode*). You are aware that under normal conditions muscular contractions are produced only at the closing (S. *Schliesung*), or opening of the current (O. *Œffnung*). Now, in order to obtain a single contraction (Z. *Zuckung*) in the normal state with the weakest possible current, say ten elements, the pole used must be the negative one, Ka, and the contraction is thus produced at the moment of closing the current. This is expressed in electro-physiological language by the formula KaSZ. To obtain a contraction with the other (the positive) pole, An, it is necessary to increase the number of elements, increase them, for example, from ten to fifteen. These results are represented thus, KaSZ > AnSZ, and form part of the formula for the normal reactions. If one finds on exploring a muscle that AnSZ can be obtained with a larger number of elements than suffice to obtain KaSZ, the result is represented by AnSZ > KaSZ. It is then said to be an inversion of the formula, which inversion forms part of the reaction of degeneration; or, in other terms, a reaction which indicates a more or less profound alteration of the muscular tissue.

We shall apply these principles in a minute to the investigation of the trophic condition of the muscles in this patient; but it should first be shown what it is that constitutes, from an electro-diagnostic point of view, simple atrophy of the muscles, and their degenerative atrophy.

1. In simple atrophy the faradic and galvanic excitability are only slightly modified. In both cases a stronger current is required to obtain a reaction than in the normal condition, but the results are parallel, there is no modification of the formula KaSZ > AnSZ. An example of these simple atrophies is seen after prolonged rest; or, in certain dynamic spinal affections developed as a consequence of articular lesions.

2. Degenerative atrophy has been studied with great care by experiments on animals, and after division of nerves. It is shown by the experiments of Erb and Ziemssen, briefly put, that absence of faradic reaction, and persistence with modification of galvanic reaction indicates a serious condition, though regeneration is possible; but, if both galvanic and faradic reactions are absent, it reveals a graver condition, a degenerative modification of either nerve or muscle, which is almost certainly irreparable.

In human pathology, gentlemen, these profound modifications of the electrical reactions, corresponding to a grave condition of muscular nutrition, are seen in affections of the peripheral nerves (division, traumatic lesions, &c.); and also in spinal disease when the lesion is so situated that the ganglionic elements, the so-called motor cells, are profoundly altered or destroyed, as, for example, in infantile paralysis after the period of possible restoration, or, again, in central diffuse myelites.

Now let us apply these data to the case of this man. The examination of the various muscles which are trophically and functionally affected gives the following results:

1. The crural nerve is faradically and galvanically excitable on both sides. The adductor muscles and the quadriceps extensor femoris also respond normally to both means of excitation.

2. In the distribution of the branches of the sacral

plexus we find normal reactions on the right side. On the left side the gluteus medius is faradically and galvanically inexcitable. This indicates that the functional shortcomings of this muscle are connected with an organic lesion, and consequently that the difficulty of standing which results, the inclination of the pelvis and of the trunk to the right, and the bending to the right side when the right foot is raised from the ground, will probably persist as permanent infirmities.

3. What has just been said about the gluteus medius can be repeated of the gluteus maximus, but this time both sides are involved. These muscles, which are supplied by the lesser sciatic, respond neither to faradism nor galvanism, a reaction of degeneration, predominating on the left. There is then scarcely a hope of procuring a re-establishment of the function of these muscles.

4. With reference to the great sciatic nerve, I shall confine myself to mentioning the facts which relate to the calf muscles, and the flexors of the leg on the thigh. On the left side faradization has no effect; galvanism only produces a slight and feeble response. On the right there is also a reaction of degeneration, but less complete (AnSZ=KSZ); here there remains some hope of ultimate restoration under appropriate electro-therapeutic treatment. The same can be said of the calf muscles; flexion of leg on thigh, and plantar flexion of the foot can without doubt be restored.

Thus, you see, electrical exploration has furnished us with data for prognosis, at the same time that it has enabled us to guess, to some extent, the degree of the spinal lesion. It certainly occupies the lower lumbar region, and viewing all the circumstances of the case is probably situated in the central grey substance. There is no reason to believe that the anterior or posterior white fibres are involved.

The posterior horns of the grey matter are not obviously affected, for there is no modification of sensibility, but the anterior horns are certainly involved to some extent in the region corresponding to the origin of the branches of the lumbar plexus. The alteration in the cells is not a profound one, possibly it is dynamic. These cells are in a state of hyperexcitability which I have proposed to designate by the name "strychninism," and which is capable of explaining the exaltation of the patellar reflexes especially on the right side.

But at the level of origin of the branches of the sacral plexus the alteration of the ganglionic elements is more profound; a certain number of the cells are modified or destroyed, which corresponds with the serious alteration in the gluteal muscles.

The spinal lesion which we have before us, developed under the influence of an injury, so far as one can judge from the evolution of a morbid phenomena, has no progressive tendency, the worst of the mischief is passed. One could almost say that the disease is now quiescent, or perhaps, in the case of certain nerve-fibres and cells, not completely destroyed, there is a tendency towards recovery.

The treatment should be directed chiefly towards favouring this restoration of the affected elements. The patient should be advised not to resume the fatiguing movements of his lower limbs which are demanded by his occupation for a long time to come. It is known in fact that old and extinct spinal lesions are sometimes re-awakened by exercise of the limbs corresponding to the affected part of the spinal centre. Thus in infantile paralysis of the left lower extremity it may happen that the right lower limb may be attacked several years later, in consequence of a forced march. As to medication, it should be chiefly directed to the trophic condition of the affected muscles. We shall also advise methodical electrization, faradic and galvanic; massage; and lastly hydrotherapy, the influence of which not only on general but also local nutrition, is undoubtedly one of the most beneficial methods of treatment.

LECTURE X.

I. DOUBLE SCIATICA IN A WOMAN AFFLICTED WITH CANCER.
II. CERVICAL PACHYMENINGITIS.

SUMMARY.—I. *Double sciatica; conditions under which this affection occurs; diabetes, certain meningo-myelites, compression of the spinal nerve-trunks at the intervertebral foramina.—The pseudo-neuralgiæ of vertebral cancer.* —II. *Hypertrophic cervical pachymeningitis; pseudo-neuralgic period; paralytic stage; spasmodic stage.—Illustrative case: recovery with retraction of the flexor muscles of the leg.—Radical cure by surgical intervention.*

I.

GENTLEMEN,—The first patient who will be presented to you to-day will take your minds back to the history of symptomatic sciatica, which occupied our attention during the last two lectures. It is a subject the practical interest of which you will not fail to perceive, and this circumstance will I hope sufficiently justify my dwelling on a few fresh features of the affection that will be unfolded as we go along.

A. The patient is a woman named D—, aged 61 years, a workwoman, whose family and previous histories present nothing worthy of note. About fifteen years ago she received a blow on the right breast, and five years later, a tumour began to develop in this region; the tumour ulcerated and eighteen months ago she underwent an operation. But, after a month the disease relapsed, and it became necessary to repeat four operations successively in the course of five or six months. But still, the growth returned. Lastly, the left breast was attacked in its turn, and the patient was admitted into that part of the Salpêtrière occupied by incurable affections, and placed in the ward reserved for cancerous cases. Over the door of this ward might well be placed the inscription which, according to Dante is found over the gates of Hell.

As a matter of fact these affections have proved, up to the present time, to be beyond the resources of our art.

I will not delay by describing to you the distorted and indurated cicatrix, and the scattered nodules, which disfigure the chest of the patient. The interest lies in another direction.

For the last four months the disease has assumed a new phase. The general health has decreased, her appetite has diminished, and she has lost flesh. But, this is the point which particularly occupies our attention, a little later, namely, about three months ago, she was attacked by pains in the lumbo-sacral region, which came on only when the patient was standing, or walking, or executing movements in bed, and which disappeared when she was at rest.

Note well, gentlemen, this influence of the erect position, and of walking, it will help us to determine the diagnosis. The pains, instead of being circumscribed, soon invaded the left lower extremity and spread along the course of the sciatic nerve, where they became continuous; but much stronger whenever the patient made any movement, or essayed to stand upright, or to walk.

Soon afterwards, they spread to the right sciatic nerve. Now it became a double sciatica; there was pain on both sides, at the buttock, at the level of the head of the fibula, and over the dorsum of the foot; it was increased by pressure over certain points; and it was on the left side that her sufferings were most acute.

(A) The patient, moreover, complained of pain in the fold of the groin, on both sides. Thus there existed a double crural neuralgia at the same time.

(B) Although the sciatica was not very intense, the pain became worse on assuming the erect posture to such a degree that walking was well-nigh impossible. Between the spontaneous pain, which was almost absent when at rest, and the pain produced by walking, there was a disproportion which is not met with in ordinary neuralgia of the sciatic nerve. Nevertheless there existed no indication of the existence of a spinal lesion; thus, when in bed movements of flexion and extension of the legs were forcible enough, there was no exaggeration of reflexes, and there was no trouble of bladder or rectum.

(c) Lastly, there is another fact which does not belong to the clinical history of ordinary sciatica. When one presses or percusses either over the sacrum or lumbar vertebræ, acute pain is produced; it is here also that the pain predominates when the patient holds herself upright, tries to walk, or moves in bed.

What is the meaning of this pain along the course of the two sciatic nerves? Is it a common sciatica, accidentally complicating the cancerous affection and, of itself without much importance? No, I believe it has quite another signification.

In the first place, the sciatic pain in bilateral. Now, all clinical observers are quite agreed that double sciatica is very suspicious of a symptomatic neuralgia, and is generally connected with a more or less serious protopathic affection. It cannot be inferred that unilateral sciatica may not sometimes also be symptomatic. In this particular case, by reason of the different anomalies that I have pointed out, it can be affirmed that the case is not one of common sciatica but of a symptomatic affection. But what is the cause?

Let us pass in review the principal affections that can give rise to double sciatica.

(A) In diabetes, it is not uncommon to observe several different nerve troubles,[1] among which should be pointed out in particular, partial hyperæsthesiæ, lightning pains, such as I have already drawn attention to, and of which several cases have been met with since,[2] and symmetrical neuralgiæ[3] occupying by preference the sciatic nerves. But, that

[1] Bernard et Féré, "Des troubles nerveux observés chez les diabetiques." 'Arch. de Neurologie,' 1882, T. IV, p. 336.

[2] Raymond, 'Gaz. méd. de Paris,' 1881, p. 627.

[3] Worms, 'Bull. de l'Acad. de Méd,' 2e série, T. IX. Drasche, "Diabetische Neuralgien" 'Wiener med. Wosch,' 1882.

diabetes is not the cause here is shown by an analysis of the urine on several occasions : it does not give the faintest trace of sugar.

(B) In certain spinal affections there exist pains along the course of the sciatic nerves on both sides.

The pains of Locomotor Ataxy do not present the same characters that are to be found here. In meningo-myelitic affections we should have a paralysis or paresis of the limbs and sphincters, and other spinal symptoms which do not exist in this case.

(C) If it is not the cord and its membranes which are affected, it must be the nerves themselves. What are the most frequent lesions which by compressing the sacral plexus, can produce a double sciatica? A tumour growing in the pelvic cavity? But an exploration of the abdomen, rectum, and bladder do not give any indication of its presence. The lesion is elsewhere, and must be looked for in the lumbar and sacral vertebræ. It is there that the cancerous infiltration has occurred, and has produced the alteration of the bones by which the nerves are compressed in the intervertebral foramina; and it is to this compression that the pains along the course of the crural and sciatic nerves must be attributed. That is a physiological and pathological problem which it is easy to elucidate; but it is more expedient to enter into certain anatomo-pathological details.

My master Cazalis insisted long ago on this point, that nothing is so common as the invasion of the bodies of the vertebræ by secondary deposits of cancer, and especially when the primitive lesion is situated in the breast, and when it takes the form of scirrhus. When these secondary deposits are limited to the bodies of the vertebræ, and are not extensive, they remain latent. But they sometimes invade the entire body of one vertebra, which in consequence becomes softened. Sometimes the articular apophyses, and the lateral masses which form the intervertebral foramina, are more or less completely infiltrated; and then the entire vertebra sinks, the intervertebral foramina become narrowed, and the nerves are compressed, although the meninges and the cord remain intact. The consequences of this sinking and compression become evident according as the nerves of the brachial plexus, the intercostal nerves, or the lumbar or sacral nerves are involved; often of one side only but sometimes of both sides together.

If we admit this condition in our case, it explains (1) the bilateral nature of the sciatica; (2) the participation of the crural nerve; (3) the exacerbation of the pain when the patient stands upright and walks; as also the tenderness to pressure or percussion in the sacral and lumbar regions. The prognosis follows as a natural consequence; it is not necessary to insist on its gravity.

Before leaving this case allow me, gentlemen, to make a few remarks relative to the clinical history of vertebral cancer.

1. It is rarely primary; in general it is a secondary manifestation of the diathesis. Very often it follows cancer of the breast, especially scirrhus, which may only manifest itself by a simple indurated depression of the skin, of which the patient is sometimes scarcely aware; though it is not exclusively after tumours of the mamma that it developes. It may supervene in subjects attacked with cancer of stomach, or of other parts.

2. If there exists a double sciatica with an undoubted carcinomous affection situated, for example, in the breasts, it is no good operating; it is a metastasis.

3. When we have to do with an intense and persistent neuralgia in a patient of the age for cancer, this persistence and intensity should attract attention, and one should always examine the state of the breast, stomach, uterus, &c.

4. These pseudo-neuralgic pains are the most frequent clinical revelation of vertebral cancer, but it should not be forgotten that it is sometimes revealed otherwise. Thus, when the body of a vertebra is invaded, it may happen that a cancerous button projects into the spinal canal, and then the cord is compressed. The result of this compression is a spasmodic paraplegia which differs in none of its essential features from that determined by Pott's disease, or by an intra-rachidian tumour. It is not generally accompanied by pseudo-neuralgic pains if the nerves themselves are not attacked.

II.

The second patient that I present to you to-day illustrates an affection known in spinal nosography under the name of *hypertrophic cervical pachymeningitis*. The interest of the case is twofold: firstly, the patient is cured; and secondly, the cure has been effected by appropriate surgical intervention. And it is precisely this useful surgical intervention, in a case of spontaneously developed spinal affection, to which I wish particularly to direct your attention.

But allow me, gentlemen, beforehand to recall to your minds in a few words the anatomical and clinical characters of this affection, as I have described them in a communication made to the Biological Society in 1871, and which are to be found described more exhaustively in the thesis of Mons. Joffroy (1873).

(*a*) The post-mortem changes are comparatively coarse. Formerly they were attributed to a hypertrophy of the spinal cord; which in fact, when covered by its membranes, presents at the autopsy a swelling 5 or 6 centimetres long, and almost completely fills the spinal canal. But the spinal cord is not really hypertrophied; the lesions consist (1) in a chronic inflammation of the dura mater, which sometimes presents a thickening of 6 or 7 centimetres; (2) in an alteration of the nerve-roots that traverse the inflamed meninges, and which are themselves more or less irritated; and (3rd) the cord itself may be attacked in some degree by a chronic inflammation, but the usual effect is a compression, and resulting therefrom a descending degeneration of the pyramidal bands, which change may be found down to the lowest point of the lumbar region.

This anatomo-pathological outline, albeit very brief, will enable you to understand the evolution of the clinical history, the principal episodes of which I shall now enter upon.

Let it be said at once that the malady is, so to speak, quite an accidental occurrence, which seems to be produced sometimes by the influence of damp cold; it is not an hereditary complaint like ataxy, and therefore there is nothing to astonish one in finding that the affection is not accompanied by constitutional diathesis.

As regards symptomatology, three periods can be distinguished :

The first period, *the neuralgic or pseudo-neuralgic period,* is distinguished by sharp pains, very severe, continuous, but with exacerbations, seated in the neck, in the posterior part of the head, and characterised by a sensation of constriction at the upper part of the thorax. These painful phenomena last four, five, or six months, and then disappear. It is the theca vertebralis which is here the cause, or rather it is the nerves passing through it, but not the spinal cord.

The second period, *paralytic period,* is characterised by loss of power in the upper limbs. *Cervical paraplegia* accompanied by *muscular atrophy,* simple atrophy in some muscles, degenerative atrophy in others. An interesting peculiarity of the atrophic paralysis is that it specially attacks those muscles supplied by the median and ulnar nerves, whereas those supplied by the radial are relatively sound. As a result of the predominant action of these last we get a special deformity of the hand, a radial deformity which we designate by the name of *the preacher's hand.* How can this be explained ? Do the nerve-tubes of the radial spring higher up or lower down than those which constitute the ulnar or the median, and are they not complicated to the same degree in the alteration ?

The third period. Sometimes matters remain in this condition, and by and by the malady ends in complete cure, sometimes indelible atrophic lesions of the muscles remain. But generally speaking the cord is more or less involved by the products of meningeal inflammation, or even becomes invaded by the inflammatory process, and a transverse myelitis supervenes leading to a secondary degeneration ; and then there results a *spasmodic paraplegia* with involvement of the bladder and rectum.

But the paralysis of the lower limbs is not an atrophic paralysis like that of the upper extremities, it is not in fact due to a lesion of the roots or anterior horns, but solely a degenerative alteration of the pyramidal bands. It is, therefore, a spasmodic paraplegia, and not an atrophic paraplegia. Note this peculiarity, that the flexion of the lower limbs is very pronounced, such as is seen specially in paraplegia due to compression.

We are now in a position to draw inferences from the actual facts. It is an ordinary case, quite typical, save on points of secondary importance. Here in two words is the patient's history. She was attacked at the age of 33, after a sojourn of several years in a cold and damp habitation ; the painful period lasted six months, the pains occupied not only the upper extremities, but also the thorax ; the dorsal part of the cord was therefore involved.

The paralytic period commenced in the upper extremities, and soon afterwards the lower extremities were attacked. There existed during more than a year an atrophic paralysis of the upper extremities with radial deformity of hand, and a spasmodic paralysis of the lower extremities with excessive flexion ; the heels touched the buttock. At the end of a year, perhaps under the influence of treatment, which chiefly consisted in the application of the cautery to the spinal region, or perhaps spontaneously, there occurred a progressive resolution of the paralytic and atrophic phenomena in the upper extremities. The movements of these limbs, both of the forearm, arm, and shoulder, returned ; the muscles increased in bulk, and the deformity of hand gradually disappeared. In the lower extremities, amelioration occurred almost concurrently ; the exaggeration of the tendon-reflexes disappeared, the muscular rigidity, or, in other words the contracture, disappeared, and free movement returned to most of the joints, excepting the knees.

At this time there was no longer a flexion of the knees to an acute angle as formerly, but flexion to an obtuse angle. And this flexion was not due to a contracture, because the movements of extreme flexion and some of the movements of extension could be produced in the joint. But when it was desired to go beyond a certain limit, one met with mechanical resistance, so to speak, whose seat appeared to be in the popliteal space. We thought that the obstacle was situated in the shortened flexor tendons, and also in the thickening, induration, and retraction of the periarticular tissues.

Whatever it was due to, complete extension was impossible, and there was an invincible obstacle to standing and walking.

There was reason to believe that an appropriate surgical operation would restore to the limbs their normal movement of extension; for I had already seen in certain cases of rigidity due to fibrous retractions supervening in a course of paraplegia from Pott's disease, good results produced by section of the fibrous bands or of the involved tendons. I then consulted my colleague Mons. Terrillon, who confirmed my opinion, and was desirous to undertake the operation. The patient was placed in his wards, which she only left a few days ago. Here is a note made by Mons. Terrillon which informs us of the principal incidents which happened while the patient was under his care.

State on admission.—The legs are in a state of semi-flexion, the skin at the level of the knee, and even the lower part of the thigh is shiny, smooth, and adherent to the deeper parts. When attempts at extension are made it is impossible to obtain more than a limited movement, and on each side of the popliteal space the tendons of the semi-membranosus and semi-tendinosus, and of the biceps, can be felt to be hard and prominent. There can also be felt in this position a considerable thickening of fibrous tissue which forms a hard non-circumscribed mass, and which appears to be the principal obstacle to the bending of the limb. The patella is firmly fixed against the condyles and is almost immovable by reason of the peri-articular fibrous induration.

From an examination of the exterior of the joint, and of the few movements which are still left in the knee, it is almost certain that there does not exist any intra-articular adhesion; and that the impossibility of bending it is due to the peri-articular fibrous deposits.

July 4th.—The patient was put under chloroform, and the tendons indicated above on both sides of the popliteal space were divided. At the same time attempts were made to gently bend the knee; but without using much force, because, in spite of the division of the tendons, the resistance of the fibrous mass occupying the popliteal space was considerable. A padded splint was then applied.

July 20th.—The patient was again anæsthetised. Forced extension was attempted and the fibrous tissues at the back of the joint gave way with a loud creaking sound, but complete extension was not accomplished for fear of injuring the popliteal artery, which was probably involved in the fibrous tissue. It was noted that the right leg was a little longer than the left. The two legs were next placed in plaster splints reaching up to the fold of the buttock.

July 30th.—Further attempts at extension were made and the splints reapplied immediately. The splint was taken off on the 15th August. From this time the patient has been able to stand upright and walk a little; and since then the progress has been uninterrupted.[1]

By way of summing up; the study of the patient who has just been presented to you furnishes us with several valuable pieces of information. I will confine myself to mentioning the following:

I. Hypertrophic cervical pachymeningitis is not incurable. The paraplegia which results, although it may be very marked and accompanied by flexion of the leg on the thigh, and of long duration, can be cured.

II. But, just as in the case of Pott's disease, and probably also in other forms of paraplegia by compression, the long persistence of the flexed position of the lower limbs has sometimes the effect of determining in the peri-articular tissues of the knee, and in the region of the popliteal space an induration, and a retraction which, although the spinal affection is cured, prevents extension of the joint.

III. Surgical intervention is necessary in such cases. It alone is able to deliver the patient from a complication which by itself would for ever prevent him standing or walking.

[1] For several months the walking continued to be difficult because of the weakness of the muscles after such prolonged inaction. Under the influence of methodical electrisation their functions have become re-established, and at the present time (May 4th, 1883) the patient is able to walk round the courtyard of the Salpêtrière and to accomplish a kilomètre without fatigue.—Ch. F.

LECTURE XI.

ON A CASE OF WORD-BLINDNESS.

SUMMARY.—*Definition of aphasia—Word-blindness (Wort-blindheit).—Case; sudden onset; right hemiplegia and motor aphasia which passed away; hemianopsia; incomplete alexia; importance of ideas furnished by movements in mental reading.*

GENTLEMEN,—In the following lectures I propose to undertake the study of aphasia from a clinical point of view.[1] It is scarcely necessary for me to remind you that in this task we shall enter upon difficulties of no ordinary kind.

In fact, the term *Aphasia,* considered in its widest acceptation, comprehends, as you know, all the many various, and at times subtile, modifications which are presented under pathological conditions by the faculty which man possesses of expressing his thoughts by signs (*Facultas signatrix* of Kant).

Now, it is scarcely necessary to mention that this faculty, or rather these faculties, which enable us to communicate with those around us, are without doubt connected with the highest functions of our central nervous system. Indeed, if if they do not, properly speaking, form an integral part of the intellect itself, they have most certainly, as their derangements show, a very decisive influence on the exercise of its functions. You will understand from this that in such a delicate analysis we shall have at each step to invoke

[1] The lectures to which allusion is here made were delivered during the summer of 1883, and were published in Italian by Dr. Rummo ('Differente forme d'afasia,' Milano, 1884); the analysis has been given by Dr. Marie in the 'Revue de Médecine,' T. III, 1883, p. 693. The thesis of M. le Dr. Bernard (Paris, 1885) contains the substance. The lectures themselves will be revised and published later on.

the aid of notions belonging to the domain of psycho-physiology, by whose help alone we can find our way along these difficult paths.

But, verily, circumstances seem to have favoured our efforts, for there is a series of cases, collected by chance in our wards at the present time, which are truly remarkable, by reason of their simplicity and freedom from complication. They will enable us to study the fundamental forms of the group of symptoms which we call aphasia, disentangled, or almost so, from every admixture and complication; and consequently in an exceptionally favorable condition for a physiological analysis.

The clinical exposition of one of these cases will form the object of our lesson to day; the further development of the subject will be postponed to another lecture. The case I allude to offers, if I am not deceived, one of the finest examples that can be seen of that form of *aphasia* which has so recently been studied as a distinct kind by certain authors under the name of *Word-blindness* (*Wortblindheit,* Kussmaul).

I shall not now undertake to define what is understood by this term; its meaning will become obvious from the description as we go along.

M. H. P—, æt. 35, is the proprietor of a linen drapers' shop at T—. He has been the head of the establishment for four years; before that he was the principal assistant in a shop of the same kind. He is a man of average culture, his education having been directed towards commerce from early life. He came into this hospital hoping to be more thoroughly examined and treated, and he has been under observation several months. He is intelligent, and he leads an active life; he speaks and writes correctly enough. As he directs his shop himself, he speaks much and writes many letters each day (twelve or fifteen per diem). He used to occupy his leisure hours in reading novels and newspaper articles; he used to read very quickly, and he had a habit of moving his lips, pronouncing his words in a low voice while he read. He has been married ten years, but he has no children.

As to his family history we have not found any nervous

antecedents in the family; his father is still living and well; his mother died of disease of the heart or chest.

Nor does his previous history offer anything of importance. He was in the Campaign of 1870, in the army of the East, and he suffered much but was never ill. He has never had articular rheumatism, nor palpitation of the heart, either before his accident or since; and at the present moment his pulse is regular (80), his heart of normal volume and without any murmur. The only affection which is worthy of being mentioned is migraine, which ever since he was 15 years of age has troubled him three or four times a month. These migraines, which have existed both before and since his accident, are sometimes sufficiently severe to oblige him to lie down for one or two hours. They present the following characters: (*a*) the pain, before it becomes general, usually occupies the right frontal region a little above the eyebrow; (*b*) it seems to be unaccompanied by any affection of vision; there is neither transient hemianopsia nor scintillating scotoma; (*c*) there does not exist any symptom of ophthalmic migraine accompanied by tingling in the arms or hands nor by temporary aphasia; (*d*) these headaches are never followed by vomiting.

So much for the pathological antecedents. You see there is nothing to note that seems to be connected with the present malady, unless perhaps it be the headache; that is a point we shall study more particularly in what follows.

Now let us pass to the history of the actual malady. On the 9th of October last, when he was out fox-hunting, he suddenly saw an animal half hidden in the cover; he took it for a fox and shot it dead. Unfortunately it was not a fox, but the dog of a friend, to which this last was much attached. There were many lamentations and tears on the part of the owner, and P— was profoundly moved by the death of the dog and at the distress of his friend. However he continued the hunt, though without interest, ate but little at luncheon and without appetite. After luncheon the shooting was resumed; a rabbit went by, P— took aim, but at that moment he fell to the ground. He was paralysed on his right side, and a few minutes afterwards lost consciousness.

The patient's recollection of what occurred immediately after the accident is very vague. He remembers that he was carried to the railway to return to T—; and during the transit, which occupied about an hour, he lost all consciousness. He regained his senses for a moment at the station of T—, which he recognised, but shortly afterwards he again became unconscious. We learn from his friends that he was put to bed immediately after arriving home, and that he slept all the night.

On the 10th October in the morning when he awoke, the right upper and lower extremities were completely paralysed; they were absolutely flaccid and powerless. He stammered in speaking and said one word for another; his wife relates that he said "I have a hand in the sun" (*paraphasia*). He could recognise at that time persons and objects, but he could not name them, nor could he even remember the name of his wife. It is impossible to ascertain if the tongue and mouth deviated to one side, or if he had any affection of sensibility.

At the end of four days (October 14th) he commenced to use the paralysed limbs well enough to be able to get up. He is quite sure that the upper extremity had become comparatively much freer than the lower. He dragged the foot for about a month.

On the 28th October an event of importance occurred. At that time he had scarcely any difficulty in speech except that he would occasionally use one word for another. His hand was free enough to enable him to write legibly. Now he wished to give an order relating to his business, took a pen and wrote. Thinking that he had forgotten something, he asked for the letter back again in order to complete it. He started to read it, and then he was aware, in all its startlingness, of the phenomenon to which I wish to draw your special attention. *He had been able to write, but it was quite impossible for him to read his own writing.*

Here then was a patient who had become all in a moment, aphasic, or rather paraphasic, and hemiplegic on the right side. At the end of several days both the aphasia and the hemiplegia had gone; he was able to write, he wrote legibly enough to give an order, but when he wanted to re-read his writing it was quite impossible for him to do so.

His writing at that time was pretty much the same as it was fifteen [? five] days later, that is about three weeks after the accident. Here is a specimen of it. The letter, dated the 1st November, and addressed to his mothor, is very interesting to compare with another letter dated the 22nd of November, 1880—three years before. The first differs from the second only by a slight change in the style of writing, the letters being more vertical, and of a more juvenile form; and by a few faults of orthography which consist principally in forgetting the s's and the x's at the ends of words, and in forgetting the word *chez*.

We find that, in the letters written four, five, and six months afterwards, these faults had disappeared, and the writing had resumed its usual character.

Ever since about the same time it was noticed that it was quite as impossible for him to read a printed page as to read a written one.

An incident may be mentioned, which is interesting in some respects, but which I will only note in passing because it does not seem to be directly connected with the main symptoms of the case. Two weeks after the accident, about the 24th of October, he experienced shooting pain in one ear, lasting about two days, and followed by a constant buzzing, which was exacerbated when he was spoken to, or if he experienced any emotion.

But here is a feature which you will probably regard as more important, although it does not strictly speaking belong to the category of derangements of language. About the 9th of November, that is to say about a month after the accident, he wished to try and play a game of billiards. He is a right-handed man, his right hand was perfectly free, and with it he grasped the cue; but he perceived at once that it was impossible for him to play and that this impossibility was due to the fact that his field of vision was lost on the right side, so that he only saw half of the green cloth and half of the board, and that the ball was entirely lost to view when it entered the right half of the field of vision. This is the first mention that we find in the history of the patient of a right lateral hemianopsia, which since then has been studied by us very regularly, and which exists at the present time although in a less degree.

When the patient came to consult us on the 3rd of March, 1883, he had no paralysis, and no motor aphasia; he could write fluently and clearly, but it was impossible for him to read either a written or a printed page; and he had right hemianopsia.

Let us study his condition when he came to us the first time a little more closely. We noted that he was an intelligent man with a quick eye, firm step, easy gesture, presenting none of that embarrassed stupid manner that is so common with aphasics. He then told us his history, aided here and there by his wife, who was present; and he accomplished this task without difficulty, without our noticing any slowness of speech, any substitution of words, and without the least stammering. We then assured ourselves that as a matter of fact although he could write freely, he could not read. We shall go into this subject in more detail in a minute. For the moment we may mention the following facts which were observed at the time of his admission. There was no deviation of the face or tongue, no trace of paralysis of the upper or lower extremities. The walk was normal and he could support himself equally well on either foot.

Dynamometric force.

March 3rd.—Right hand 60 kil.
Left hand 50 „
April 5th.—Right hand 75 „
Left hand 59 „

No affection of tactile sensibility was discovered, no analgesia, no alteration of muscular sensation. He was able to appreciate weight and temperature perfectly. No modification of taste, hearing, or smell; vision alone was altered. No modification of the patella-reflexes on either side.

The existence of right lateral homonymous hemianopsia is easily detected in the most summary manner; but a more systematic study of the vision, and the ophthalmoscopic examination furnishes us with more precise information.

1. There is no modification in the ophthalmoscopic appearances. 2. The right lateral homonymous hemianopsia is limited by a perfectly vertical line passing through the point of fixation. It is therefore a typical hemianopsia such as is usually met with in a lesion of the optic tract. 3. No diminution in the acuteness of vision in the healthy part of the field. 4. No modification in the perception of colours.

Now we must concentrate our attention on his faculty for writing and reading.

I ought to say at the outset that our patient presents no difficulty of movement in the tongue or lips in the articulation of words; and there is no notable alteration in the intelligence. All his troubles belong to the category of signs (*Facultas signatrix*). Besides the impossibility, or rather the difficulty, of reading, it should be noticed that he has some forgetfulness of a certain number of substantives and proper names, though he recollects the names of persons who are closely connected with him. He has not yet been able to recollect the names of the streets in Paris which he formerly frequented, although he sees these streets in his mind (visual memory), and when he passes along them he recognises quite well the places by which he passes, the house for example where he has decided to stop; but as he cannot read the names of the streets, and since he has for the most part forgotten them, he hesitates to go out alone. He recognises perfectly well ordinary objects and names them correctly when they are presented to him.

In reference to his reading and writing this is the summary of the examinations which we have made almost daily. The patient's condition is very notably ameliorated at the present time, but two periods should be distinguished, one from the 3rd to the 30th March, the second from the 1st to the 15th April.

He can write his name and address without hesitation, a long phrase, and even a long letter, without obvious faults in the orthography, and without omitting words. "I write," he says, "as though I had my eyes shut, I cannot read what I write." As a matter of fact he does write equally well with his eyes shut.

He has just written his name and we ask him to read it. "I know well enough," he replies, "that it is my name that I have written, but is impossible for me to read it." He has just written the name of this Infirmary and I, in my turn, write it on another sheet of paper and give it to him to read. He is unable to do so at first ; but he makes further efforts to do it and while he is accomplishing the task we notice that he traces, with the end of his right index finger, one of the letters which constitute the word, and with much trouble he says "La Salpêtrière." We write, "Rue d'Aboukir," the address of his friend. He traces with his finger in space the letters which compose the word, and after a moment or two says, "It is the Rue d'Aboukir, the address of my friend."

Thus you see the alexia is not complete for written characters. But the reading of them is extremely difficult to him, and is only possible with the aid of ideas furnished by movements executed by the hand in the act of writing. Evidently it is the muscular sense which is here brought into play, and it is the ideas furnished by it which alone enable the patient to verify the vague notions which he gets by vision.

We give him a printed page and he says immediately, "I can read printing less well than writing, because in writing it is easier for me to mentally reproduce the letter with my right hand, whereas it is more difficult to reproduce the printed characters." In fact he has never been accustomed to trace printed characters with his hand, as a painter of letters would be. We made him read a line of printed characters; he takes eight minutes to decipher it and three minutes only to read the same line in written characters. It is noticed that in reading he always traces the characters in space with his right hand ; and even after placing his hands behind his back and telling him to read, one sees that he traces the letters with his index finger on the nail of the thumb. When reading printed matter it is convenient for him to have a pen in his hand ; with the aid of this he is better able to accomplish the task.

Each day since March 5th, we have given him a task to read. He reads it without writing the words down, but always by the aid of tracing the characters in space. It is to be observed that under the influence of treatment he is making daily progress. Here is a Table which shows the gradual progression which he was making.

March 21st	one line in	1	minute	43	seconds.
23rd	"	1	"	53	"
24th	"	2	"	11	"
25th	"	1	"	36	"
26th	"	1	"	47	"
27th	"	1	"	20	"
28th	"	1	"	36	"
31st	"	1	"	21	"
April 1st	"	1	"	20	"
2nd	"	40 seconds.			
3rd	"	30 "			
4th	"	35 "			
7th	"	38 "			
8th	"	36 "			
10th	"	35 "			
12th	"	27 "			

After electrization of the great sympathetic in the neck—

April 13th	one line in	31 seconds.
14th	"	30 "
15th	"	39 "
16th	"	25 "

So as to thoroughly comprehend the importance of the notions furnished by muscular movements in the mental reading of written signs, we made the patient shut his eyes, placed a pen in his hand and communicated to his hand passive movements, making him write on paper "Tours, Paris;" he said immediately, "Tours, Paris," and the same results occurred if passive movements were executed in space without a pen.

In reference to his faculty of reading, the following points should also be noticed. In reading printed matter the patient does not now move his lips or speak in a low tone, although it was his habit to do so in a state of health. He is content to write only those letters which he does not know well by sight, or to trace them with his finger in space. He knows all the letters of the alphabet except q, r, s, t, and especially x, y, z; and singularly enough these last three letters which he does not recognise, and which he cannot decipher when they are isolated, he nevertheless writes easily enough when they form part of a word. Thus he can write quickly the words "Xavier, Yvan, Zèbre." He has more difficulty in writing when he is hungry than after a meal. After 15 or 20 minutes' reading he feels fatigued. If he is questioned on the subject of what he has just been reading with so much difficulty, he remembers very few of the details except in the case of figures. Thus, he only vaguely recollects, that in an article which he read yesterday the question of a statue of the Republic was discussed, which it was proposed to make of colossal size, but he recollected very well the figures 400,000 and 200,000 francs mentioned in the journal. He has since made progress in this respect.

He knows figures very well, he can *see* them very well. He can add and multiply well enough, though he occasionally makes faults if the multiplication is a little complicated.

When the signification of a word is known to him, he can read it more quickly than when it is not known, thus:

République	. .	4 or 5 seconds.
Indépendance	. .	1 minute.
Ptérigoïdiens	. .	4 minutes.

He frequently repeats, "When I commence to read, although I have much improved, it seems to me as if it were the first time."

At the same time that his education is making progress by daily application, the hemianopsia is concurrently undergoing a progressive modification.

To recapitulate, you see that in this patient the notions furnished by vision in the act of reading are vague, and insufficient for the comprehension of the text; and this it is which constitutes "*word-blindness.*" If he reads it is with the aid of an artifice; the series of movements which go to form a graphic representation of a letter, or of a word, are alone able to awake in him a precise recollection of the letter or the word respectively. Briefly put, one can say of him *that he reads only in the act of writing.*

By way of contrast I shall call your attention in the next lecture to the case of another aphasic man whom I will show you to-day, and who, though absolutely incapable of pronouncing a single word, hears all, understands all, reads mentally with perfect facility, writes freely, and understands perfectly all that he writes and all that he reads.

You will realise at once from this parallel how profoundly distinct from one another are the different forms of aphasia, when they occur, as they so rarely do in nature, quite disentangled from all complication.

LECTURE XII.

ON WORD-BLINDNESS (*continued*).

SUMMARY.—*History of word-blindness; MM. Gendrin, Trousseau, Kussmaul, Magnan, &c.—Study of sixteen cases.—Clinical cases.—Cases followed by autopsy.—Localisation.—Frequency of hemianopsia.—Nature of the lesion.*

GENTLEMEN,—You have not forgotten the account that I gave you in last lecture of a man who suffers from a partial aberration of the faculty of expressing himself by language. In this patient, the acuteness of vision has not undergone any modification in the left half of the visual field in the two eyes, but he experiences great difficulty in spelling out the words, although he can see them perfectly well, and although he can render his thoughts freely and correctly in writing.

This affection, I told you, has been of late years considered as constituting a special kind of aphasia, and has been described under the names of *verbal-blindness, word-blindness, Wortblindheit.* This designation was suggested by M. Kussmaul, one of the first who initiated the study, not yet very common amongst us, of this clinical form. It should be added that our case is distinguished from most others of the same kind that have yet been published, in that the phenomenon of word-blindness is to be found more disentangled from every admixture or complication.

It will be useful, I think, in order to bring out the interesting points of the case more clearly, to compare it with some of the cases belonging to the same group which have appeared in different publications.

The nosographical history of word-blindness is not very exhaustive. It was, I believe, Professor Kussmaul[1] who

[1] Kussmaul, 'Die Störungen der Sprache,' Leipzig, 1877.

first described it as a distinct affection, in 1877. It was Mons. Wernicke[1] who first gave the description of another form of aphasia to which I shall draw your attention in a future lecture, and which he has called by the name of *sensorial aphasia;* though M. Kussmaul in his systematic survey of the affection has described it under the name of *word-deafness, Worttaubeit.*

However, it must not be believed that word-blindness has only recently been observed, for curiously enough, in his 'Médecine Pratique,' which was written forty years ago, M. Gendrin[2] speaks of patients who "found it impossible to read, but who could write by a sort of memory of the movements of the fingers necessary to trace the word; and yet when the letter was once written, the patient was not able to recognise it."

One of the cases of which Trousseau[3] speaks in his clinical lectures belongs to this category. "Here," said this great observer, "is a patient who cannot read, yet who can speak wonderfully well. He cannot even decipher the heading of a journal, he cannot put syllables together; yet he is not amblyopic, and he is capable of picking up a pin from the ground. What is most astonishing about this man is that he cannot read what he himself has written, although it is written correctly enough." His patient, like ours, had been hemiplegic and aphasic for several days.

But, as I said, it was M. Kussmaul who pointed out that blindness for words is capable of being met with clinically as an isolated condition, and that it represents the pathological condition of a special faculty that may be called, as we shall soon explain, *visual memory of the signs of language.*

These views of M. Kaussmaul have not been admitted without opposition in France; they have even been the

[1] Wernicke, 'Der aphasische Symptomen-complex.' Breslau, 1874; 'Ueber den wissenschaftlichen Standpunkt in der Psychiatrie.' Kassel, 1880; 'Lehrbuch der Gehirnkrankheiten.' Kassel, 1881, Bd. I, p. 206; 'Fortschritte der Medicin,' Bd. I, 1883.

[2] Gendrin, 'Traité philosophique de Médecine pratique,' T. I, p. 432, 1838.

[3] Peter, "De l'aphasie d'après les leçons cliniques du Professor Trousseau." Arch. gén. de Méd.,' 1865.

object of some very severe criticism on the part of MM. Mathieu[1] and Dreyfus-Brisac.[2] On the other hand, they have been favorably supported by M. Magnan, and accepted in his teaching at the Asylum of St. Anne ; and one of his pupils, Mlle. Skwortzoff, has published in her thesis[3] a special chapter devoted to word-blindness, which includes the description of a dozen cases, of which one belonged to the author, and two others to M. Magnan.

Since the publication of this work five new cases have been published, three followed by autopsy, into the details of which we shall enter further on, and two other cases very very well described, but confined to the clinical aspect, one belonging to M. Armaignac,[4] and another to M. Bertholle,[5] who designates the disease by the name "*Asyllabia*," [*Asyllabie*].

The study and comparison of these seventeen cases furnishes us with some very interesting clinical information about the subject of word-blindness.

(1) Generally speaking, the onset of the affection is sudden, and at its commencement there occurs a certain degree of right hemiplegia, which soon, however, disappears, such as was seen in our patient. In the early days there is mostly a certain degree of motor aphasia, which little by little disappears, leaving in some of the cases the condition of word-blindness in a state of isolation. All these circumstances, you see, are to be found in our patient. But it is important to mention that primary word-blindness may occur, isolated from the very commencement (cases by Armaignac and Guéneau de Mussy),[6] and without the complication of hemiplegia.

[1] Mathieu, 'Arch. gén. de Méd.,' 1879, 1881.

[2] Dreyfus-Brisac, "De la surdité et de la cécité verbales," 'Gazette Hebdomadaire de Méd. et de Chir.,' 1881, p. 477.

[3] Skwortzoff, "De la cécité et de la surdité des mots dans l'aphasie," 'Thèse de Paris,' 1881.

[4] Armaignac, 'Revue Clinique du Sud-Ouest,' 1882.

[5] Bertholle, "Asyllabie ou amnésie partielle et isolée de la lecture" ('Gaz. Hebd. de Méd. et de Chir.,' 1881, p. 280).

[6] Guéneau de Mussy, 'Recueil d'ophthalmologie,' 1879, p. 129.

(2) Certain visual troubles are vaguely described in some of the cases; hemianopsia, such as existed in our patient, is to be found mentioned in one observation only, that of M. Westphal.[1]

(3) This same observation of M. Westphal contains another fact which interests us very much. You have not forgotten how, in our patient, when he made efforts to read either written or printed characters, he practically wrote the letters and the words, or at any rate traced them in space, with the index finger of his right hand. The ideas furnished by these movements of the fingers appeared to be indispensable to give value and precision to the vague notions presented by visual images. In other words, the patient could only read while writing. Now this same feature is to be found in M. Westphal's case, and in one recorded by Mlle. Skwortzoff.

(4) In our case these instinctive movements of the fingers which came to the aid of the patient in visual reading have been utilised, you will remember, as a means of treatment. Every day did our patient perform a task which was set him to read a certain number of lines, aiding himself by the instinctive movements of the fingers, and thus revivifying, as it were, his visual memories. We have seen how much improvement he has made lately in this respect. In the case of Mlle. Skwortzoff the patient was hemiplegic on the right side, and could only receive, through the intervention of the fingers of his left hand, but imperfect notions. Mlle. Skwortzoff, acting on the advice of M. Magnan, had recourse to another expedient. The patient learned to recognise by their touch large raised letters, and when he was sufficiently instructed in this way, he obliged himself to read with his eyes at the same time that he aided himself by his tactile perception of the raised letters; but at the end of several months the patient could only read very short words in this way.

(5) Now I come to the cases followed by autopsy. These cases are three in number. One belongs to M. Déjerine,[2] another belongs to M. Chauffard,[3] a third to MM. d'Heilly

[1] Westphal, 'Zeitschrift für Ethnologie,' 1874, 4 Mai, p. 94.

[2] Skwortzoff, loc. cit., p. 52.

[3] Chauffard, 'Revue de Médecine,' T. I, 1881, p. 393.

and Chantemesse.[1] Unfortunately the clinical history of all these cases leaves something to be desired, because the word-blindness is only to be found complicated to a very considerable degree by word-deafness. However, these three cases, the only ones, if I am not deceived, on which one could found a supposition as to localisation, agree perfectly on one point. In all the lesion predominates in the inferior parietal lobule, with or without participation of the angular gyrus and the first temporal convolution.

It is therefore in the inferior parietal lobule, with or without participation of the angular gyrus, where the lesion would be situated upon which depends the word-blindness that we observe in our patient. It should be well understood that this localisation is mentioned with every reserve, and is only indicated as the most probable one in the present state of our knowledge.

Moreover, this localisation will perhaps enable us to explain in a certain degree the existence of the phenomenon which plays a very important part in the history of our case, I mean the symptom of hemianopsia, the existence of which has been made out with so much precision. It is, as you know, a right lateral homonymous hemianopsia. Without entering for the moment into a formal discussion of the question of cerebral hemianopsia, which to be properly treated would require a long time, I will confine myself to-day to pointing out that there are a certain number of cases, seven or eight perhaps, followed by autopsies, which seem to establish pretty clearly that the phenomonon of lateral hemianopsia may be produced by lesion of certain definite parts of the cerebral cortex.[2]

Now, it seems to be clear from these cases, that the lesion in hemianopsia of cortical cerebral origin pretty constantly occupies approximately the same region as that which we have indicated as being the seat of lesions attended with word-blindness. You will observe that we have made no mention of the data afforded by experimentation on animals relative to the visual centre, because at the

[1] D'Heilly et Chantemesse, 'Progrès Médical,' 1883.

[2] Ch. Féré, 'Contribution à l' étude des troubles fonctionnels de la vision par lésions cérébrales (amblyopie croisée et hémianopsie),' 1882.

present time there exists considerable contradiction among authors who are occupied with the question. Moreover, supposing that they were all agreed as to the seat of the visual centre in animals, even in the case of the monkey, it would require further proof to determine if these results were veritably applicable to man.

However, the information we possess relative to cerebral hemianopsia in man will serve to enable us to understand how, in our case, there is a coincidence between lateral hemianopsia and word-blindness. The same interpretation can be applied to the case of M. Westphal.

But you will realise at once the difficulty which here presents itself. If word-blindness and cerebral hemianopsia occupy the same seat in the brain—that is to say, the inferior parietal lobule—the two clinical phenomena ought almost always to occur associated together. However, that does not seem to be the case, for it is possible to cite examples of cerebral hemianopsia without word-blindness, and cases of word-blindness without cerebral hemianopsia.

However, it is well to note that the phenomenon of hemianopsia, in cases where it is not so accentuated as it is in our patient,—in cases, for example, where the line which limits the visual defect is at some distance from the point of fixation,—might perfectly well pass undetected unless a systematic search was made. Future observations will alone enable us to settle this point. Moreover, the inferior parietal lobule is sufficiently extensive for the two kinds of lesion to find place without their being necessarily superposed.

I would remind you in passing that in our patient, whether spontaneously or under the influence of treatment it is difficult to say, the hemianopsia has become very remarkably modified, proportionately as the symptoms of word-blindness have improved. At the commencement, the hemianopsia differed in absolutely nothing from the clearly defined hemianopsia which results from a lesion of the optic tract, for the line of demarcation passed exactly through the point of fixation (fig. 23). But at the present time it is no longer so. The limit of the defect has moved little by little from the point of fixation, and the extent of the visual field has gradually increased (Figs. 23, 24, and 25).

An amendment of this kind is a rare circumstance, and quite exceptional in the hemianopsia which depends on a lesion of the tract. Nevertheless, it is quite capable of being one of the clinical features of hemianopsia from a cerebral cause.

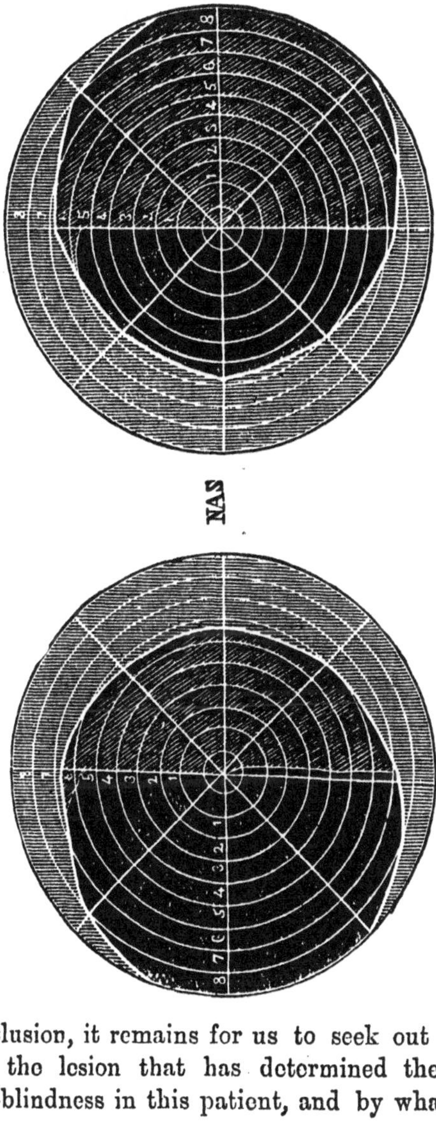

FIG. 23.—Extent of the visual field of P—, 21st February, 1883.

In conclusion, it remains for us to seek out what is the nature of the lesion that has determined the hemianopsia and word-blindness in this patient, and by what mechanism it is developed. Here again, we find ourselves confronted only with hypotheses more or less probable. Though, alas! it should be recognised that in cerebral pathology, even in

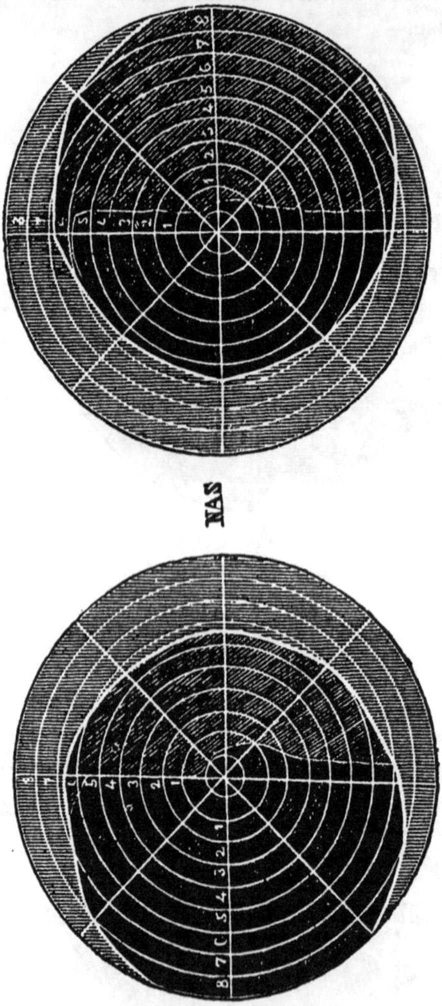

FIG. 24.—Extent of the visual field of P—, 3rd March, 1883.

the present day, we are not unfrequently reduced to this condition.

I need scarcely remind you that the sylvian artery, which I do not hesitate to point to as the cause here, furnishes branches both to Broca's convolution, the seat of the lesion in aphasia, and also to the regions which seem to be the seat of the disease in word-blindness and hemianopsia. Disease of these arterial branches is the chief cause of a more or less

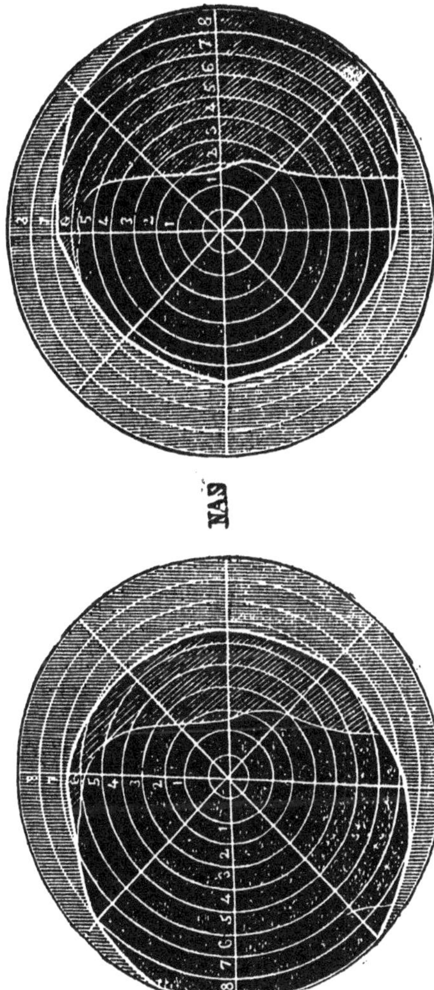

FIG. 25.—Extent of the visual field of P—, 3rd April, 1883.

pronounced alteration in the cerebral tissue, but of what does this vascular lesion consist? Is it spasm, thrombosis, or embolism?

That, I fear, cannot be exactly determined. The existence of frequent and severe migraines would induce us perhaps to suppose, according to Latham's theory, the former existence of repeated vascular spasms in the area supplied by the sylvian as a predisposing cause.

It seems, in fact, that the repetition of a vascular spasm may at length bring about, in certain cases, profound modification in the vascular walls; since, in ophthalmic migraine at any rate, we sometimes see that hemianopsia, or sometimes aphasia, at first transitory, becomes established by-and-by as a more or less permanent symptom. But we are not in a position to state that the migraine of which our patient suffered was true ophthalmic migraine.

The hypothesis of thrombosis consequent on arteritis, or an embolism, can only be accepted with reserve, the first by reason of the age of the subject, the second because of the fact that there exists no organic disease of the heart.

I must therefore, in conclusion, content myself with the following statement. It is probable that the origin of the trunk of the sylvian artery has been obliterated. This will explain the aphasia, amnesia, and the paralysis of the two limbs of the right side, from which the patient suffered at the outset of the disease. But the circulation soon became re-established in the area supplied by the first three branches, and thus the hemiplegia and even the aphasia disappeared. However, the ischæmia in the area supplied by the parietal artery has persisted, and consequently the nerve-tissue in this region has undergone more or less profound alteration; and it is for this reason that the hemianopsia and word-blindness have become established in a permanent condition for nearly six months.

Nevertheless, the lesion, whatever it may be, is not absolutely incurable; for we have seen that, under the influence of very simple treatment, the disease has tended day by day to improve. If this amendment continues, as indeed we have reason to hope, the patient is much to be congratulated, because, to judge from the history of other cases that have been published, word-blindness when once established scarcely ever improves, and more often remains with the patient as a permanent infirmity.

LECTURE XIII.

ON A CASE OF SUDDEN AND ISOLATED SUPPRESSION OF THE MENTAL VISION OF SIGNS AND OBJECTS (FORMS AND COLOURS).[1]

SUMMARY.—*Gall, Gratiolet, Ribot, on partial memories.—Partial destruction of the different forms of memory.—Visual memory.—Galton's observations.—Case of sudden suppression of the visual memory.—Its effects.—Substitution by auditory images.—Verbal amnesia does not correspond to a simple pathological condition.—The condition is a complex one [complexus]; in educated persons four fundamental elements can be recognised in it; the commemorative auditive image; the visual image; and two motor elements, to wit, the motor image of articulation, and the motor image of writing.*

GENTLEMEN,—In an important work, which is devoted to the study of diseases of the memory,[2] M. Th. Ribot has well pointed out that at the present time, in psychology, the distinction of partial forms of memory, for the first time indicated by Gall,[3] has become an established truth. And in this respect he points out that Gratiolet[4] had already recognised that each sense corresponds to a memory which is its correlative; and that the intellect, like the body, has temperaments, which result in the preponderance of this or that order of sensations in the natural workings of the mind.

"In truth," adds M. Ribot, "the system of faculties, in psychology, has been established so long that the memory has

[1] Lecture edited by M. Bernard.

[2] 'Les maladies de la mémoire,' Paris, 1881, p. 111, 112.

[3] 'Fonctions du cerveau,' T. I.

[4] 'Anatomie Comparée,' T. II, p. 460.

come to be considered as an indivisible whole [*une unité*], and the existence of partial memories has been completely forgotten, or regarded as an anomaly." But in psychology, as in more material science, it is experience to which we defer for ultimate decision. By the light of this experience it has been shown that "in reality, in an ultimate analysis there exists special memories, or, as certain authors express it, local memories." Now, if it be true that in the normal state "the different forms of memory," quoting still from M. Ribot, "have a relative independence, it is only natural that in a morbid state, although one form may be lost, the others may quite well remain intact. It is a fact which should now appear simple enough, and should require no explanation, since it results from the very nature of memory."

I shall call your attention to-day to a remarkable pathological condition, which is well calculated to throw some additional light once more on the existence in pathology of this isolated suppression of one of the forms of memory. The case is one of loss of *mental vision for objects* (*Mental Imagery of Galton*[1])—forms and colours—supervening suddenly in a gentleman, who was capable, as it was proved, even after the occurrence which deprived him of one of his most brilliant faculties, of great intellectual activity. The case is so interesting from many different points of view that it is worth narrating *in extenso*.[2]

M. X—, a merchant at A—, was born in Vienna. He is a well-educated man, and is a thorough master of German, Spanish, French, and also Latin and Greek. Up to the time of the commencement of the affection which brought him before us, he could read the works of Homer quite fluently; he knew the first book of the Iliad, and he could repeat without hesitation a passage of which the first line was recited to him. He knew modern Greek well enough to correspond on commercial matters in this language. He was very familiar with Virgil and Horace.

[1] Francis Galton, "Inquiries into Human Faculty," 'Mental Imagery,' p. 83, London, 1883.

[2] The notes of this case were taken by Dr. Bernard (of Marseilles), then my clinical clerk.

His father, a professor of Oriental languages at S—, possesses a very remarkable memory. So also does his brother, professor of law at W—. One of his sisters is a distinguished painter. His own son, who is only seven years old, is already well up in the most minute historical dates.

M. X— enjoyed for several years an equally remarkable memory. Like that of his father and his son it was especially a *visual memory*. *Mental vision* would give him in an instant a picture of the features of persons, and the form and colour of objects with as much clearness and intensity, he assures us, as the reality itself.

If he wished to recall some fact or figures mentioned in his voluminous correspondence, made in several languages, he could do so immediately, and the precise wording of the very letters themselves would appear before him with the smallest details, mistakes, and erasures in their drafting.

If he wished to recite a lesson when he was at school, or a piece of a favourite author later in life, two or three readings sufficed to fix in his memory the page with its lines and its letters, and he could recite it, reading in his mind's eye the desired passage, which in an instant would appear before him with forcible clearness.

In adding up figures, M. X— had but to run through the different columns of figures exhibited before him, however long they might be, and he filled in the total without any hesitation at once, without being obliged to go into minute details, figure by figure, such as is usually done. In a similar manner he would execute various other operations of arithmetic.

He had but to recall a passage from a play at the theatre which he had seen performed, and it at once called up all the details of the scenery, the performance of the actors, and the spectacle presented by the audience.

M. X— has travelled much. He liked to *sketch* places and scenes which struck him. He drew fairly well, and his memory would offer to him at will the most exact panoramas. Did he but remember a conversation, or recall a discourse, or a given word; immediataly the place of conversation, the physiognomy of the interlocutor—in a word the entire scene, of which he recalled only one detail—would reappear before him in all its completeness. *The auditive memory* constantly failed M. X—, or at least it never occupied in his mind any but a secondary position. Moreover, he has never had any taste for music.

About a year and a half ago he was seized with grave apprehensions on account of certain important debts, of which the payment seemed to be somewhat uncertain. He lost appetite and sleep. Events did not justify his fears; but the emotion was so severe that he did not become calm again, as he had hoped, and one day M. X— was astonished to find that a sudden and profound change had come over him. At first everything was complete confusion, and from that time he was aware of an immense contrast between his new and his former condition. M. X— feared at the time that he was threatened with mental derangement, so many things around him seemed new and strange. He had become nervous and irritable. In every instance the visual memory of forms and colours had completely disappeared, yet he could perceive them when present without difficulty, and the knowledge of this somewhat reassured him as to his mental condition. He realised, moreover, little by little, that he could by other means, by invoking the aid of other forms of memory, continue to successfully direct his business affairs. And thus, at the present time, he has become reconciled to the new situation, the difference of which from that of M. X—'s former condition, as described above, will be easily detected.

Every time that M. X— returned to A—, whence his business frequently took him for long distances, it seemed to him as though he entered an unknown town. He looked with astonishment at its monuments, houses, and streets, as though he had arrived there for the first time. Paris, which he has frequented quite as much, produces the same effect on him, though the remembrance returns to him by degrees, and finally he is able to find his way amongst the labyrinth of streets. We ask him for a description of the principal square of A—, of its arcades, of its statue; "I know," says he, "that all those exist, but I cannot picture them to myself, and I cannot tell you anything about them." On several former occasions he had sketched a ground plan of A—, but to-day he tries in vain to reproduce the principal routes, and completely fails.

Asked to draw a minaret, he reflected, and after having said that it was a high, square tower, he traced on paper four lines, two long equal vertical ones, two shorter horizontal ones. The upper one united the extremity of the two vertical ones, and the inferior one was prolonged on each side to represent the ground. It is a very elementary sort of drawing. "You want an arcade? I hope that I shall succeed in drawing it, because I remember that a rounded arch is formed of a half circle, that a pointed arch is formed by two arcs meeting together at an acute angle, but I cannot really see in my mind's eye any of these things."

The profile of a man's head which M. X— drew at our request might be the work of a child; and he confesses to being aided in this drawing by the faces of persons who are around him. A shapeless scrawl represents a tree that we asked him to draw. "I don't know, I don't know at all, how it is done," says he.

He finds the visual recollection of his wife and his children impossible. He cannot remember them any better than the roads and streets of A—, and even when they are before him they seem fresh to him; he seems to see new traits in them, and new characteristics in their physiognomies.

He cannot even recall his own face. Recently in a public gallery his path seemed to be stopped by a person to whom he was about to offer his excuses, but it was merely his own image reflected in a glass.

During our investigations M. X— has complained bitterly on several occasions of his loss of colour vision. It seems to occupy his mind more than his other losses. "My wife has dark hair, I know it quite positively, yet it is impossible for me to find the colour in my memory. It has as completely gone as her face and features."

This visual amnesia applies quite as much to the objects of youth as to more recent images. M. X— cannot represent in his mind's eye [*visuellement*] his paternal home. Formerly he often evoked this memory, and it was a very vivid one.

The examination of the eye is completely negative. M.

X— is strongly myopic to the extent of −7 D. As the result of the examination of M. X—'s eyes, which has been made with the greatest care by M. le Docteur Parinaud in the ophthalmological room of the Clinique, we find that no ocular lesions nor functional troubles can be discovered, excepting perhaps a slight diminution of chromatic sensibility equally involving all colours.

It should be added that no somatic symptom has ever preceded, accompanied, or followed the destruction of mental vision that is found in our patient. At the present time M. X— is able, like other people, to open his letter press-copy book, and find there the information which he desires; and he can turn over the pages just as well, in order to arrive at the place he seeks. He cannot remember more than the first few verses of the Iliad now, and his quotations from Homer, Virgil, and Horace are but very feeble attempts.

He pronounces in a low voice the figures that he adds up, and only proceeds by small imperfect calculations.

When he recalls a conversation, when he wishes to remember a statement made to him, he knows quite well that it is the auditive memory that he must now consult, which is of course an effort to him. *Words and speech [when] recalled*[1] *seem to resound in his ear, with a sensation altogether new to him.*

He is obliged to make efforts of audition in order to reproduce in writing two lines from a daily journal that we have given him to read. In reading, moreover, he executes movements with his lips of which he is conscious; and, deprived of his *mental vision*, it has become necessary for him to have recourse to *internal speech* and to *articular movements of his tongue and lips* in order to comprehend the lines which he reads. M. X— seems to have analysed very thoroughly all the mechanisms of his memory, and all the different observations that we have made about him, he had for the most part already made on his own behalf.

Since this great change has come over him, M. X— is obliged, in order to learn a thing by heart, a series of phrases for example, *to read these phrases in a loud voice several times*, and thus affect his ear. And by-and-by when he wishes to

[1] [Retrouvés, literally, met with again.]

repeat the passage learned, he is very conscious of a sensation of *interior audition*, which precedes the enunciation of the words, and which is a sensation that he never knew before.

M. X— speaks French very well and fluently, nevertheless he declares that he cannot think in French, and that he only speaks this language by translating his thoughts from Spanish or from German, the first languages which he learnt when a child.

It is an interesting detail that *in his dreams* M. X— has no longer the visual representation of objects. The representation of words alone remains to him, and these belong almost exclusively to the Spanish language.

Besides the loss of the faculty of the visual representation of objects, *word-blindness* also exists in the patient to some extent. When asked to write the Greek and German alphabets he omits several letters from the alphabet; thus in Greek θ, ς, σ, ζ, φ, ψ, χ. If these letters are traced before him, he recognises them only after having traced them himself, after several mistakes, and after having compared them one with the other. If Greek words, into whose composition these letters enter, are dictated to him, he understands and writes them clearly and deliberately, whereas, to read the same words written by another person he is obliged in the first place to write them himself. From this, one sees that he is obliged to compensate by the aid of his hand the defect of his visual memory for words, with which he is affected to a certain degree, in some languages.

However, notions belonging to the category of muscular sense, furnished by movements of the hand in the act of writing, are not in him of an exceptional intensity. In fact, if when his eyes are shut one communicates to his hand the movements necessary to write—the word Vienna, for example, —he is incapable of detecting the word which he has been made to write; he is obliged to see the word and to read it in order to name it.

The following letter which the patient has written in reply to me will complete on several points the case that has just been related, and will enable you better to understand the temporary derangement, and the permanent destruction, of faculty which has been produced in the patient in consequence of this loss of mental vision.

"I hasten to reply to your letter, and to ask you to be good enough to excuse my imperfect knowledge of the French language, an imperfection which renders the exact expression of what I wish to submit to you a little difficult. As I have already told you, I possessed at one time a grand faculty of picturing to myself [representer intérieurement] persons who interested me, colours and objects of every kind, in a word, everything that is reflected in the eye.

"Allow me to remind you that I made use of this faculty extensively in my studies. I read anything I wanted to learn, and then shutting my eyes I saw again quite clearly the letters with their every detail; thus it was also with the physiognomies of people; the appearance of countries or towns that I have visited in my many voyages; and, as I just now mentioned, of every object that I had seen with my eyes.

"All of a sudden this internal vision absolutely disappeared. Now, even with the strongest desire in the world, I cannot picture to myself the features of my children or my wife, or any other object of my daily surroundings. Hence, when you realise that I have absolutely lost this power of mental vision, you will readily understand that my impressions are changed in a corresponding fashion. No longer being able to represent visible objects, and yet having completely preserved my abstract memory, I daily experience astonishment at seeing things which I have known so well for a long time. My sensations, or rather my impressions, being made new an indefinite number of times, it seems to me that a complete change has come over my existence, and naturally my character is modified in a remarkable way. Formerly I was impressionable, enthusiastic, and I possessed a vivid imagination; to-day I am calm, phlegmatic, and my imagination never leads me astray.

"The faculty of picturing objects within myself being absolutely wanting, my dreams are correspondingly modified. At the present time I dream simply of speech, whereas I formerly possessed a visual perception in my dreams.

"As an example, which may be more convincing, if you

were to ask me to represent the towers of Notre-Dame, a browsing sheep, or a ship in distress in the open sea, I should have to reply to you that although I know perfectly well how to distinguish these three different objects, and perfectly well know all about them, they have for me no meaning at all as regards mental vision.

"A singular result of the loss of this mental faculty, as I said before, is a great change in my character and my impressions. I am much less affected by grief or disappointment. I may mention that having lately lost one of my relatives, for whom I had a sincere attachment, I experienced a much less intense grief than if I had still possessed the power of representing, by my internal vision, the face of the relative, the phases of the disease through which he had gone; and especially, if I had been able to picture within myself the outward effects produced by his premature death on the other members of our family.

"I know not if I clearly explain what I experience, but I may tell you that I possessed at one time in no ordinary degree the mental vision which is now so completely lost. It exists at the present time in my brother, a professor of law in the University of X—, in my father, a professor of Oriental languages, well known in the scientific world, and in my sister, a painter possessed of much talent.

"In conclusion, I beg you to remark that I am obliged at the present time *to say things which I wish to retain in my memory, whereas formerly it was sufficient for me to photograph them in my eye.*—Paris, 11 July, 1883."

By way of comparison I should like to mention another case that I have recently met with of an artist, 56 years of age, who has noticed, to his great grief, that for several months he has lost the faculty of picturing things to himself, or of imagining objects, and that he is no longer good at painting, except for copying; and even for this kind of work he is obliged to keep the original constantly before his eyes in such a way as not to lose sight of it for an instant.

The case of M. X— needs but little comment. We will confine ourselves to a few brief remarks on this subject.

It has been seen that the powerful memory which M. X— enjoyed only eighteen months ago depended chiefly on his faculty of representation by mental vision, a faculty which in him had reached an extɹeme development.

In this respect he belonged to that class of individuals of whom M. Galton[1] speaks, and who read, as it were mentally, each word that they pronounce, as though they really saw them printed; and who consequently, when it is desired to express an idea by a sign of language, evoke the *visual equivalent* of the word and not its *auditive equivalent*;—in whom the visual representation of objects is sometimes so powerful that they are capable of projecting on the paper, so to speak, the internal image, and there fixing it by drawing. When it is thus developed, this faculty seems, according to M. Galton, to be an hereditary gift; and as a matter of fact the brother, the sister, and the father of M. X— possessed it in a very remarkable degree.

It is very remarkable that this complete suppression of internal vision (which prevents M. X— from picturing anything to himself, or of figuring objects or faces to such an extent that the faces he has seen many times always appear to him as new, and that he can no longer draw from memory, &c.) has not had the effect of profoundly modifying his faculty of expression by language, since the visual representation of signs is wanting in him as well as that of objects, of faces, of countries, &c.

But it should be noted in this respect that from the moment when he perceived that he was deprived of visual memory, M. X— was led, instinctively so to speak, to use his auditive memory, which he had as it would seem sadly neglected up to that time. Formerly, when he wished to learn a series of phrases by heart, it was sufficient for him to have *seen* them once or twice; but now in order to obtain the same result he is obliged to *read* the phrases several times in a *loud voice*, and when the time comes for him to repeat the passage learned, he has very clearly the sensation (new to him) of interior audition which precedes the enunciation of the words. That is to say, being actually deprived of the visual image of signs, he has learned to evoke his

[1] Loc. cit., pp. 96, 99.

auditive image; or, in other terms, his *auditive equivalent* for words replaces his *visual equivalent*. It is then a fresh example of those "substitutions" [suppléances] which are met with no doubt at each step in the history of aphasia by those who examine the subject attentively.

You know that in my recent lectures on "aphasia,"[1] founded on a clinical analysis of a certain number of appropriate cases, I endeavoured to show that what is known as verbal amnesia, contrary to the opinion very generally held, does not correspond to a simple pathological condition [*unité*]. The word indeed is a *complexus* [applied to a class having several varieties]. One is able to recognise, in educated individuals, at least four fundamental elements in this condition:—The commemorative auditive image: the visual image: and lastly, two motor elements belonging to the category of muscular sense, that is to say, the *motor image*[2] *of articulation*, and the *graphic motor image*; the former being developed by the repetition of the movements of the tongue and lips necessary to pronounce a word, the latter by a repetition of the movements of the hand and fingers necessary in writing.

It should be remarked, moreover, that verbal amnesia, whether auditive or visual, represents, so to speak, the early stages of affections which, when they are carried to a higher degree, constitute either word-deafness or word-blindness as the case may be. Thus when, the idea being present, one is not able to evoke either the auditive image or the visual image of a given word, there is said to be *verbal auditive amnesia* in the first case, or *verbal visual amnesia* in the second; but when the written words which are seen, or which resound in the ear, are not recognised, it is said that there is either word-blindness, or, in the latter case, word-deafness. We should be able, following out the same principle, to say that there is *verbal motor amnesia*—of a more or less accentuated form, according to the case—when the motor images, either of articulation or of writing are wanting.

[1] See p. 130, note 1.

[2] Image motrice; *Bewegungsbilder*, in the nomenclature of M. Kussmaul.

Finally, it must not be forgotten that, in reference to the [physiological] mechanism of recalling a word, there would seem to exist fairly well-marked individual varieties. In some kinds—and these perhaps form the greatest number—when it is desired to render an idea by the corresponding sign, the auditive element exclusively is evoked; in others the visual element alone; and in other varieties the individuals have recourse directly to one or other of the motor elements. These three chief types, moreover, are exclusive of mixed transitional forms.

If, for the sake of convenience, one were to designate summarily the representatives of each of these great [physiological] types by the name of *visuals, auditives,* and *motors,* the patient, M. X—, would undoubtedly have been a *visual.* From this reasoning one would suppose that the suppression in him, or at any rate the clouding, of internal vision of signs ought, necessarily, to bring with it serious disorder in the expression by language.

But it is just here where the phenomenon of "substitution" [suppléance] mentioned above comes in. Thanks to the persistence of the auditive and motor elements of a word, the compensation has been established to the extent that, in M. X—, the destruction only betrays itself in reality by delicate, scarcely perceptible shades, and the function of language operates very nearly as under normal conditions. On the other hand, the absence of the visual element in the constitution of the idea, seems to be a flaw that will be with difficulty reparable.

However that may be, it should be well understood in the present day, that such conditions are quite possible, and that examples do actually occur in which there is suppression of a whole group of memories, or a whole category of commemorative images, without participation of other groups or other categories; and that this is an established fact in pathology as well as in cerebral physiology. This necessarily leads one to admit that the different groups of memories have their seat in certain circumscribed regions of the encephalon. And this in turn becomes added to the proofs which go to establish that the hemispheres of the brain consist of a number of differentiated "organs," each of which possesses its proper function, though each one remains in the most intimate connection with the others. Moreover, this last proposition is generally admitted in the present day by those who study the functions of the brain, not only in animals in the laboratory, but also, and especially, in man, by the processes of the anatomo-clinical method.

LECTURE XIV.[1]

NOSOGRAPHICAL REVISION OF THE AMYOTROPHIES.

SUMMARY.—*Deuteropathic amyotrophies.—Protopathic amyotrophies.—Primary myopathies.—Pseudo-hypertrophic paralysis.—Juvenile form of Erb.—Myopathy without change of volume in the muscles, Leyden's form.—Analogies between pseudo-hypertrophic paralysis and Erb's juvenile form.—Hereditary infantile variety of Duchenne (de Boulogne).—Its characters.—This last variety is analogous to the preceding ones.—Pseudo-hypertrophic paralysis, juvenile form of Erb, Leyden's form, hereditary infantile form of Duchenne (of Boulogne); are but varieties of primary progressive myopathy.*

GENTLEMEN,—By the chances of clinical work we have at this moment, collected in our wards, an interesting series of cases[2] which represent the different aspects under which *progressive muscular atrophy* may present itself to the physician.

I propose, therefore, to avail myself of this opportunity, and in to-day's lecture to take up the subject of muscular atrophies, or perhaps better, *progressive amyotrophies*.

As a matter of fact, during the last few years this subject has reached a somewhat critical phase. The nosographical history of progressive amyotrophies requires to be revised by the light of recent observations; even to be reconstituted in part on new principles. To-day I can but offer you an

[1] This lecture is edited by MM. Marie and Guinon.

[2] These cases have been reported *in extenso* in a publication by MM. Marie and Guinon "On some of the clinical varieties of Primary Progressive Myopathy," ('Revue de Médecine,' October, 1885).

attempt, a mere sketch of such reconstitution, reserving for a future occasion the task of presenting to you a more detailed and more settled plan.

In the domain of progressive amyotrophies matters are rather more complex than one would at first imagine. Refering for a moment to my teaching of ten years ago; the clinical group of progressive muscular atrophies, as we then divided it, comprised different affections which were connected solely by exterior, superficial resemblances; but which nevertheless all had this in common, that they were of spinal origin; that they depended in other terms on a lesion of the spinal cord, and more particularly of the anterior horns of its grey substance. However, we were enabled to establish at least two fundamental divisions, viz.

I. *Deuteropathic*[1] spinal amyotrophies, in which the lesion of the grey substance is secondary.

II. *Protopathic*[1] spinal amyotrophies, in which the lesion of the grey substance was the only feature, or at least the primary and fundamental one.

In this first group, that of Deuteropathic Amyotrophies, we may establish the following distinctions.

In the *first* place there are the cases in which the lesion of the grey substance is an accessory occurrence, accidental so to speak, to conditions such as the diffuse myelites, disseminated sclerosis, tumours of the spinal cord, locomotor ataxy, &c. This class of spinal amyotrophies can be eliminated from our present studies, for they can more conveniently be grouped, clinically, with the diseases on which they depend.

In the *second* place there are cases in which the lesion of the white columns is primary, but always, and necessarily, followed by a lesion of the grey matter. In these cases it is the pyramidal bands which are first attacked and then subsequently the anterior horns, whose participation nevertheless is a necessary factor. When the disease occurs in its complete form we have the ordinary symptoms of progressive muscular atrophy, to which is superadded a spasmodic element, by means of which it is distinguished from other

[1] Vide note p. 26.

kinds. This group is nosologically distinct, and is of perfectly legitimate constitution. There is at the present time nothing to add to it, nothing to withdraw.

As for the other great class of spinal amyotrophies, we have proposed to designate it *clinically* by the name *progressive muscular atrophy of the Duchenne-Aran type.* The lesion of the grey motor centres, spinal or bulbar, is the unique fact, or at least is the primary one. If the white columns participate, it is but a secondary or accessory feature. It is this class which can be anatomically characterised by the denomination *protopathic spinal amyotrophy;* or perhaps better, *chronic anterior poliomyelitis.* It should be recognised that the constitution of this second class is less homogeneous than that of the first. It is this one that is so much discussed at the present time, and which is in danger of being shaken to its very base; it is against this one that the strictures of the critics, so often just, are really directed. It is in this category that the alterations, and legitimate separations, have to be made.

It is not that the efforts made in this direction tend really to compromise the existence of the Duchenne-Aran nosographical type. There does undoubtedly exist a kind of progressive muscular atrophy, characterised, anatomically, by an isolated lesion of the anterior horns of the grey matter of the cord, and, clinically, by amyotrophy. One certainly meets with cases in which the onset, occurring after twenty years of age, is manifested by an atrophy of the upper extremities, of the hands, more especially of the thenar and hypothenar eminences; and by the progressive spreading of these alterations to the rest of the limb. Fibrillar twitchings are met with in these cases, and the reaction of degeneration in some of the atrophied muscles. It is distinguished clinically from amyotrophic lateral sclerosis in that the participation of the bulb, though it may exist, is more rare than in the last-named affection, and especially, by the fact of the complete absence of the spasmodic element, and later on, of contracture.

Formerly this category of amyotrophies was very vast, but the number of cases which constitute it appear to become fewer and fewer under the influence of newer and more precise investigation. In this way a certain number of distinct varieties are separated from it, such as has been done in the case of amyotrophic lateral sclerosis. As a result of this, its extent, already much narrowed, is from time to time becoming more and more limited, in proportion as the heterogeneous elements which were annexed to it have become withdrawn. Now, what the cases are which modern research is detaching every day from the Duchenne-Aran type is precisely what we are about to investigate. Under what now guise will these cases appear to us; in what nosographical category shall we find them, or where can we place them?

Gentlemen, besides the amyotrophies of spinal origin there exists a large and increasing class in which progressive myopathy is more or less generalised, and which is independent of all lesion in the nerve centres or peripheral nerves. Here we have a protopathic disease of muscle, a *primary myopathy*. As an example of this kind of affection one can mention the *pseudo-hypertrophic paralysis* or *myosclerosis* of Duchenne (de Boulogne). It was shown by Eulenberg and Cohnheim in 1866, and by myself in 1871, that in these cases the lesion of muscle is completely independent of any lesion of the cord or nerves. And in reference to this matter I might remind you that I protested at that time against the then reigning tendency to connect all these progressive myopathies with lesions of the nerve centres. There are, I declared, undoubtedly cases of primary myopathy; and all the later observations have shown this statement to be correct, and also that these primary myopathies are more numerous and more varied in their clinical manifestations than was at first supposed.

But this form of myopathy, this pseudo-hypertrophic paralysis which was described by Duchenne (of Boulogne), that great worker in neuro-nosography, is so different in its clinical characters from the progressive spinal amyotrophies that they have rarely been confused clinically. Pseudo-hypertrophic paralysis is a disease of early youth. It is scarcely ever met with after twenty years of age. It is noticed that the child becomes clumsy in his walk, that he is more easily fatigued than the other children of his age; for it is always, quoting from Duchenne's description, in the lower extremities where it commences. Then the upper extremities may be attacked in their turn; but, whatever be the degree of the affection, the hands are generally absolved. Finally the muscles attacked, or at least a great number of them, present an augmentation of volume, an enormous increase in size, giving to the limb, or a segment of the limb, Herculean proportions. Anatomically this hypertrophy is characterised by lesions of the interstitial tissue, such as does not exist in the same degree in spinal amyotrophies. Moreover, and this is a peculiarity which is not found in Duchenne-Aran disease, heredity plays a great part in the development of pseudo-hypertrophic paralysis of the muscles. It often happens that several children are attacked in one family, and that some of their relatives may present the same affection.

The man named Gai— is now 19 years old. The affection from which he suffers, and which displays all the clinical features of the myosclerotic paralysis of Duchenne, commenced during childhood. You observe the enormous size, the athletic proportions of the muscles of the calf; they present in a state of repose a marked increase over the normal consistence, and during contraction they are as hard as a stone. The quadriceps extensors are large, projecting, and knotty, during the contractions. But if you test the strength of contraction of these muscles, you will observe that although they are Herculean in size, they are far from being so in power. There exists an undoubted functional weakness, not a paralytic weakness, that is to say it is not of nervous origin; but it more or less exactly corresponds to the degree of alteration of the muscular fibres. Side by side with this hypertrophy you will observe in the patient a notable diminution of volume and also of force in the upper extremities, particularly the muscles of the arm. This last is the only point of resemblance which connects the myosclerotic paralysis to the progressive amyotrophy of spinal origin, and which might possibly lead to confusion, although they are really so distinct from each other.

There is another form of muscular atrophy apparently unconnected with nerve lesions which attacks young people or infants; and which Professor Erb (of Heidelberg) has recently described under the name of *juvenile form of progressive muscular atrophy*, and which he rightly considers to be quite distinct from the spinal forms that had been described up to that time.[1] The variety in question is not perhaps altogether a new discovery, but the description undoubtedly contains new facts, or at any rate such as have not been hitherto brought out conspicuously enough. The disease presents certain striking analogies with pseudo-hypertrophic paralysis, which are well revealed in Erb's description. It commences generally before the twentieth year, more rarely in infancy. It may sometimes present intermissions of improvement, due possibly to the efficiency of treatment, although its course is generally progressive. Nevertheless, it allows patients to live on, who are perfectly able to procreate, and as a general rule to reproduce amyotrophic subjects like to themselves. It starts in the upper extremities, the arms in particular, and the muscles of the shoulder girdle (Schultergürtel), never in the thenar and hypothenar (Fig. 26).

The lower extremities may be attacked in their turn. The calf, as in pseudo-hypertrophic paralysis, remaining in general free from any diminution of volume. It is atrophy which appears to be the leading feature; hypertrophy is rare, although M. Erb has observed it sometimes in the deltoids, the triceps, and the muscles of the calf. It is the diminution of volume of muscles which sometimes leads to Erb's variety being confounded with the Duchenne-Aran disease. In fact, if one examines the cases that have been collected by Duchenne in his 'Treatise on Localised Electrization,' one finds, as M. Erb pointed out, that a certain number of them very well correspond with the juvenile form. But Erb's disease is distinguished from progressive muscular atrophy of spinal origin by certain distinctive characteristics. Amongst others there are, the mode of invasion which, in

[1] Prof. W. Erb, "Ueber die Juvenile Form der Progressiven Muskelatrophie, &c." ('Deutsch. Archiv. für klin. Med.,' 1884).

the juvenile form, never takes place in the hands (thenar and hypothenar eminences); the absence of fibrillar twitchings in the atrophied muscles; the results of electrical

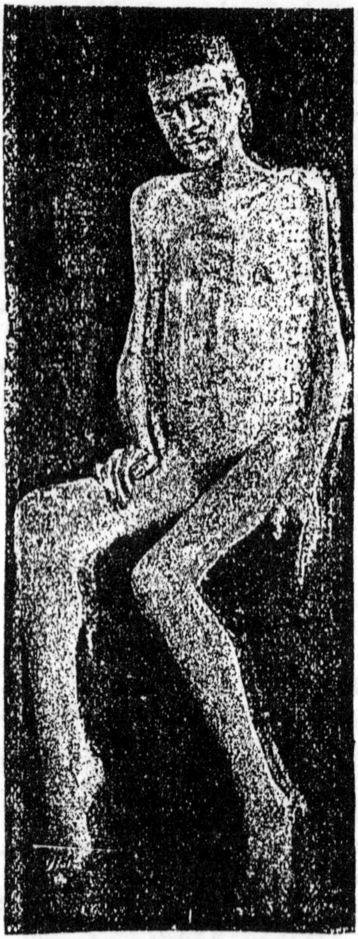

FIG. 26.

examination of the same muscles which never give the reaction of degeneration; the age of onset, which is always before twenty years of age; and finally, from an anatomo-pathological point of view, the complete absence of all spinal lesion.

The juvenile form described by Professor Erb is therefore quite distinct from amyotrophies of spinal origin. But is it equally distinct from pseudo-hypertrophic paralysis? I do not think it is, and here I agree with the opinion expressed, although with certain reserves, by M. Erb himself in his work, which appears to me to throw so much light on the question now before us. The apparent hypertrophy in one case, the apparent atrophy in another, is the only point of difference. But it should be recognised, I think, that this distinctive character is not fundamental. The hypertrophy is not, on the whole, an essential element in the constitution of the affection called pseudo-hypertrophic paralysis. I am about to show you a case which marks, in a sense, the transition between the juvenile form with amyotrophy on the one hand, and pseudo-hypertrophic paralysis on the other.

In the child L—, who is now before you (Fig. 27), *functional weakness is the leading feature; and as to the modification in the volume of the muscles, either increase or decrease, it does not exist*, a fact with which my Chef de Clinique, M. Marie, was particularly struck when he first saw the patient. This case so to speak reproduces, in respect of alteration of motor power, Erb's juvenile form of atrophy without the atrophy, and pseudo-hypertrophic paralysis without the hypertrophy. It is quite possible to suppose that the alteration of the muscular fibres, which is the chief cause of the weakness, can occur without modification of volume in the muscle. In Lang—, who is now 11 years old, the disease commenced *during infancy*. The little patient presents the arching of the back, and the walk so characteristic of pseudo-hypertrophic paralysis. If he is made to lie down on the ground on his back, he cannot get up again without the aid of his hands, which, supporting themselves on his knees, climb, so to speak, along the thighs until he reaches the vertical position, in a manner quite characteristic of this disease.

Now, in the next place look at the muscular masses; not

one of you will be able to discover either atrophy or hypertrophy. It is not meant to say that this child is very muscular, but there is no striking modification of volume in the muscles. The only clinical fact, therefore, which strikes

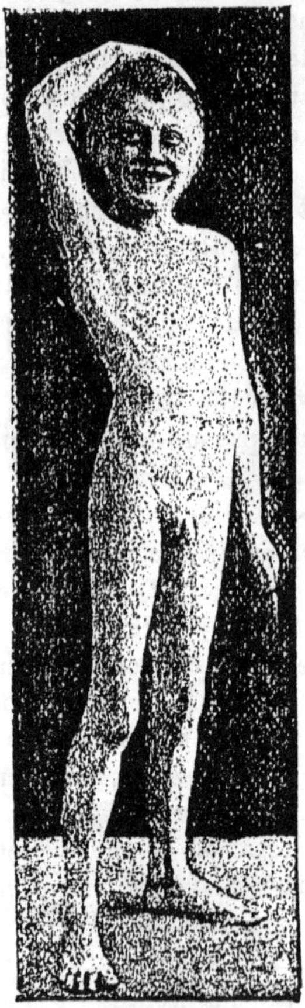

FIG. 27.

one about him is the diminution of force of his muscles, which are in the appearance normal as regarded their volume.

Where should this case be classed? Among the cases of

Erb's juvenile form, or, with the pseudo-hypertrophic paralysis of Duchenne? No, gentlemen, neither with the one nor the other precisely. It seems to belong, not to a distinct morbid species, but simply to a variety representing the different modes of evolution of one and the same affection, *primitive progressive myopathy.*

Thus we have seen that there are a certain number of cases which can be abstracted from the Duchenne-Aran group, but these are not all. I am now going to show you two other kinds of muscular atrophy which formerly belonged to the too extensive class of Duchenne-Aran's disease, but which now we shall be able to sort out, so as to place them in their true position, that is to say, among the primitive myopathies.

Here is a young woman of 24 years of age, named Dall—, who had been attacked with amyotrophy of the lower extremities, or more correctly of the legs. This atrophy is very pronounced; the patient is scarcely able to walk without support, and if one examines the gait attentively it is seen to be very peculiar. In fact, as a consequence of the feebleness of the muscles of the leg, the point of the foot falls when the patient, in walking, raises the leg so as to carry it forward. As a result of this she is obliged to flex the knee to an unnecessary extent so as not to allow the point of the foot to trail on the ground, imitating the movements of a *high-stepping* horse. It is analogous to what is observed whenever the muscles which produce dorsal flexion of the foot are atrophied, as in alcoholic paralysis for example, a case of which I recently had the opportunity of showing you. The disease commenced at the age of fourteen, in the lower extremities; then the upper extremities were attacked in their turn at the age of twenty; and at the present time it may be seen that there is, besides a certain functional weakness of the arms, a slight degree of atrophy of the hands, which are flattened on the palmar surfaces on account of the diminution of volume of the thenar and hypothenar eminences.

Albeit that there is here no trace of heredity, and although the patient has neither brothers nor sisters subject to the same complaint, this case appears to me[1] to belong to the variety described by Professor Leyden under the name *hereditary variety of progressive muscular atrophy;* and of which one of the characters is its commencement in the lower extremities. This form, moreover, is not strikingly different, as it seems to me, from the juvenile amyotrophy of Erb; and it is highly probable that, like this, it can be classed amongst the primary progressive myopathies of non-spinal origin.

Here, then, we already have three clinical varieties, namely, pseudo-hypertrophic paralysis; the juvenile form of Erb; and the hereditary variety of Leyden; which although possessing certain distinctive characters, can perfectly well be regarded as identical in their essence.

Now let us pass to another form, which Duchenne (de Boulogne) described as representing a variety of progressive muscular atrophy and to which he gave the name *infantile form of progressive muscular atrophy.* It must be somewhat rare, for it is scarcely mentioned in standard works. Duchenne, in his 'Treatise on Localised Electrization,' said that he had met with a score of cases, and in the 'Revue Photographique des Hôpitaux' are to be found photographs, made by Duchenne himself, which represent the faces of several patients, who are the subjects of this affection.

Here the disease begins in the face according to Duchenne's description, and particularly in the orbicularis oris; the lips becoming everted in such a manner as to simulate the habitual aspect of these organs in strumous people. Then the limbs are attacked consecutively, the arms first and then the trunk. It is important to note that this infantile form is hereditary, and one sees in the same family atrophic parents begetting sons and daughters attacked by an amyotrophy, commencing in the face. From his account it would be quite natural to conclude that the amyotrophy is

[1] The full report of this case is to be found in the memoir by MM. Charcot and Marie, "Sur une forme spéciale d'atrophie musculaire progressive débutant par les jambes et distincte de la forme de Leyden" ('Revue de Médecine,' February, 1886).

here connected with a spinal lesion, as in the cases of the Duchenne-Aran type; of which indeed according to Duchenne himself they only represent a simple variety. But this supposition is not correct. MM. Landouzy and Déjerine presented to the Academy of Sciences last year reports of typical cases of the infantile progressive muscular atrophy of Duchenne; and in one of these cases the autopsy proved that there existed no lesion, either in the spinal cord or in the peripheral nerves. Here again, then, we have cases of primary myopathy. I can show you a patient who exactly reproduces most of the characters of the description given by Duchenne.

Mdlle Lavr— is now 16 years old. In her the malady commenced in earliest infancy by a complete immobility of the upper lip, which was especially marked during laughter or crying (Figs. 28 and 29). She has never been

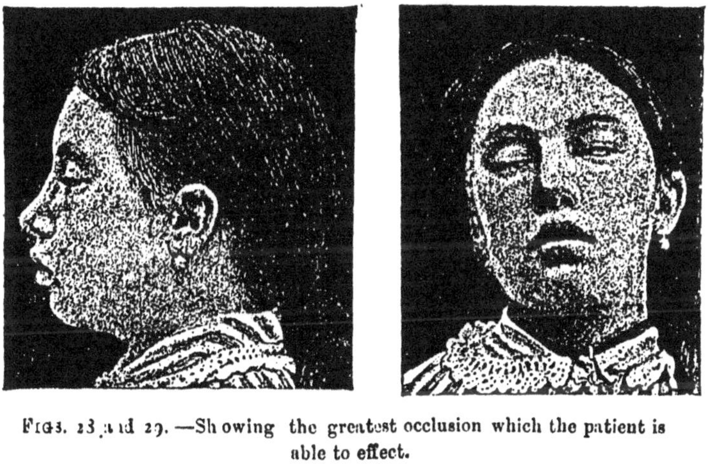

FIGS. 28 and 29.—Showing the greatest occlusion which the patient is able to effect.

able to whistle, and if she was asked to accomplish the act, it would be noticed that the upper lip, which did not contract, floated like an empty sail in the wind. She has at the present time a certain disturbance of the faculty of speech. Certain letters are particularly ill-pronounced, and she speaks as though she had a ball in her mouth. This paralysis of the orbicularis gives to the physiognomy quite a special character.

The lips are thick, everted, and elongated into the form of a snout, recalling the aspect of the lips in strumous people.

But besides this there is a symptom in our patient which has not been noted I believe by Duchenne in his general description; the upper part of the face is also attacked. The little patient cannot wrinkle her forehead, or elevate her eyebrows; she sleeps habitually with the eyes half open, and even in the waking state the most energetic contraction of the orbicularis palpebrarum will not suffice to produce complete closure. There is always a chink of

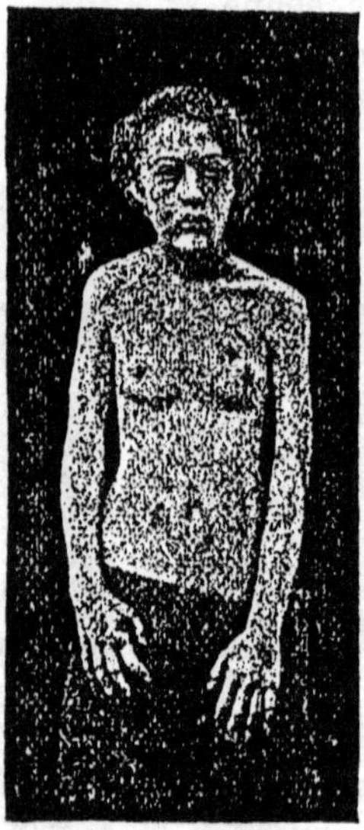

FIG. 30.

several millimetres between the free borders of the eyelids, through which the globe of the eye can be seen. This condition has been observed from her earliest years. At the age of 14, the upper extremities began to be attacked in their turn (Fig. 30), and atrophy soon appeared—and here the description of the muscular affection corresponds absolutely with that of the juvenile form of Erb. The atrophy of the muscles of the arms is considerable, resistance both to flexion and extension is impossible. The patient cannot raise her arm by a contraction of the elevator muscles of the limb, as in the act of blowing the nose. She is obliged to throw her hand violently upwards

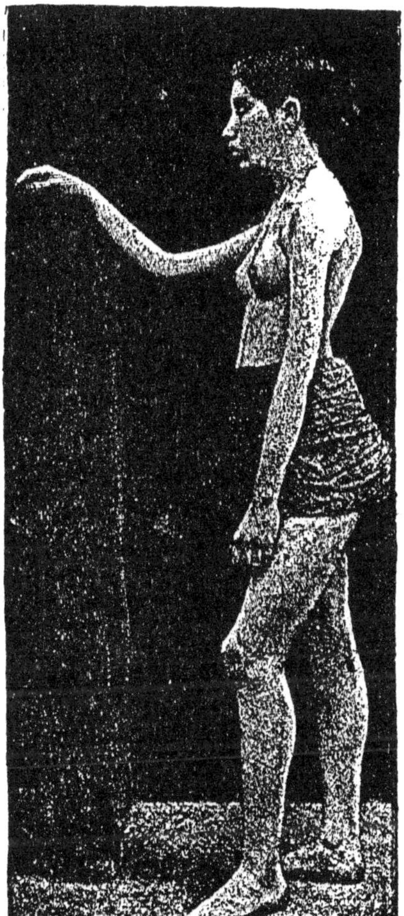

FIG. 31.

and outwards from the trunk, a movement so striking that it attracts one's attention directly (Fig. 31). When she walks,—which act is typically that of pseudo-hypertrophic paralysis and includes the arching of the back,—the arms swing inertly beside the body.

12

I am able to present to you the father of this girl. He is 44 years of age and is attacked with the same affection. Between the father and the daughter you see the resemblance is very striking. In him as in her, the face and the upper extremities, are atrophied. Not the least trace of hypertrophy of the muscles has ever been discovered either in him or in her. He cannot wrinkle his forehead, and the occlusion of the eyelids is always incomplete. He cannot whistle, and when he tries to do so, the orbicularis contracts unequally and forms a sort of knot in the right half of the upper lip, at the only point where the contraction takes place. As in his daughter, there is complete integrity of the muscles of the hand. It may be remarked in passing, that the muscles of the tongue, and those of deglutition, are normal; and one does not find, in a word, any of the bulbar symptoms which sometimes exist in progressive muscular atrophy of spinal origin.

This, gentlemen, is a most original variety, one possessing strong individualities, the commencement in the face particularly. But is that a specific characteristic, and should one on that account create a special group for it? I do not think so. If you abstract the participation of the face you have in these patients the very image of the juvenile form of Erb. It is, then, very probable that there exist numerous points of contact, to say no more, between these two varieties; and consequently an analogy with pseudo-hypertrophic paralysis.

This proposition would be proved, partially at any rate, if it were found that in some of the cases the onset occurred in the limbs (juvenile variety), and the face was attacked only late in the disease; and that there were other cases in which several members of the same family presented, either associated in the same individual, or occurring in separate subjects, some of the different varieties that we have just been describing. Well, such conditions are to be met with. There is a case described by M. Remak[1] where the outset was that of the ordinary juvenile variety, that is to say where the upper extremities were invaded first of all,

[1] Mendel's 'Centralblatt,' 1884, No. 15.

whereas the face was also attacked, only much later in the disease, at the age of twenty-nine. And again, Mr. F. Zimmerlin[1] has published the history of a family in which two of the children presented the juvenile variety, the onset occurring in the upper extremities; whereas a third child was attacked by the variety where the face is first involved, and the lower extremities with pseudo-hypertrophy. Hence, it follows that the commencement in the face, or simply the involvement of the face, is not a characteristic worthy of forming a special class, but simply a variety.

While bearing in mind these cases of transition, the different forms which we have enumerated, though distinct undoubtedly in appearance, become fused together into a uniform group which alone is worthy of forming a class. If matters are really thus, they are undoubtedly much less complicated than they seemed to be at first; and the progressive amyotrophies are divided quite simply into two great classes; the *first class* is represented by the *amyotrophy of spinal origin*, which comprise the following *groups*:

(1) Lateral Amyotrophic Sclerosis.

(2) Progressive Muscular Atrophy of the Duchenne-Aran type. But this last, let it be understood, may be reduced to a much narrower extent, and disengaged from all foreign elements which do not belong to it, but which belong to the following class of cases.

The *second class* consists of *Primary Progressive Amyotrophies*, which include, though only under the head of *varieties*, the following:

(1) Pseudo-hypertrophic paralysis.

(2) Juvenile form of progressive muscular atrophy, described by Erb.

(3) Infantile progressive muscular atrophy of Duchenne (of Boulogne).

(4) Those transitional cases, such as the one I have shown you, where muscular weakness was the leading feature; and where one finds in fact, neither atrophy nor hypertrophy. Finally—

(5) Hereditary form of progressive muscular atrophy described by Leyden, commencing in the lower extremities.

[1] Mendel's Centralblatt,' 1885, No. 3.

The mixed, or transitional, forms allow us to draw these different varieties closer together; or even, it may be, to group them together. Perhaps in the cases described by M. Erb, a thoroughly searching examination of the muscles of the mouth and eyes would have enabled him to find some of the signs of Duchenne's infantile form. In nearly all our patients, in fact, even in that one which showed neither atrophy nor hypertrophy, there exists some difficulty of movement of the muscles of the face. But in the slighter cases these symptoms are not very striking. It is necessary to look very carefully in order to find them. We have under observation at this time two other patients, whom, unfortunately, it is not possible for us to show you to-day, which are typical cases of the infantile form described by Duchenne

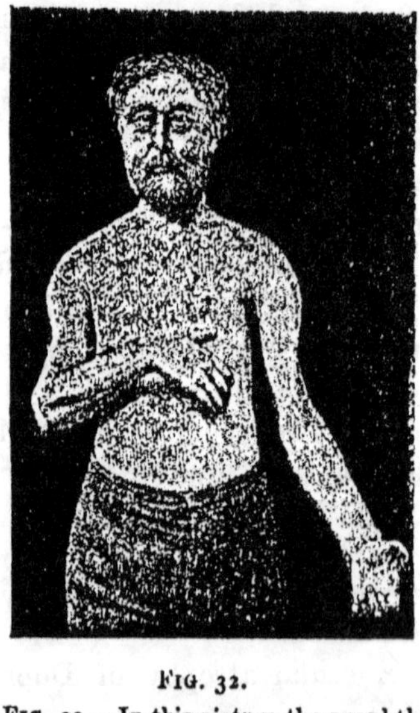

FIG. 32.

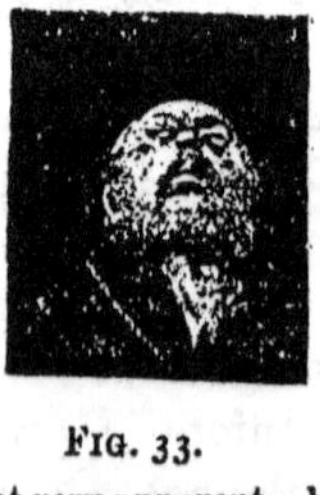

FIG. 33.

FIG. 32.—In this picture the exophthalmos is not very apparent; but the preservation of the deltoid, and the atrophy of the biceps and thenar muscles are well seen.

FIG. 33.—Shows the incomplete occlusion of the eyes, and the asymmetry of the lips when the patient attempts to whistle. (The head in this photograph is forcibly pushed back.)

(of Boulogne). The father and the son (Figs. 32 and 33) are both affected in the same manner; and in both, the participation of the orbicularis oris, and of the orbicularis palpebrarum, would perhaps have remained undetected if one had not examined them very carefully.

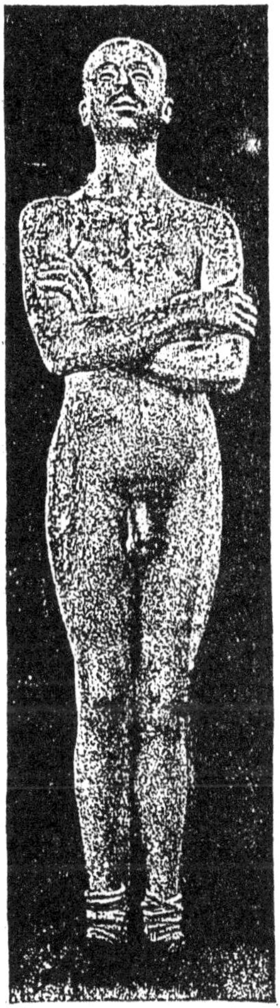

FIG. 34.

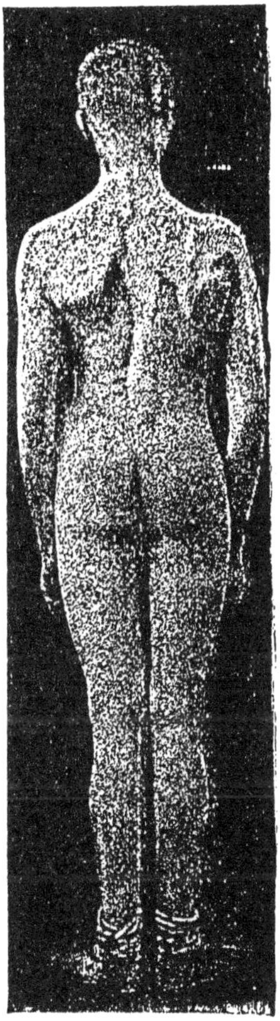

FIG. 35.

FIG. 34.—Shows the incomplete occlusion of the eyes, and, to some extent, the asymmetry of the lips. It is also well seen that the shoulders are too forward.

FIG. 35.—This shows the deviation of the spinal column and of the shoulders.

The son is an example of *those cases of transition* of which I spoke just now (Figs. 34 and 35). There exists in him a very pronounced weakness of the muscles of the upper extremities, without atrophy or hypertrophy, whereas the quadriceps extensor of both sides is more voluminous and harder than under normal conditions.

Thus, all these varieties, so different in appearance, are nevertheless all linked together, and all constitute one great class, one morbid entity, *primary progressive myopathy.*

Such then, gentlemen, is the outline of this large subject, as far as I have been able to lay it before you to-day. It certainly merits being developed and discussed at greater length, under the light of the long series of publications which bear upon this important question. But that is a task which I hope to be able to fulful on some future occasion.

LECTURE XV.

TREMORS AND CHOREÏFORM MOVEMENTS.—RHYTHMICAL CHOREA.[1]

SUMMARY.—*Tremors of disseminated sclerosis; oscillations of large extent.—Tremors of paralysis agitans, and senile tremors.—Tremors with small oscillations; rapid oscillations, or vibratile tremors.—Hysterical tremors.—Alcoholic and mercurial tremors.—Tremors of general paralysis and of Basedow's disease.*

Chorea; characters of the involuntary movements of the chorea of Sydenham.—Chorea and hemi-chorea, pre- and post-hemiplegic.—Athetosis and hemi-athetosis.

Rhythmical chorea; characters of the movements; they appear in crises; they are rhythmical, systematic, and reproduce more or less faithfully the movements of ordinary life or of professional gesture (dancing chorea, hammering chorea).—The disease is generally allied to hysteria.—Prognosis varies in different cases.

GENTLEMEN,—In connection with the cases of disseminated sclerosis that I have shown you in the last few lectures, I wish to speak to you to-day about the various involuntary movements with which the tremors, so characteristic of this affection, may be confounded. I have insisted on the peculiar characters of the tremors of disseminated sclerosis, and have already shown you that they only become manifest on occasions of voluntary movement of a certain force (intentional tremors, *Intentionzittern* of German authors); that it ceases to exist when the patients assume a condition of complete repose, by lying down on the bed, for example.

If they are only seated, then the muscles of the neck and

[1] This lecture was edited by M. Guinon, Interne des Hôpitaux.

the trunk are called in requisition to maintain the vertical position of the body, and they produce oscillations of the head and of the trunk, although the limbs are in repose. If you wish to make the trembling reappear in the limb, you have only to ask the patient to carry a glass or a spoon to his mouth. This act requires a voluntary movement of sufficient force, which is a necessary condition to bring on the trembling; for the tremor does not habitually manifest itself in the smaller movements, such as threading a needle, &c.

At the moment of grasping the glass the oscillations are but little marked, yet they progressively increase, and reach their maximum at the moment when the glass approaches the mouth. This special character of the tremors of disseminated sclerosis is easily revealed by the tracing given by a registering apparatus. No. 1 of Fig. 36 represents the intentional tremor of disseminated sclerosis.

The line A B indicates the state of repose. The point B represents the moment of commencing the voluntary movement; B C represents the duration of the movement, and the trembling is represented by the wavy line *x y z*, of which each oscillation is larger the farther we get from B.

Such are the tremors of disseminated sclerosis. In order to bring out more clearly the special characters which distinguish it, I wish to employ the method of contrasts. In other words, I wish to show you this tremor side by side with other tremors belonging to very different maladies; although several of them have been confounded with it up to the last few years.

Let us commence with paralysis agitans. Like that of disseminated sclerosis, the tremor of Parkinson's disease is composed of rhythmical oscillations, but of small extent and of short duration. You can make out these characters in the patient whom I will show you now. Notice that the hands and fingers tremble individually, but fix well in your memory the altogether peculiar attitude of the hand.

The phalanges are stretched one along the other, but the fingers are flexed on the metacarpus. The pulp of the thumb is pressed against the index finger, imitating thus the position of the hand in the act of holding a pen. The movements, which agitate all the parts, remind one sometimes of the act of rolling up a ball of paper, or of crumbling bread. This tremor is continuous, and is manifested—this is the important point—independent of any voluntary movement. If you tell the patient to carry the glass to his mouth, you will see perhaps that the tremors augment a little in amplitude, but he will never produce those oscillations of large extent, which are characteristic of disseminated sclerosis. This character is well revealed by tracings taken with the aid

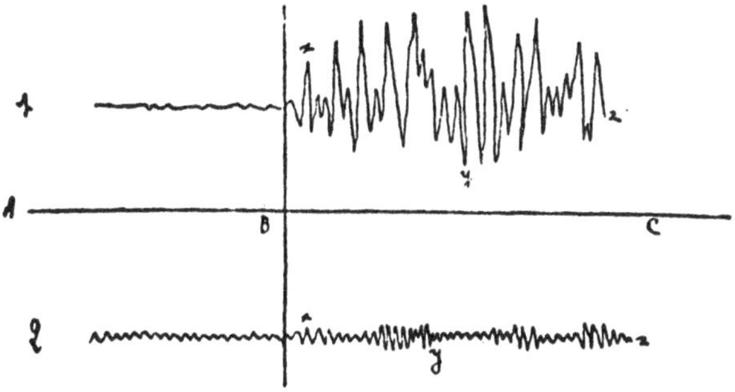

FIG. 36.—This figure is a semi-diagrammatic reproduction of tracings obtained by the graphic method in two patients now in the wards.

of the registering apparatus. No. 2 in the figure represents the tremors of paralysis agitans. You see at once on looking at this diagram how the two tracings differ in the portion B C. The segment under the line A B represents the time of repose. It is cut up by little waves corresponding to the continuous trembling. At point B voluntary movement commences. From this point the components of the wavy line *x y z* are a little longer and more irregular than in the period of repose, but they are never so much so as in disseminated sclerosis.

Bear in mind also that in paralysis agitans the tremor does not in general attack the head, and if this seems to participate in the involuntary movements it is in reality but the seat of communicated movements.

The tremors of disseminated sclerosis and of Parkinson's disease are *slow oscillations*, with an average of four or five to the second. This same slowness of oscillations is found again in what is called senile tremor. Here are two women who are affected with this tremor. In one, the woman named La— (now 73 years of age), the disease came on at the age of 60 in the index finger of the left hand, after an injury. In the other, the woman named Les—, 80 years of age, it came on fourteen years ago, during the siege of Paris, after violent emotion. In this woman the hands and the fingers tremble individually as in Parkinson's disease. The head participates in the shaking, on its own account; the movements, which are both vertical and horizontal, succeed each other with regularity, and in these the patient seems, by her gesture, to say yes or no. These movements are absolutely characteristic of the oscillations of the head in so-called senile tremor.

Before passing to the subject of tremors of rapid oscillation, I wish to mention a kind of trembling that seems to occupy a place between the two kinds, I mean hysterical trembling. We have at the present time in our wards two men who are thus affected. In one the number of oscillations is five, in the other it is seven per second. I will only mention this kind of trembling just in passing, as I propose to come back to the subject later on in more detail. I mention the fact only provisionally just now from the point of view of rapidity of the jerks, which constitute in this respect a variety intermediate between the group of slow oscillations and the one we are about to consider.

The second class includes those tremors having a rapid oscillation, which I propose to call *vibratile tremors*. The number of jerks in these cases amounts to eight or nine per second, and this feature appears to be the only difference which separates the first and second groups. We include in it:

(1) Alcoholic trembling.
(2) Mercurial trembling,
(3) That of general paralysis, and, lastly,
(4) That of Basedow's disease.

A further distinction that can probably be made between

the first three and the last-named, rests on the fact that whereas in the former the fingers tremble individually, in the latter there is no trembling of the fingers themselves. This distinction can be easily demonstrated by the aid of a graphic method such as that which M. Marie has employed. If a caoutchouc bag, communicating by a tube with the reaction drum of a registering apparatus, be placed in the hand of the patient, one sees that in cases where the fingers tremble of themselves the tracing is very undulatory, whereas in other cases, in Basedow's disease, for instance, we obtain a straight line, or at least one only interrupted by very slight undulations.

In connection with the subject of muscular tremblings, that is to say, tremors having a rhythmical oscillation, which we have just been considering, there is another variety of involuntary movement which can be, and which as a matter of fact often is, confounded with the tremors of disseminated sclerosis. I refer to chorea, or rather *choreïform movements* in general. Here we have to do, not with rhythmical oscillations, but rather with gestures, of larger, unnecessary, and purposeless extent. These gestures do not present any kind of cadence, and they are altogether without signification, that is to say, they do not imitate any expressive or professional movements.

They continue, like the preceding ones, during muscular repose, and become exaggerated during voluntary movement. But these useless gesticulations pervert the general direction of the movements, and cause the patient to miss the mark, whereas in disseminated sclerosis, and in the other tremblings of which I have just been speaking, the general direction of the movement, although interrupted by the jerkings which shake the limb, is as a whole always preserved. Well, gentlemen, in spite of the fundamental differences which exist between choreiform movements and the movements of disseminated sclerosis, it happens that the most distinguished physicians for a long time regarded disseminated sclerosis as a sort of chorea. Duchenne (de Boulogne), who had well differentiated the collection of symptoms belonging to disseminated sclerosis, but who did not recognise it from an anatomo-pathological point of view, called it choreïform paralysis. I will therefore say a few words on the subject of these choreïform movements.

In the first place we have *ordinary chorea*, so-called rheumatic; comprising *chorea minor*, which might also be called the *chorea of Sydenham*, and which should be clearly distinguished from the true dance of Saint Guy, the great epidemic chorea, *chorea major*.

It principally affects, as you know, children from five to fourteen years of age, more rarely adults and old people. You doubtless remember the girl named Flon—, whom I have already presented to you as illustrating ordinary chorea. In this girl the disease is dying away, and the intervals of repose which separate the involuntary movements are, at the present time, fairly long. But sometimes, under the influence of an emotion, the doctor's examination, for example, or sometimes spontaneously, small jerks, more or less accentuated, become manifest in the upper extremity of the left side. The patient brings her hand abruptly to the side of her body, or, making alternative movements of pronation and supination, rubs her hand against her thigh. In her, by way of exception, a voluntary act does not increase the jerkings, and if you ask her to carry a glass or spoon to her mouth, the movement is fairly well directed, and the goal is reached with sufficient accuracy, such as by no means always exists in chorea. The face on the left side is also affected with involuntary movements, and thus she makes grimaces continually.

In the same group of inco-ordinate choreïform movements should also be placed *pre- and post-hemiplegic chorea*. Here the movements are in fact of the same nature, the only essential difference rests in the pathology, the disease being in such cases connected with cerebral lesions, localised in a certain manner.

In the same way, gentlemen, *athetosis*, in a natural classification, should be grouped with chorea and with post-hemiplegic chorea. In athetosis there is no rest, and the movements are equally inco-ordinate. I need not stop to describe to you the contortions of the fingers and their alternate flexion and extension. I have shown you already several examples of athetosis, I should only like to remark that it differs notably from chorea in that the movements are slower (said to be like the movements of the tentacles of an octopus), and less abrupt than in this last malady; and that they are limited to the fingers and the wrists, to the feet, and to the toes, although sometimes they have been observed in the face and eyelids. The patient is unable to hold anything in his hand or carry anything to his mouth; anything placed in his hands is immediately allowed to fall. In cases of double athetosis these phenomena sometimes present a rough analogy with the movements of disseminated sclerosis.

These, gentlemen, constitute the first two groups of tremblings or involuntary movements; but I must now speak to you of an affection which constitutes our third group. It also bears the name of chorea, although it differs considerably, as you will see, from the chorea of Sydenham and the allied affections. The study of these movements will make us digress somewhat from disseminated sclerosis, but I fear, if I delay, to miss the occasion of showing you a number of cases which one rarely has the chance of finding collected together,—for it is a very rare affection.

In *rhythmical chorea* we find neither oscillations nor vibrations, as in the tremors, nor the inconsistent and purposeless gesticulations of ordinary chorea. But if this affection is also characterised by involuntary impulsive movements, these movements are more complex, and furthermore they often assume a *regular rhythm* or *cadence*. They have not, you understand, the regular character of the choreïform movements that I have just been describing to you. They might, indeed, be called *systematic* because they seem to be co-ordinated on a definite plan, imitating, for example:

(1) Certain *movements of expression* such as those of the dance, and particularly character dances (*dancing chorea*).[1]

[1] [*Chorée Saltatoire*, which it would be more correct etymologically to render *gesticulating chorea*.]

(2) Certain *professional acts,* such as the movements of an oarsman or a blacksmith (*hammering chorea*) [chorée malléatoire].

In a word, we have here a more or less faithful reproduction of voluntary or purposive movements.

The disease in question seems to be most frequently allied to hysteria, or to be even of hysterical origin; although it may exist in some cases by itself, independent of all phenomena indicative of hysteria. You will be able to see for yourselves, moreover, how a transition may take place between the two conditions, for without dwelling more on theoretical considerations I will now place successively before you three patients who present the symptoms of rhythmical chorea in different degrees.

The first one, a girl named Flor—,[1] is known to you already. But you only saw her casually and she merits a more attentive study. She has been in the wards more than six months, and formed the subject of a lecture last year. From this you may infer that it is a very rebellious affection, of which it is very difficult to relieve your patient. This young woman is 26 years of age. She has been married twice, first at the age of eighteen, and then at twenty. She has had three children. She is of an irritable temper. She was married to a workman, a fine fellow withal, but the frequent disagreements between them gave rise to much discord in the home.

Nothing of interest is to be found in the hereditary antecedents, nor in the history of the patient herself. Three years ago, after her last confinement, she began to exhibit the following symptoms. She often experienced after dinner, in the region of the stomach, a sort of swelling and pulsation, followed by a sensation of a ball in the throat. Then she fell into a kind of syncopal or lethargic condition, and these symptoms finally terminated by a fit of crying. About the same time she had expectoration or vomiting of blood (neuropathic hæmorrhages of Parrot). It should be added also that at about the same period there was right hemianæsthesia, though not very pronounced. At the present time

[1] A more detailed account of this patient is to be seen in the Appendix.

this has passed over to the left side, without modification in the visual field, or any other sensorial affection: she has never presented the ovarian phenomenon [ovarie]. These represent, gentlemen, the stigmata of the great neurosis. They have almost completely disappeared at the present time; but their past existence enables us to affirm their more or less hysterical nature, or at least the hysterical origin of the affection from which she suffers now.

The onset of the attacks of rhythmical movement took place on the 15th of May 1884, that is to say, last year. They occurred for the first time during the menstrual period, on the occasion of a dispute, and after one of the attacks which she habitually had after dinner. Then the chorea became permanently established, the attacks coming on at any time, except during sleep. The seizures would last from one hour to an hour and a half, separated by intervals which were at first short, but which at the end of a few weeks became gradually longer, until at the present time they rarely occur spontaneously. We have discovered, however, that they can be provoked with certainty by certain manipulations.

Static electricity appears to have produced the amendment which has lately occurred. It is undoubtedly under its influence that the hemianæsthesia was at first shifted, and then disappeared; but I am afraid that the patient is far from being completely cured yet. I remember a young Polish girl who had attacks of hammering movements in the arm, coming on in seizures lasting from one to two hours, several times a day, which had continued ever since the age of seven. I know not if she be actually cured yet; and furthermore, I shall presently show you a patient in whom the attacks have lasted for thirty years.

The condition of Flor—, at the present time is as follows. I have already told you that she had both spontaneous attacks and such as were provoked. The former usually come on after a meal, and are as it were a sort of relic of the original hysterical attacks of the ordinary type. The patient experiences pain and palpitation in the epigastrium combined with a feeling as of repletion. Then the right upper extremity begins to move, and is soon followed by the left, and then by the lower extremities. Then you witness a succession of various and very complex acts, in which you can recognise the characteristics of rhythm, or cadence, and of a perfect imitation of certain voluntary purposive movements, such as I mentioned in the general description with which I commenced. When it is started spontaneously, the attack begins without any other aura than a blinking of the right eyelid.

The induced attacks can be obtained by pulling on the left arm, or by striking with a hammer on one or other patella tendon such as I am now doing. When you have excited the attack by means of pulling the left arm, that arm immediately commences performing rapid rhythmical movements in which the patient seems to be whipping eggs. Then she bends her fingers, applying their tips to the thumb; and raising her arm, makes the gesticulation of an orator who is demonstrating. From time to time the whole of the upper extremity performs extensive movements of circumduction. The lower extremities are also affected by movements in their turn, and if the patient is in the erect position she dances alternately on each foot, very nearly imitating a jig or dance of the Tsiganes, or of the Zingari of Andalusia. During the whole time of the attack the patient is perfectly conscious; and strange to say, when anyone is placed close to her when she is executing some of these violent movements, which would have the result of violently striking the person near her, she warns them to take care before the commencement of the gesture. It would appear then, and this is an important feature from a psychological point of view, that the act is preceded by a mental representation which warns the patient of what is about to happen.

You can question her during the attack and she will reply to you that she does not suffer; that she is simply fatigued, and inconvenienced by violent palpitations. After awhile she stops and rests for a minute; you think that the attack is past; but no, soon it all recommences, and the same phases are reproduced. The total duration of an attack varies from one to two hours. She then lies down and it is all finished. When she gets up again she feels somewhat tired.

Now you will be able to see an attack very similar to this produced in another patient after similar manipulations. It is in this woman, named Deb—, that the chorea has lasted for more than thirty years; though the malady has lately undergone some amelioration in that the spontaneous attacks have become extremely rare. One scarcely ever sees them in her now unless they are provoked.

She is now 67 years old. The menopause occurred a long while ago, and one cannot therefore count on it to put an end to her symptoms. I could show you several examples of this kind in the category of hystero-epilepsy. At the present time there does not remain any permanent sign of hysteria in this patient; and there is nothing else to be discovered in her except a great susceptibility to emotion, and the attacks of rhythmical chorea. The attacks are easily produced either by pulling on the arm, or percussing the patella tendon, as in our first patient.

But before giving rise to one of these attacks I should like to indicate summarily the history of her case. The onset occurred at the age of thirty-six. About this time, when out driving in a carriage with her husband, she fell over a precipice with the horse and carriage. After the great fright which she had thus experienced she lost consciousness for three hours. This was followed by a convulsive seizure of hysteria major [grande attaque hystérique], by rigidity of the limbs of the right side, and cries like the barking of a dog. It was only after several months that the rhythmical crises made their appearance, such as we see to-day, only at the beginning they were more intense and of longer duration.

Now look at this patient. It will not be necessary for us to intervene, for the emotion that she has experienced at finding herself before so many people in the lecture room will save us the trouble of provoking an attack. In the first phase, rhythmical jerkings of the right arm, like the movements of hammering, occur. The patient has her eyes closed. Then after this period there succeeds a period of tonic spasms, and of contortions of the arm and head,

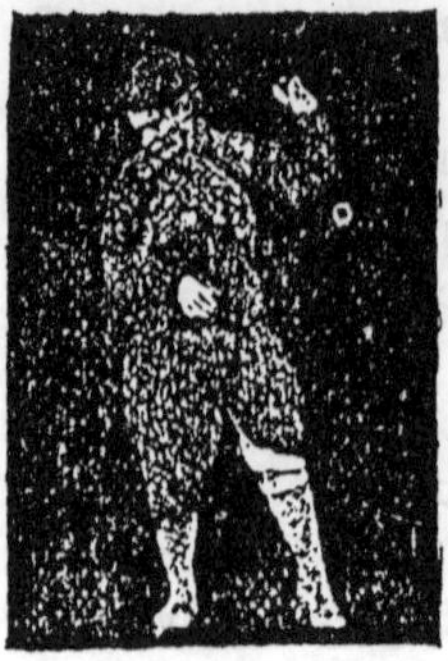

FIG. 37.[1]

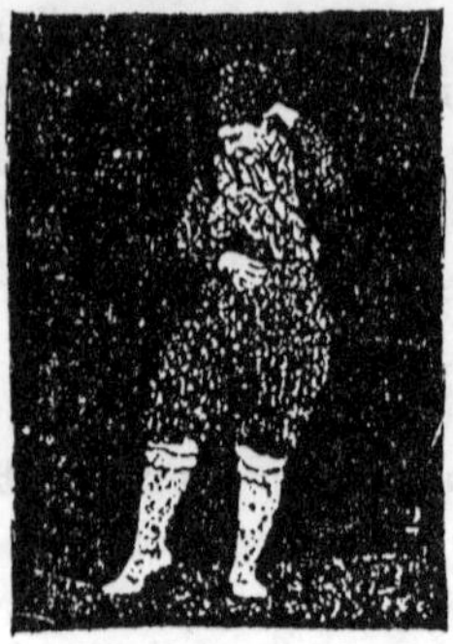

FIG. 38.

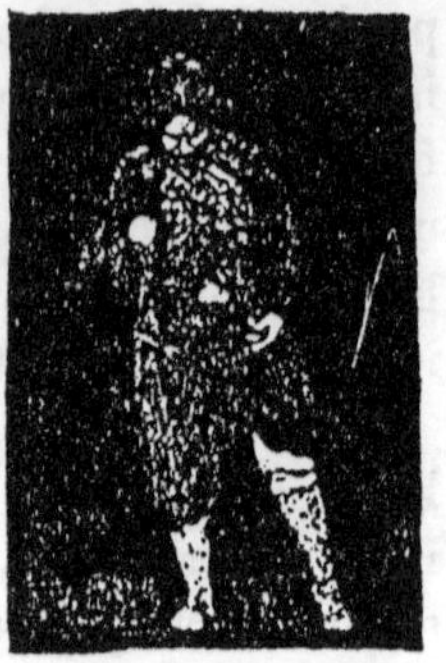

FIG. 39.

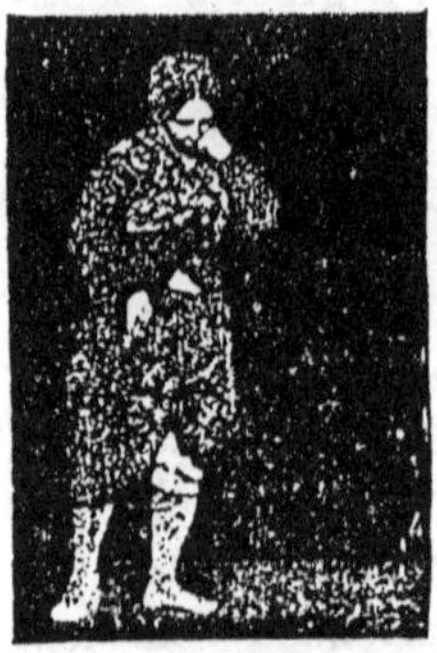

FIG. 40.

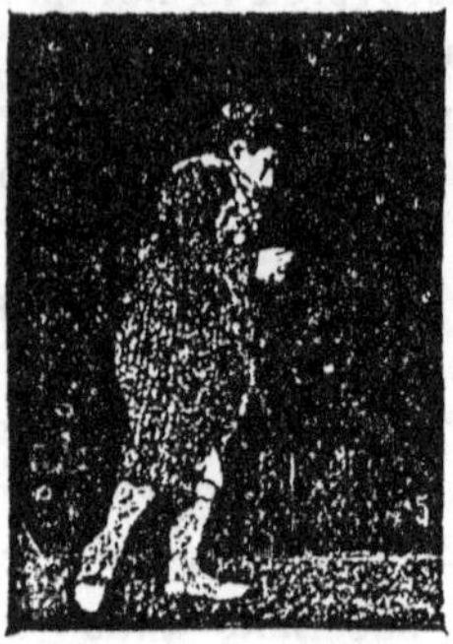

FIG. 41.

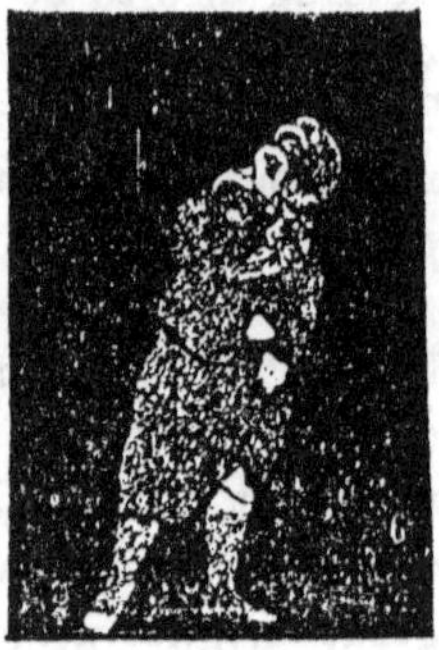

FIG. 42.

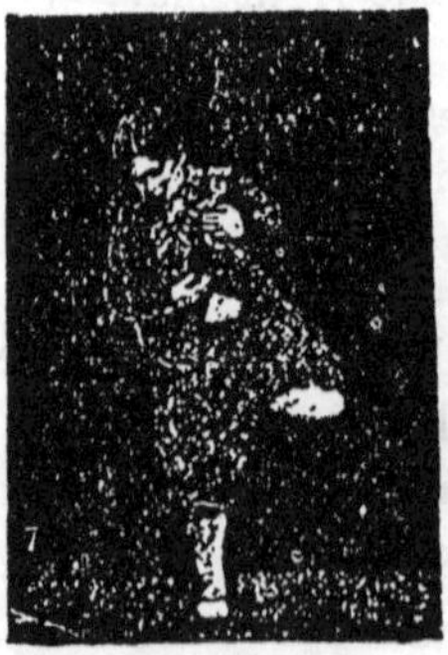

FIG. 43.

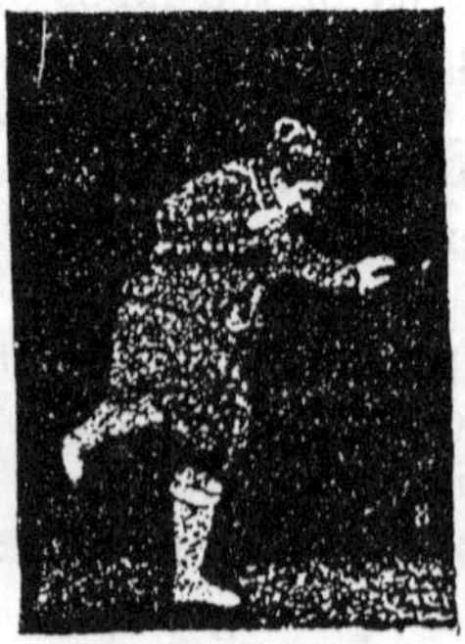

FIG. 44.

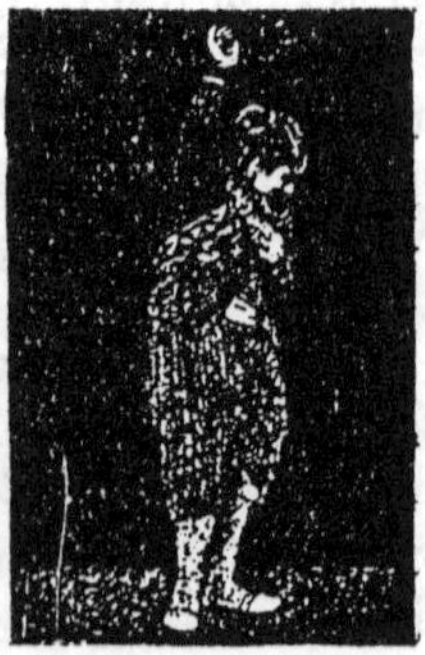

FIG. 45.

[1] The photographs here reproduced have been made by M. Londe in the laboratory of the Salpêtrière.

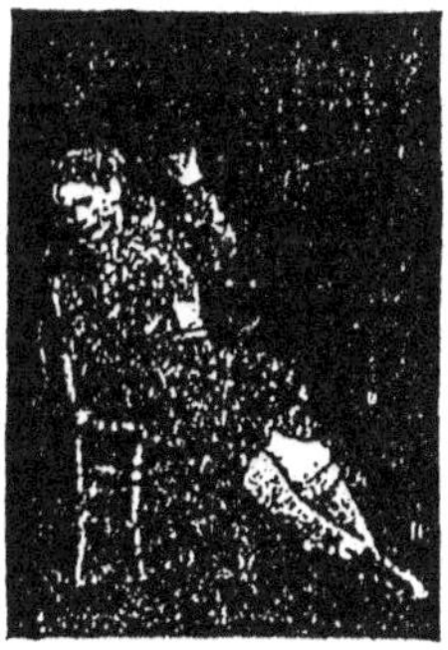

FIG. 46.

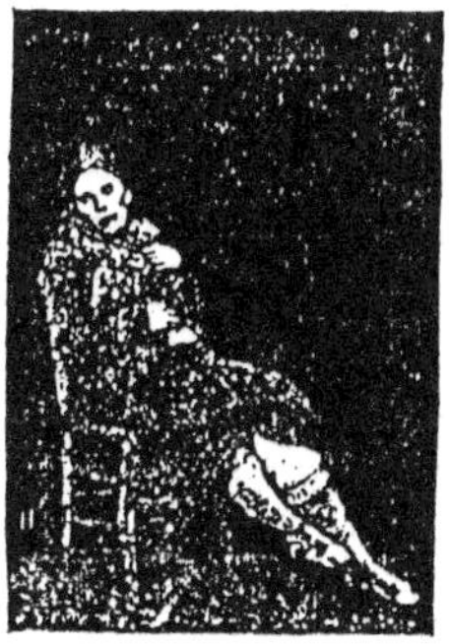

FIG. 47.

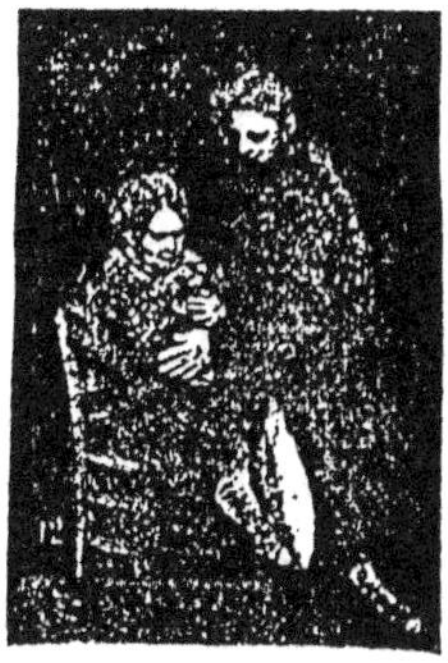

FIG. 48.

recalling partial epilepsy. Here probably is a remnant of the convulsive hysterical attack. Finally, measured movements of the head to the right and the left occur; rapid movements defying all interpretation, for I ask you, what do they correspond to in the region of physiological acts? At the same time the patient utters a cry, or rather a kind of plaintive wail, always the same. And here again we find that character of co-ordination, that apparent adaptation, which belongs as a peculiar feature to rhythmical chorea. The attack ceases spontaneously. During all the time the patient has not lost consciousness for a single instant.

You see by this example that rhythmical chorea may be in certain cases a grave affection. Not that it directly menaces life, but that it may persist over a very long period of time, and become a most distressing infirmity; preventing the patient from following any occupation, and obliging her to live apart from the world by reason of the fear which these attacks inspire in those around, and the sentiment of repulsion of which these unfortunates feel themselves the object.

Happily, gentlemen, matters are not always so dark in the history of rhythmical chorea. And I can, by way of contrast with the last two patients, present to you a third, in whom the rhythmical choreïc movements exist, though in a rudimentary condition, and presenting in an early stage the recurrent attacks, both spontaneous and provoked, which we have seen in the other two cases. But here they are always intermingled with the phenomena of ordinary convulsive hysteria. In a word, the rhythmical chorea which assumes a hammering form in this third case, is an accompaniment of the hysterical attack from which it cannot be altogether dissociated.

The woman Bac—, 29 years of age, a needle woman, has been in the wards since the 6th January, 1885. There is no trace of nerve disease to be found either in the hereditary or personal antecedents. At the age of twenty-two years, after a severe grief caused by the death of a relative, she suffered from undoubted hysterical attacks, in which even then choreïc movements like those of the present time were manifest. From 1878 to 1884 she had but four or five attacks, and those only as a consequence of annoyances. I may note in passing, several blennorrhagic arthrites in the right wrist and the left knee, as having co-operated more or less in producing a return of the present symptoms. There does not exist any sensorial trouble, no modification of sensibility other than imperfect perception of cold on the left side. An ovarian point exists on the right side; and thus the ovarian phenomena and the hemianæsthesia are crossed in a way that sometimes occurs.

When the attacks supervene spontaneously they commence by a sensation of uneasiness in the epigastric region, and by palpitations of the heart; sometimes the sensation of a ball occurs. There is never any cephalic aura. One can, moreover, provoke the attacks by pulling on the left arm, and by jerking it at the same time, so as to imitate the movements of hammering chorea. At first the left arm commences to execute hammering movements, which the right arm soon after executes also. At the same time the whole body becomes stiff, the head and lower extremities remaining immobile. At other times the legs begin to shake, the eyes being closed and the eyelids flickering. Every few seconds the patient interrupts the monotony of the attack by making the arc of a circle. Pressure over the right ovarian region causes the attack to stop, and then for a moment the patient remains without speaking, or without being able to put out the tongue. Here the hysterical origin is much more clearly revealed than in the case of our first two patients. The rhythmical malady cannot be altogether detached as a separate affection. Hence, the case is I hope less grave. In short, the case of this woman, apart from the hammering phenomena, is one of ordinary fits belonging rather to hysteria minor than to hysteria major; the attacks occurring only rarely on the occasion of an emotion. One can hope that under the influence of appropriate treatment, these attacks will disappear at the same time as the rhythmical choreïform movements which accompany them.

LECTURE XVI.

SPIRITUALISM AND HYSTERIA.[1]

SUMMARY.—*The influence of intellectual stimuli on the development of hysteria.—Belief in the supernatural, in the marvellous; practices of spiritualism.*

Narration of an epidemic of hysteria which attacked three children of one family, living in a military penitentiary, and addicted to spiritualism.

Nervous and rheumatic antecedents.—Description of the attacks; hallucinations of vision; permanent and transient stigmata.—Conclusion.

GENTLEMEN,—It is undoubtedly true that whatever forcibly strikes the mind, whatever strongly impresses the imagination, is singularly favorable, in subjects predisposed, to the development of hysteria. Among all the different means of affecting the cerebral functions perhaps nothing is more efficacious, and nothing whose action may not be more frequently detected, than the belief in the marvellous and the supernatural which is fostered and exaggerated by excessive religious exercises, and the related order of ideas, spirtualism and its practices.

It is sufficient to recall certain well-established facts, as, for example, in former times, the incident of the "*Possédée de Louviers*,"[2] whose imagination had been held, before the "possession," in a constant state of tension by the wicked spirit which *returned* each night to the house where she lived.

[1] This lecture was edited by M. Gilles de la Tourette.

[2] Full report, taken down at the time, relating to the deliverance of a girl possessed of the devil at Louviers (1591), office of the 'Progrès Médical;' 'Bibliothèque Diabolique' (1883).

And more recently the epidemic of hysteria which attacked the six children of the same Breton family, who had been satiated with fantastic stories, where sorcerers and apparitions played the principal parts.[1]

We have had the opportunity of observing one of these little epidemics, of which I am able to present to you the principal actors, and which merits a detailed description, both on account of its mode of development and the means which it affords of studying hysteria in children, particularly in little boys. It was in a military penitentiary that the following incidents occurred.

Life in a penitentiary cannot be very gay. Moreover, in consequence of the arrangements necessary in such an establishment, the apartments even of the directing officials are considerably imbued with the sadness and discipline of the place. The rooms occupied by M. X—, a sub-lieutenant, are situated on the third floor. They are reached by a dark staircase; and the apartments themselves are badly lighted; for all the windows look on to the central court, a large one, it is true, but they are situated beyond the reach of the sun, are narrow, and permit very little light to enter.

M. X—, who has lived in the penitentiary three and a half years, is 43 years of age. He has pursued his military career with much indifference, though he appears fairly intelligent. I shall refer again to his mental condition. He has always enjoyed good health, and there are no pathological antecedents of importance, excepting that at the age of thirteen he suffered from an affection which started with febrile symptoms and was followed by *delirium lasting for six months.*

Madame X— is 36 years of age, and has been married since 1879. She is of a neurotic disposition. She is impatient, lively, very emotional, but she has never had any convulsive attacks. On the other hand, her mother, who died in the month of March, 1884, at the age of seventy-two, of a cerebro-spinal affection, was the subject of very

[1] "Les possédés de Plédran," par le Dr. Baratoux, 'Progrès Médical,' No. 23, 1881, p. 550.

characteristic hysterical attacks on two or three occasions. It may be noted also that her father was a confirmed invalid from rheumatism.

M. and Mdme. X— have had four children, three of whom are living, the fourth died, probably of asthenia, at the age of two and a half years.

The child before you now, Julie, is the eldest of the three surviving, and is 13½ years old. She was born prematurely at seven and a half months, and in the early years of her life was very delicate, having been brought up by hand. From the age of three she was boarded out with someone in the neighbourhood of the penitentiary. Ever since an early age she has always been exceedingly nervous. In the convent, as at home, she was always disobedient, difficult to manage, crying and laughing without cause. In 1883 she menstruated for the first time; the first periods being accompanied by violent abdominal pain, and since then they have not returned. Every year she passed her holidays in the penitentiary with her parents. It should be mentioned that she never witnessed a convulsive fit.

Now I present to you the youngest of the boys, François, aged 11, who is pale and anæmic like his sister. When fourteen months old he had convulsions, and at the age of two he suffered from rheumatic pains in the joints of his lower extremities, the knees and the feet. These pains, which since that time have returned on different occasions, have been severe enough to keep him in bed. He was boarded at a pension in the neighbourhood of the penitentiary, but returned every evening to sleep in the apartments of his parents.

The eldest of the boys, Jacques, 12 years old, also anæmic, lived the same life as his brother. For several years he has had different varieties of "tic," situated chiefly round the mouth, such as you can see for yourselves to-day.

In the month of August last the whole family was reunited for the holidays, the father and the mother following their usual avocation, the children playing together in the courtyard of the penitentiary, almost always alone, because among the other officers' families there was only one child, four years old.

Life in the interior of a house of detention is undoubtedly, as I said, terribly monotonous. Beyond the ordinary routine, there is scarcely any distraction. Hence it happened that in order to find relief from this monotony, the wives of the officers devoted themselves with much earnestness, for more than a year, to spiritualistic séances, at which a friend of one of them came to preside every other day. This form of distraction was very popular, and spiritualism counted many devotees, amongst whom in particular were M. and Mdme. X—. Madame, moreover, in addition to the séances, devoted herself with much fervour to reading books which treated of occult sciences; books which she did not hesitate to place in the hands of her daughter. As for M. X—, at first he was very indifferent to spiritualism, but since the month of March, 1883, he had never omitted to indulge, *every Friday*, in table-turning. This day was specially marked out by him, because on a Friday he had been promised a *medium*, by the aid of which he could call up the spirit of his mother.

Julie had already been allowed to be present at a spiritualistic meeting during the Easter holidays, though it had not affected her. The holidays began on the 19th of August. She had already taken part in several meetings, in which she had only been allowed to place her hands on a table; but on Friday, the 29th, her father attempted afresh to learn if it had not come to his turn to be a medium. He asked the table, and that article, instead of indicating him, as he had hoped, replied, "*Julie will be the medium.*" The whole of Friday was devoted to an almost uninterrupted séance. The next day, at 9 o'clock in the morning, they again met and called up different persons, and about 3 o'clock in the afternoon the table ordered Julie to write. She took a pencil, but at the same moment her arms became rigid and her look fixed. The father, being frightened, threw a glass of water in her face; she came to herself, and her mother, fearing danger, would have forbidden her any more table-turning. But this did not suit the convenience of the neighbour, the spirit of whose friend was present at the séance.

Desirous of questioning the soul of a certain person, who it seemed was her sister, she took Julie home with her, and the séance recommenced. About 7 o'clock the table rapped, the spirit appeared, and Julie said to it, "*Please to sign your name.*" Immediately she herself, in the capacity of medium, and under the inspiration of the spirit, seized a pencil, and with trembling hand signed, convulsively, "*Paul Denis,*" with a flourish. The writing was that of a man; the P and the D, moreover, presented most curious characters, such as the little girl has never been able to reproduce since that occasion. The signature was no sooner made than the hand which had written it became convulsed, and then Julie, bursting out into a laugh, stood upright, and rushed about the house as though she were mad or delirious, giving utterance to inarticulate cries. Soon afterwards she rolled on the ground, presenting a series of hysterical attacks, which were characterised chiefly by clownish acts [clownisme].

The next and the following days she had a great number of attacks, twenty to thirty a day. Matters went on thus till the 15th of November, Julie continuing to have fits which were scarcely modified by the application of different means of treatment, and particularly of hydrotherapy.

A few days before this François, the youngest of the boys, who like his brother had taken very little interest in the spiritualistic performance, had been seized with pains in his joints which necessitated his staying in bed. All of a sudden, on the 15th October, he sat up in bed, cried out that he could see lions and wolves; then he got up, knocked at the doors, saw his father dead, attempted to kill imaginary brigands with a sword, rolled about on the ground, crawled along on his belly, and produced some very characteristic passionate attitudes.

Two days later, Jacques was taken with an exacerbation of the tic in the face. Then, seeing his mother crying, he called out, "I will kill myself if you weep." And after that, transient attacks of delirium supervened, during which he muttered, pronounced incoherent words, saw brigands and assassins whom he wished to strike.

It was on December the 9th that the distracted father

and mother, who had tried a lot of ineffectual treatment, brought their children up to Salpêtrière.

Isolation at any rate had become an absolute necessity, for when one of them was seized with a fit the other two immediately followed the example.

Julie, whose previous history you already know, and who is 13½, is a tall girl, well built and well developed, although, as I told you, the catamenia, which had appeared for the first time in 1883, have not become permanently established. In spite of what we learned from her mother, she appears to be of an amiable and tranquil disposition. On the early days of her arrival, and daily since then, she has had several attacks which in general possess the following characteristics. All of a sudden, sometimes after an *aura* of very brief duration and very varying kind, she throws herself backwards, the arms become stretched out from the trunk, the hands assume a position of pronation, and the fingers are strongly flexed. Not unfrequently she performs one or more semicircular bendings of the body, generally in a lateral direction, and finally the clonic stage occurs, characterised by somersaults forwards and backwards, the head touching the pelvis; or else the upper extremities are thrown about in the air, the head resting on the bed. During the attack Julie groans, laughs, but never speaks. The seizure, which is composed of a series of fits analogous to those I have just described, lasts sometimes three quarters of an hour, one hour, and even an hour and a half. It can be stopped or provoked at will by pressing on one of the hysterogenic points which the patient possesses. In fact Julie presents some of the permanent hysterical stigmata. Although she has neither cutaneous anæsthesia, nor the ovarian phenomena [ovarie], she has numerous hysterogenic zones situated at the same level of the two breasts, on the outer side of the two flanks, the two calves of the legs, two external malleoli, and on the inner side of the right elbow-joint. An examination of the eyes made by M. Parinaud gives very characteristic results. On the right side there is a very marked retraction of the visual field; moreover, not only is the red field situated within the blue, but it is very perceptibly more extensive than that for white light. The same phenomena exist on the left side, although less accentuated. The other special senses are intact.

François, the youngest of the boys, 11 years old, also presents some permanent stigmata, in addition to the attacks I am about to describe. Thus the day after his admission we discovered an anæsthetic area which included the whole of the face. This area was somewhat variable, for during the next few days the insensibility was confined to the middle part of the forehead, and the nose. The integument beyond this is notably hyperæsthesic. All the special senses are affected; the taste is totally abolished; there is complete insensibility of the tongue; and the pharyngeal reflex does not exist. The mucous lining of the nose, and the sense of smell, share the general condition; the external auditory canal is insensible, and hearing is very deficient. An examination of the visual field is very instructive. There is very accentuated retraction on the left side, and not only is the red circle outside the blue circle, but here again it is larger than the field for white. On the right side the retraction is less marked, and there does not exist the transposition of colours. François has one to five attacks every day, some of which last as long as two hours. He presents very clearly the series of phenomena of hysteria minor and hysteria major [petit et grand mal hystérique]. In him the first consists of a contracture of the two orbicularis palpebrarum muscles, which lasts from three to five minutes without loss of consciousness; or again, the child strikes out with his fist, or with his foot, utters a few incoherent words and then it is all over. But more frequently the preceding symptoms are followed by a series of fits constituting an attack. Then the child stiffens his upper and lower limbs, shuts his eyes, throws himself into semicircles; then he flings himself on the ground, crawls on his belly, strikes the earth, calling out about an assassin, and kicks at and defends himself against imaginary beings. Then the tonic phase commences again, and thus the attack is constituted by a series of fits, with confusion, or a very varying predominance, of one or other phenomenon. Curiously enough, when the left hand with its outstretched fingers is squeezed, the attack stops instantly; but it cannot be provoked in this way. The skin in this position presents no affection of sensibility.

Jacques 12 years of age, pale and anæmic like his brother and sister, is the least serious case of the three. Although he has one, two, and sometimes three or four attacks a day, he does not present any permanent stigmata, and there is a marked predominance of hysteria minor over hysteria major in his case. We know that before this illness he was subject to "tic" in the face. This becomes greatly exaggerated at the outset of the attack. He makes grimaces, the labial commissures are drawn outwards, he mutters, shuts his eyes, pronounces a few incoherent words, and then perhaps all is finished. But sometimes, following on these symptoms, or even at the very outset, the eyes close, the body becomes stiff, and assumes the position of an arc of a circle. Then the child runs or walks, talks aloud, calls out about a thief, and finally goes and throws himself on his bed, where either the attack ends, or else a fresh series of fits recommence, lasting rarely more than a quarter of an hour.

These facts seem to me to merit your earnest attention. The symptoms which these children present are not the transient phenomena of hysteria. Julie has been ill for four months, and although isolation seems to have had a calming effect on her attacks, such as it has had on her brothers, it is nevertheless true that her symptoms threaten to persist for a long time still; because one dare not put the children together again without immediately bringing on an attack in all three.

The complete narration of the epidemic occurring in this little household is most instructive in many ways. It will enable you to understand the genesis and evolution of the complaint in a "nervous" and "arthritic" family, and is a contribution therefore to the two diatheses, between which an alliance is so frequent and so potent. It will show you the influences which may be exercised by different modes of life, and surrounding conditions. Finally, it clearly indicates to you the danger, especially in those predisposed to this class of disease, of superstitious practices, which have unfortunately so great an attraction for those very individuals. It reveals the danger of the constant tension of mind which necessarily exists in those who are addicted to spiritualism, or, to gratifying a love of the marvellous—a love that has such a remarkable hold on the minds of children.

LECTURE XVII.

ISOLATION IN THE TREATMENT OF HYSTERIA.[1]

SUMMARY.—*Recapitulation of the epidemic of hysteria.—The treatment comprises two parts:*

(A) *Moral or psychical treatment:* 1, *Removal from the place where the disease originated;* 2, *Complete separation of the persons attacked;* 3, *Suppression of all visits from relations or friends.*

(B) *Medical treatment:* 1, *To modify the diathesis, if one exist; rheumatism, for example;* 2, *Static electricity;* 3, *Methodical hydrotherapy.*

Preponderating influence of isolation.—Cases.—The treatment has been adopted, not invented, in Germany or in England.

GENTLEMEN,—Before coming to the principal subject of our lecture to-day, I think it may be useful to give you the latest particulars of the three children belonging to one family, whom I presented to you on the 19th December last. I do not intend to again relate all the history of this little epidemic of hysteria, which originated under the influence of spiritualistic practices. You will find all the particulars set forth in the preceding lecture. It is only necessary for me to remind you of certain details as to the state of the children at that time, so that you may be better able to judge of the modifications which have been produced in their condition under the influence of the measures which we have adopted for their treatment.

The family, I may remind you, consists of three children; two boys and a girl. In this last named, who is 13½ years old, the affection started on the 28th April, 1884, after a

[1] Lecture edited by M. Gilles de la Tourette.

spiritualistic séance which had lasted from nine o'clock in the morning to seven in the evening, and in which the patient *Julie* played the part of medium. At the conclusion of the séance she was seized with convulsive fits, which recurred fifteen or twenty times a day up to the time of admission of the family into the Salpêtrière on the 9th December, 1884.

Shortly afterwards the two brothers followed the bad example which had been set them by their elder sister. On the 15th November, that is, about six weeks after the famous spiritualistic séance, *François*, the younger of the two, 11 years of age, who was not, however, directly affected by the séance, was seized with an hysterical fit, accompanied by delirium, at a time when he was laid up in bed with an attack of rheumatism.

Two days later, on the 17th, the elder of the boys, *Jacques*, was in his turn seized with a delirious attack, accompanied by hallucinations.

From that time it was impossible for the children to meet in the house without being seized with these attacks. The little girl would begin, and then the brothers followed her example. This might happen several times a day, and the position consequently became unbearable. Then it was that the parents besought us to intervene, and we suggested to them that we should take the children into the Infirmary, in which course they gladly acquiesced.

The proposition thus made to the parents contained in itself a series of therapeutic considerations, which I can now explain.

The admission into the Infirmary would enable us to effect:

(1) The *removal* of the patients from the place where their malady had originated.

(2) The *absence of the father and mother*, who had themselves become very nervous; and whose presence, according to my former experience, which dates now from a good many years ago, would effectually check all treatment.

(3) The *separation* of the three children from one another.

The little girl was placed in one of the female wards of the Clinique. The two boys were placed in the only men's ward which we possessed at that time. Thus, the respective isolation of the three patients was not quite perfect; though we had at any rate prevented their all being together. Such in my judgment should be the fundamental conditions of treatment. The parents consented that they should only see their children with my authorisation; and then I thought we should probably be able in a few months to send them back home, completely cured.

This was the treatment so far as the *moral or psychic* side was concerned. We did not, however, propose to lose sight of the more strictly *medical* treatment. The children who were confided to our care were all three pale and anæmic, therefore we prescribed for them tonics, amongst which iron and bitters held the chief place. One could also endeavour to modify the rheumatic diathesis, which was so accentuated in at least two of them.

As for the agent specially directed to the hysterical condition, we depended upon the employment of *static electricity*, which daily renders us great service in these cases; especially bearing in mind that we could not employ *methodical hydrotherapy* as the hydrotherapeutic establishment of the Salpêtrière was not yet completely arranged. We did not place any hope in the employment of *bromides*. The experience we have had for some time past has tended to show that this class of remedies, which acts almost always in a greater or less degree in epilepsy, remains completely inert not only in hysteria proper, but also in that form of hysteria which most nearly resembles epilepsy, that is to say, hysteria of an epileptic form, or hystero-epilepsy. I do not allude to opium in large doses, nor to the numerous other anti-spasmodics, whose employment I do not absolutely condemn, but which, it seemed to me, would lead to no result under the conditions we then had to deal with.

But, gentlemen, I must confess that among all the therapeutic agents which it was possible to employ, I relied chiefly on *Isolation;* that is to say, on moral treatment, although it was necessarily incomplete. It was possible, no doubt, that the children might meet in going about the Infirmary, such as not unfrequently did actually happen. Moreover, the two brothers lived in the same ward; and, like their sister, they were doubtless able to see the manifestations of convulsive hysteria from time to time as they went about the place. But we had no choice, and in my opinion it was better for them to live under such conditions, than to remain under the parental roof in perpetual contact with their father and mother, and in actual communication with each other all the time.

It would not be possible for me to insist too much on the capital importance which attaches to Isolation in the treatment of hysteria. Without doubt, the psychic element plays a very important part in most of the cases of this malady, even when it is not the predominating feature. I have held firmly to this doctrine for nearly fifteen years, and all that I have seen during that time—everything that I have observed day by day—tends only to confirm me in that opinion. Yes, it is necessary to separate both children and adults from their father and their mother, whose influence, as experience teaches, is particularly pernicious.

Experience shows repeatedly, though it is not always easy to understand the reason, that it is the mothers whose influence is so deleterious, who will hear no argument, and will only yield in general to the last extremity.

In private practice, Isolation, such as I understand by the use of the term, is practised daily for cases of this kind under excellent conditions. In Paris, during the last fifteen years, establishments of hydrotherapy take patients who are so disposed in hand with much success. In the provinces, Isolation is more difficult to effect, because conveniently arranged establishments are more frequently wanting. One can, no doubt, create artificial private asylums, but it may be readily understood that the arrangements are often seriously defective.

The patients are placed under the direction of competent and experienced persons. They are generally religious people who by long practice have become very expert in the management of this sort of patient. A kind but firm hand, a calm demeanour, and much patience, are here indispensable conditions. The parents are systematically excluded up to the time that a notable amelioration occurs; and then the patients are allowed, as *a sort of recompense*, to see them ; at first at long intervals, and then more and more frequently in proportion as the improvement becomes more obvious. Time and hydrotherapy, without counting any internal medication, perform the rest. For my part, I am firmly convinced that hysteria, recently acquired, especially in young subjects and particularly in males, could often be stifled at the outset if it were possible to persuade the parents to undertake energetic measures at the beginning, and not to wait until the disease had taken deep root and become developed from having been a long time abandoned to itself.

In order to render more apparent this remarkable influence which Isolation has in the treatment of hysteria in young subjects, including young and marriageable girls, I might quote a number of cases where it has proved itself most efficacious. But not being able to enter here into lengthy detail I will confine myself to the following anecdote, which seems to be quite a case in point. It relates to a young girl of Angoulême, thirteen or fourteen years of age, who had grown very fast for five or six months, but who then systematically refused all kind of nourishment, although she was not troubled with any affection of deglutition nor any disorder of the stomach.

It was indeed one of those cases bordering on hysteria, but which do not always properly belong to it, and which have been so admirably described by Lasègue in France, and by Sir William Gull in England, under the name of *nervous anorexia* or *anexoria hysterica*. The patients eat nothing, they do not wish to, they cannot eat, although they have no mechanical obstacle in the primæ viæ, and although there is no reason against the food remaining in the stomach when they have taken it. Sometimes they take nourishment in secret, but not always as it has been supposed ; and, although the parents themselves foster this deceit by providing them with food which they prefer because they can consume it in secret, alimentation always remains insufficient. Weeks and months pass by, and it is always hoped that the desire for food will reappear. Prayers, entreaties, violence, are unable to overcome their resistance. Then emaciation soon comes on; it reaches truly extravagant proportions; and the patients, without exaggeration, become nothing but living skeletons. And what a life! Cerebral torpor has succeeded to the fictitious agitation that existed at the outset. For some while walking, and even standing upright, have become impossible. The patients are confined to bed and they are scarcely able to move. The muscles of the neck are paralysed, the head rolls like an inert mass on the pillow. The extremities are cold and cyanosed, and one is tempted to ask how life is carried on in the midst of such decay.

The parents have been alarmed for some time, but the alarm reaches a very high degree when matters have come to this point. It is indeed quite justifiable, for a fatal termination seems to threaten, and I myself know at least four cases where it has actually occurred.

Such was very nearly the situation in the case of the little patient from Angoulême, when I received a letter from the father depicting this lamentable condition, and beseeching me to come and see his child. "It is unnecessary for me to come," I replied; "I can, without seeing the patient, give you appropriate advice. Bring the child to Paris, place her in one of our hydrotherapeutic establishments, leave her there, or at least when you go away make her believe that you have quitted the capital, inform me of it, and I will do the rest." My letter remained without reply.

Six weeks later, a medical man from Angoulême arrived at my house one morning, in great haste, and apprised me that the little girl, who was his patient, was in Paris installed in one of the establishments that I had indicated; that she was going from bad to worse, and that very probably she had but a few days to live. I asked him why I had not been informed sooner of the arrival of the little girl. He answered that the parents had avoided doing so because they were resolved not to be separated from their child. In reply I told him that the principal element, the *sine quâ non* of my prescription, had been misunderstood, and I must decline all responsibility in the unfortunate affair. However, at his request, I went to the establishment indicated, and there I saw a lamentable sight. She was a tall girl, 14 years of age, who had reached the last stage of emaciation, in a dorsal decubitus, with weak voice, extremities cold and blue, and the head drooping, reproducing in a word the main features of the picture I have just sketched to you. There was indeed every reason to be uneasy, very uneasy.

I took the parents aside, and after having addressed to them a blunt remonstrance, I told them that there remained, in my judgment, but one chance of success. It was that they should go away, or pretend to go away, which amounted to the same thing, as quickly as possible. They could tell their child that they were obliged for a special reason to return to Angoulême. They could lay their departure to my door, a matter which was of little importance provided that the girl was persuaded that they were gone, and that they went immediately.

Their acquiescence was difficult to obtain in spite of all my remonstrances. The father especially failed to understand how the doctor could require a father to leave his child in the moment of danger. The mother said as much, but I was animated by my conviction. Perhaps I was eloquent, for the mother yielded first, and the father followed, *uttering maledictions*, and having I believe but little confidence in the prospect of success.

Isolation was established; its results were rapid and marvellous. The child, left alone with the nun who acted as nurse, and the doctor of the house, wept a little at first, though an hour later she became much less desolate than one would have expected. The very same evening, in spite of her repugnance, she consented to take half a little biscuit, dipped in wine. On the following days she took a little milk, some wine, soup, and then a little meat. The nutrition became improved, progressively but slowly.

At the end of fifteen days she was relatively well. Energy returned and a general improvement in nutrition, so far that at the end of the month I saw the child seated on a sofa, and capable of lifting her head from the pillow. Then she was able to walk a little. Then hydrotherapy was brought into play and two months from the date of the commencement of the treatment she could be considered as almost completely cured. Power, nourishment, appetite, left very little more to be desired.

It was then that the girl, when questioned, made the following confession to me: "As long as papa and mamma had not gone—in other words, as long as you had not triumphed (for I saw that you wished to shut me up), I was afraid that my illness was not serious, and as I had a horror of eating, I did not eat. *But when I saw that you were determined to be master, I was afraid,* and in spite of my repugnance I tried to eat, and I was able to, little by little." I thanked the child for her confidence, which as you will understand is a lesson in itself.

I should easily be able to multiply examples which clearly show the favorable influence of isolation, properly carried out, in the treatment of certain nervous affections not coming under the head of mental alienation, but of hysteria, or of neurasthenia.

In fact, what I have just said in reference to nervous anorexia can be repeated in relation to most of the other forms of the hysterical neurosis, but it will suffice for the moment to have aroused your attention to the curative influence of isolation. It is a subject on which I shall have occasion to return many times without doubt in the course of these lectures. I have spoken of it every year for nearly fifteen years, and several of the lectures that have been devoted to it have been published. The method has, moreover, made some progress, for I see that in Germany principally, and also in England and America, its efficacy has begun to be loudly proclaimed. But I think that we may claim priority, for if I am not deceived it belongs legitimately to us, at least as far as relates to the treatment of hysteria and allied affections. It is, in fact, Isolation which represents the chief feature in the method that was described a few years ago by Drs. Weir Mitchell in America, Playfair in England, Burkart[1] in Germany, in the treatment of neurasthenia and of certain forms of hysteria.[2]

[1] R. Burkart, "Zur Behandlung schwerer Formen von Hysterie und Neurasthenie" (Volkmann's 'Sammlung,' 8 Octobre, 1884).

[2] The isolation of hysterical patients has for a long time been considered

But I see that it is time to come back to our young patients. I wish to show you what course their affection has followed during the last six weeks, since the time when the treatment, in which isolation has played the principal part, was initiated. An amelioration has occurred in all three, commencing in the boys.

The youngest, *François*, may perhaps be considered as cured. He has not had any fits for a fortnight, and yesterday he celebrated the event at home with his father; from which trial he has emerged triumphant.

It is not quite the same with his elder brother *Jacques*. He was, you will remember, attacked the last. The serious fits have completely disappeared in his case. However, they have been replaced by small attacks of vertigo, like enough in their form to epileptic vertigo, though these even have become very rare for the last two weeks; however, when he went to see his father in company with his brother he had one of these little vertigos which I have been in the habit of describing under the name of *le petit mal hystérique*.

The girl did not take part in this expedition; she remained at the Salpêtrière, for we were much less sure about her than about her brothers. She is not yet cured, although day by day the crises diminish in frequency, in duration, and intensity.

Her progress would certainly have been much faster in the ward which she occupies, if she had not been in constant intercourse with subjects of hysteria major in whom she saw attacks daily.

But we have not been able to do better, not having an isolation ward at our disposal. Nevertheless, the situation

as the chief part of their treatment. The following quotation from Jean Weir (1564) is sufficient to prove this: "For the rest, if there be several bewitched or possessed of the devil in one place, such as may sometimes happen in monasteries, principally by means of girls (as being the more convenient agents for the wiles of the devil), it is necessary above all things that they should be separated, and that each should be sent away to his relations or elsewhere; to the end that they may be more conveniently trained and cured, always having regard to the necessities of each. And so that all may not be booted from the same last, as the saying is." (Jean Weir, 'Histoires, disputes, et discours des illusions et impostures des diables, &c.,' II, pp. 173, 174, Édition Bourneville, Paris, 1885.)

is very much improved, for here is a significant fact, the children have been several times all three together in the electro-therapeutic room without any fits having occurred.

I am now going to present to you the boys first and afterwards the girl, for, as I have said, I am not quite so sure of her, and I fear that the sight of so large an assemblage may affect her to the extent of provoking some crises. Then in the case of the boys first, and also in the girl, I want you to observe that the hysterical stigmata, as we call them, have become modified in the same way as the spasmodic and deliriant crises. That is a very important point, because I do not believe that one should consider an hysterical patient cured as long as the permanent stigmata persist.

Here then is little *François*, 11 years old. It is in him that the cure is most advanced. You will notice in the first place that he has a much better aspect than he formerly had. The tonic medication and the regimen of the hospital, albeit not of an ideal kind, has done him much good in this respect. As for the stigmata, I would remind you that in him they consisted of an anæsthesia limited to the face, and especially to the forehead, like a mask. He could not perceive odours, nor was the nasal mucous membrane influenced in any way by ammonia or acetic acid. Hearing was blunted, and one could introduce into the external auditory canal little paper spills without producing any sensation. The general sensibility of the tongue and the taste were completely abolished. One could put sulphate of quinine, or aloes, on the tongue of the patient without his having the least perception.

In reference to this last point, about fifteen days ago I presented this little patient to my distinguished colleague from London, Dr. Russell Reynolds, who was passing through Paris, proposing to make him acquainted with the troubles of gustation. I confess to you that I was very agreeably surprised at finding that the little fellow drew in his tongue, and made an ugly grimace; for it indicated to me that our method of treatment had been attended with good results, and that the patient was on the road to cure. As far as the taste is concerned, the symptoms have not completely gone, as you will be able to judge for yourselves.

Vision, you know, in this child presented special characters. It is true that they do not belong absolutely to hysteria, but they are met with so frequently that one can attach to them a great diagnostic importance. The retraction of the visual field was very accentuated on both sides; but although on the right side there did not exist a transposition of colours, on the left the red circle was not only outside the blue circle but it was even more extensive than the white one. A fresh campimetric examination made by M. Parinaud two days ago has shown that these troubles were disappearing and that the vision was becoming normal.

I have already told you that the crises had completely disappeared. Allow me to remind you that he had an average of three a day, amounting to a total of twenty to twenty-five per week.

Now I present to you little *Jacques*, the eldest of the boys, 12 years old, who was attacked last in order, though less seriously than his brother, and who did not present permanent hysterical stigmata. In him the attacks of hysteria minor [petit mal hystérique] occurred much more frequently than the attacks of hysteria major [grande mal]. Nevertheless he has had fifteen attacks in seventeen days. For fifteen days he has only had two attacks of vertigo, and one of those occurred yesterday, under circumstances of which you are aware. In connection with this question, I may mention once again that it is but an imitation of the vertigo of petit mal épileptique and nothing more. It is but epilepsy in appearance, not in reality; and, in fact, the petit mal épileptique and petit mal hystérique are two phenomena radically and fundamentally distinct.[1] You will remark moreover, that the general condition of this child has improved, though there is still much to be desired in many respects.

Here is the little girl *Julie*, the eldest of the three. She appears to me to have grown and developed during the month. In any case her general condition has become more satisfactory. As for the hysteria, you will remember that she had on

[1] See upon this subject (1) Bourneville et Regnard, 'Iconogr. photogr. de la Salpêtrière,' vol. i, p. 49, and vol. ii, p. 202, and (2) Bourneville, 'Recherches clin. et thérap. sur l'épilepsie, l'hystérie, &c.,' Compte rendu du service des enfants de Bicêtre pour 1883, p. 100.

an average four or five attacks, or rather series of attacks, every day, which lasted from one hour to one hour and a half. For the last fortnight the attacks have not appeared more than two or three times a week. They are less violent, and last for scarcely a quarter of an hour. You know that there exist in her some very well-marked hysterogenic points, situated at the same level on the two breasts, the external part of the two flanks, the two calves, the two external malleoli, and the inner side of the right elbow. The zones of the two breasts, of the calves, and of the right elbow, have disappeared. The ovarian phenomenon did not exist, but instead of this we discovered several anæsthetic areæ irregularly scattered on the left side. The hysterical amblyopia, which was very well marked in her, has not been discovered for the last ten days. And lastly, as I have already said, she is able to meet her brothers without incurring an attack.

Such is the situation now, and there is every reason to hope that his little family drama, or as one ought to say, this little comedy, for there is nothing really sombre in all these occurrences, will soon be ended. In ten days or so more, we shall send the elder of the boys home to his parents; the younger will leave us to-day, and the girl will join them later on.[1]

I will leave you to meditate on the teaching which the history of these children implies. I believe that by the aid of the means which I have explained, one can very frequently manage to quench an attack of nascent, or infantile hysteria, at its outset, especially in the male. I speak now only of this kind; for when this neurosis has become inveterate, and occurs in adults, the chances of success, although still great, are much more problematical. As far as concerns these children, I believe that in spite of the neurotic disposition which seems to be in them so accentuated, they will henceforth be free from hysterical manifes-

[1] The younger of the boys is now completely cured. For more than fifteen days the little girl has only had one slight attack and that was during a visit of her parents to the Salpêtrière.

tations for a long while, if not for always. The parents, taught by experience, will certainly for the future avoid spiritualistic practices, and, knowing the weak side of their children, will be enabled, I hope, by the aid of physical, moral, and intellectual hygiene to prevent a return of similar accidents.

LECTURE XVIII.

CONCERNING SIX CASES OF HYSTERIA IN THE MALE.[1]

SUMMARY.—*Hysteria in the male is not so rare as is thought.—The part played by injuries in the development of the affection : railway-spine.—Permanence of hysterical stigmata in well-marked cases of both sexes.*

An account of three typical and complete cases of hystero-epilepsy occurring in men.—Striking similarity of these cases to each other, and to corresponding cases in women.

GENTLEMEN,—Our attention will be occupied to-day with hysteria in the male, and in order to bring the subject within more definite limits, we will consider more particularly hysteria as it occurs in adolescence, or in the prime of life, that is, in men from twenty to forty years of age; and, moreover, we shall specially examine that intense form which corresponds to what is called in women hysteria major [la grande hystérie], or hystero-epilepsy, with mixed fits. I am induced to approach this subject, which I have already referred to on several occasions, because we have in the wards, at this moment, a truly remarkable collection of patients which I can show you and study with you. My object, above all, is to make you thoroughly comprehend the identity of this great neurosis in the two sexes. Because, in the comparisons which we shall draw as we go along of the symptoms of hystero-epilepsy in woman and in man, we shall everywhere come across the most striking analogies, and here and there only certain differences which, as you will see, are of minor importance.

Moreover, this question of hysteria in the male is in a

[1] Lecture edited by M. Georges Guinon, interne du service.

sense the order of the day just now. In France, of late years, it has much occupied the attention of medical men. Between 1875 and 1880, five inaugural dissertations on hysteria in the male have been presented to the Faculty of Paris, and M. Klein, who under the direction of Dr. Oliver is the author of one of these theses, was able to collect eighty cases of the affection.

Since then the important publications of M. Bourneville, and his pupils, of MM. Debove, Raymond, Dreyfus, and others have appeared, and all these works tend to prove, amongst others things, that cases of male hysteria can be met with frequently enough in everyday practice. Quite recently male hysteria has been studied by Messrs. Putnam and Walton in America,[1] principally as it occurs after injuries, and especially after railway accidents. They have recognised, like Mr. Page,[2] who in England has also paid attention to this subject, that many of those nervous accidents described under the name of *Railway-spine*, and which according to them would be better described as *Railway-brain*, are in fact, whether occurring in man or woman, simply manifestations of hysteria. Hence, one can understand the interest which the practical minds of our American colleagues take in such a question. The victims of railway accidents naturally demand damages from the companies. They go to law; millions of dollars are in the scale. Now, I repeat, it is frequently hysteria which is the agent in these cases. These serious and obstinate nervous states which present themselves after collisions of this kind, and which render their victims incapable of working, or paying any attention to their avocations for many months, or even many years, are very often hysteria, nothing but hysteria. Male hysteria then, is certainly worthy of being studied and comprehended by the medico-legist, since the question arises of heavy damages claimed in a court of justice. This importance will perhaps tend to remove the discredit which is still, even in the present day, attached, from deeply

[1] Putnam, 'Am. Journ. of Neurology,' 1884, p. 507; Walton, 'Arch. of Med.,' 1883, vol. x.

[2] Page, 'Injuries of the Spine and Spinal Cord without Apparent Mechanical Lesions and Nervous Shock,' London, 1885.

rooted prejudice, to the word hysteria—a circumstance which renders our task the more difficult. A profound knowledge, not only of the malady, but also of the conditions under which it occurs, will be so much the more useful, because nervous troubles often occur in such cases apart from any traumatic lesion; and simply as a result of the psycho-nervous commotion produced by, yet frequently not appearing immediately after, the accident. Thus at a time when one of the victims of the collision who has broken his leg, for example, is cured by lying up for three or four months, another will be attacked with an outburst of nervous symptoms which will perhaps prevent him from working for six months, a year, or more; and which may not even then have attained its full intensity. One sees in such cases how difficult is the mission of the medico-legist, and it is this side of the question which seems to have revived amongst our American colleagues, the study of the hysterical neurosis, till recently somewhat neglected.

In proportion as the malady has become more studied and better known, the cases, as generally happens under like circumstances, have become apparently more and more frequent, and at the same time more easy of analysis. I told you just now that M. Klein, in his thesis, four or five years ago, had collected eighty cases of hysteria in the male; but at the present time M. Batault, who is preparing in our clinique a special work on the subject, has been able to collect 218 cases, of which nine are in my wards.[1]

Hence we may conclude that male hysteria is far from being a rare disease. Well then, gentlemen, if I may judge from what I daily see around me, these cases are often unrecognised, even by very distinguished physicians. One can conceive that it may be possible for a young effeminate man, after excesses, disappointments, profound emotions, to present hysterical phenomena, but that a vigorous artisan, well built, not enervated by high culture, the stoker of an engine for example, not previously emotional, at least to all appearance, should, after an accident to the train, by a collision or running off the rails, become hysterical for the same reason as a woman, is what surpasses our imagination.

[1] E. Batault, 'Contribution à l'étude de l'hystérie chez l'homme,' Paris.

Yet nothing can be more clearly proved, and it is a fact which will have to be accepted. No doubt it will be with this, as it has been with so many other propositions now established in the minds of all men, after having encountered for years scepticism, and ofttimes derision.

There is a prejudice which without doubt is a serious obstacle to the diffusion of a knowledge of hysteria in the male; to wit, the false comparison which is generally made between the clinical picture of this neurosis in woman and in man.

In the male, no doubt, the malady often presents itself as an affection remarkable for the permanence and obstinacy of the symptoms which characterise it. On the other hand, in the female, what is believed to be the characteristic feature of hysteria is the instability, the mobility of the symptoms; and it is this, without doubt which seems to constitute the important difference between the two sexes in the minds of those who are not thoroughly acquainted with hysteria in the female.

In hysteria, say they, founding the statement naturally on observations made in women, the phenomena are mobile, fleeting, and the capricious course of the disease is frequently interrupted by the most unexpected events. Well now, gentlemen, this changeableness, this evanescence, is, as I have shown you by numerous examples, far from being an invariable characteristic of hysterical affections, even in women.

Yes, even among women there occur cases of hysteria where the phenomena are unchanging, permanent, extremely difficult to modify, and which sometimes defy all medical interference. And cases of this kind are numerous, very numerous, even if it be true that they do not constitute the majority. This is a point to which I shall return, but for the moment, I am content simply to impress upon you that the permanence and obstinacy of hysterical symptoms often prevent their being recognised for what they are. Some people, in presence of phenomena which resist all therapeutic agents, believe, in cases where there are sensorial derangements with nervous fits, simulating epilepsy more or less, that these must be due to a central organic lesion, an intracranial neoplasm; or, if paraplegia be present, then that there exists an intraspinal lesion. Others will willingly acknowledge, or even affirm that we have to deal here not with an organic lesion, but simply with a dynamic alteration; but, that inasmuch as the tenacity of the symptoms does not correspond with the stereotyped description of hysteria they have in their minds, they believe the case to be one of a special disease, not yet described, and which merits a special place.

An error of this kind seems to me to have been committed by Messrs. Oppenheim and Thomson, of Berlin,[1] in a memoir which contains a large number of interesting and well observed, if not always well interpreted, facts.

These gentlemen observed sensitive and sensorial hemianæsthesia, like in all points to hysteria, in seven cases analogous to those of Messrs. Putnam and Walton. It occurred in stokers, engine-drivers, victims of railway or other accidents, who had received a blow on the head, severe shaking, or general shock. Neither alcoholism, nor plumbism, existed in these cases, and it is acknowledged that in all probability no organic lesion existed in these subjects.

They were, then, patients exactly resembling those of Messrs. Putnam and Walton; but differing from these gentlemen, the German authors are unwilling to recognise that we have to do with hysteria. They regard it as some special, I know not what, hitherto undescribed pathological condition, for which they would find an unoccupied place in our nosological tables. The principal arguments which Messrs. Oppenheim and Thomson furnish in support of their theory are the following:—1. The anæsthesia is obstinate; one does not see in it those capricious changes which are so *characteristic* (?) of hysteria. Its duration is a matter of months, or years. 2. Another reason is found in the mental condition of these patients not being that of hysterics. The patients are depressed, permanently melancholic, and without much fluctuation in any direction.

It is impossible, gentlemen, for me to subscribe to the conclusions of Messrs. Oppenheim and Thomson, and I hope

[1] 'Arch. de Westphal.,' Bd. xv, Heft 2 and 3.

to show you—1stly. That the sensorial troubles of hysteria can, even in the woman, present a remarkable tenacity; and 2ndly. It is particularly in the male that we commonly observe a melancholic tendency in cases of most marked and most undoubted hysteria. It is true we do not usually see in men those caprices, those changes of mind and temper, which more generally, though by no means necessarily, belong to hysteria in woman; but one cannot regard this as a distinctive character of the highest order.

But it is time, gentlemen, to stop these preliminaries, and to come to the principal object of our lecture to-day. We will commence by clinical demonstration, studying together, and with some detail, a certain number of perfectly characteristic cases of male hysteria. As we go along we shall reveal the analogies and differences which exist between the hysterical phenomena observed in men, and those which we daily see in the corresponding form of the ailment in women. Lastly, I will present to you, by way of summary, a few general considerations on hystero-epilepsy [la grande hystérie] as it occurs in the male sex.

But before coming to the male cases, I should like to briefly recall to your minds, by two examples, the extent to which in women the established symptoms of hysteria, the hysterical stigmata as we are in the habit of calling them for convenience' sake, can show themselves fixed, obstinate, and wholly free from that proverbial mobility which is applied to them, and which, it is pretended, forms the characteristic feature of the malady.

I need scarcely recall to your minds six or eight hystero-epileptics now collected in our wards. Some of them have presented for months, or years even, anæsthesia on one or both sides which all the most appropriate therapeutic agents can but influence for a few hours. I will confine myself to bringing to your notice two women, truly veterans in hystero-epilepsy, who, delivered some years ago from their great attacks, now hold the position of servants in the Infirmary. The first one named L—, well known in the annals of hystero-epilepsy, and celebrated on account of the "demoniacal" character her convulsive fits presented, is now 63 years old. She came to the Salpêtrière in 1846, and she has been continually under our observation since 1871. At that time she was affected, as she is still, with right hemianæsthesia, all sensitive and sensorial impressions being completely absent, and with an ovarian hysterogenic point of the same side; and neither of these, during the long period of fifteen years, has been modified *even temporarily*, whether by the many times tried æsthiogenic agents, whether by progressing years, or by the advent of the menopause. Five or six years ago, at a time when our attention was particularly drawn to the modifications which the field of vision undergoes in the subjects of hysteria, we discovered in her the existence of a very marked retraction of the visual field, on both sides, but much more pronounced on the right. An examination repeated once or twice a year has never failed to recognise the permanence of this retraction.

The other patient, a women named Aurel—, now 62 years of age, in whom the great attacks, replaced sometimes by symptoms of angina pectoris, have continued for a dozen years, presented even in the year 1851—as a valuable note taken at that time establishes—left hemianæsthesia, complete, absolute, sensitive and sensorial, which as you can now see for yourselves, still exists to-day, that is to say, after the long period of thirty-four years! This patient has been under our observation for fifteen years and the hemianæsthesia has never ceased, during our oft-repeated examinations, to be present. The double retraction of the visual field, well marked on both sides, though more pronounced on the left, which campimetric examination still discovers, existed in her five years ago.

This is enough, I think, to show you how stable in women the stigmata, of which no one doubts the hysterical nature, may prove to be; how permanent, and how little they correspond with the idea, a false one when too much generalised, which is usually held concerning the course of the symptoms in this ailment.

I come now to the study of our male hysterical subjects.

CASE I.—The man named Rig—, a shop-assistant, æt. 46, came into the Salpêtrière the 12th May, 1884, little short of a year ago. He is a big man, strong and well developed; he was formerly a cooper and stood hard work without fatigue. The *family antecedents* of this patient are very remarkable. His *father* is still alive and aged seventy-six years. From thirty-eight to forty-four years of age, in consequence of disappointments and monetary losses, he suffered from "*nervous attacks*," as to the nature of which our patient can but imperfectly inform us. His mother, a sufferer from asthma, died at sixty-five. The *great uncle* of his mother was *epileptic*, and died in consequence of a fall into the fire during an attack. Two *daughters of this uncle* were also epileptic. Rig— has had seven brothers and sisters who have not presented nervous ailments. Four are dead, and of the remaining three one sister is asthmatic. He himself has had nine children, of whom four died in early life. Of the five who are still alive, *one girl fifteen years old has nervous fits; another ten years old has hystero-epileptic fits*, which M. Marie has seen in this hospital; *another daughter is of weak intellect;* and lastly, two sons present nothing peculiar to note.

In his *personal antecedents* we find the following facts. At nineteen and at twenty-nine years of age the patient had attacks of acute articular rheumatism without cardiac mischief. The last attack continued for six months, and it is perhaps to rheumatism that we must attribute the deformities which exist in his hands. When a child, he was timid, and his sleep was disturbed by dreams and nightmares, and moreover he was a somnambulist. He often got up at night, worked, and on the morrow was very astonished to find his work done. This condition of things lasted twelve or fifteen years, and he married at the age of twenty-eight. One finds in his previous history neither syphilis, nor alcoholism, although the patient was a cooper. When thirty-two years old he came to Paris, working first with his father, afterwards employed as a shop-assistant in an oil-purifying factory.

In 1876, he being then thirty-two years old, his first accident occurred. He cut himself rather deeply with a razor which he was sharpening, as some people are in the habit of doing, on the anterior surface of the forearm. A vein was severed, the blood spouted out; and what with the hæmorrhage and fright together the patient fell to the ground, deprived of sensation and movement. He was a long while recovering, and remained for two months profoundly anæmic, pale, and unable to work.

In 1882, three years ago, he was lowering a barrel of wine into the cellar when the cord which held it broke; the barrel rolled down the steps, and he would infallibly have been crushed, had he not had just time to jump on one side. However, he could not do it quickly enough to avoid a slight wound of the left hand. In spite of the fright he had received he was able to get up, and help raise the barrel; but, five minutes later he had a loss of consciousness which lasted twenty minutes. On coming to, he was unable to walk, so feeble were his legs, and they were obliged to take him home in a cab. For two days he was quite unable to work, at night his sleep was disturbed by fearful dreams, and broken by cries of "Come to me, I am being killed!" and he saw in his dreams again the scene of the cellar. He did, however, recommence his work; but *ten days after the accident*, in the middle of the night, he had his *first attack of hystero-epilepsy*. Since that time the attacks have returned almost regularly every alternate month, sometimes in the interval; and during the night, whether at the moment of his first sleep, or at the time of waking, he was sorely troubled by visions of ferocious animals.

Formerly, in coming out of his fits he would remember what he had dreamed during the attack, but this is not so now. He would be in a forest pursued by brigands or frightful looking animals; or again, the scene of the cellar was enacted before his eyes; or he would see casks rolling towards him, and threatening to crush him. Never, he states, either during the attacks, or in the interval, has he had dreams or hallucinations of a cheerful or agreeable character.

About this time he sought advice at St. Anne. They gave him bromide of potassium, and this medicine, note well, has never had the least influence over the attacks, although the drug has been administered in a continuous manner and in large doses.

These were the circumstances under which Rig— entered our wards, and the following was his state on admission:

The patient is pale, anæmic, has but little appetite, especially for meat, preferring acid dishes, and his general condition is unsatisfactory. The hysterical stigmata in him are well marked. They consist of very extensive patches of anæsthesia on both sides of the body, both for pain (pricking or pinching) and for cold. Sensorial anæsthesia exists in general but to a small degree; taste and smell are normal, but the hearing is markedly defective, especially on the left side, nor does he hear any better when a sonorous body is applied to the cranium. As to vision the symptoms are much clearer and would suffice in themselves to allow us to affirm the hysterical nature of the affection.

He presents on both sides a *well-marked retraction of the field of vision*, more marked, however, on the right. He can distinguish all colours, but the visual field for blue is more retracted than that for red, and passes within the latter, a phenomenon which when met with is altogether characteristic of the visual field of hysterics, as far as I know, and of which I have shown you examples a great many times. And finally, to finish with the permanent stigmata, there exist in Rig— two *hysterogenic points*, one cutaneous, seated beneath the lower false ribs of the right side, the other a deeper one, is near the right popliteal space, at the point where the patient has a very painful cystic tumour. The point in the testicle does not exist in Rig—. Pressure on these spasmogenic points, whether accidentally or purposely, produce in the patient all the phenomena of an hysterical aura: precordial pain, constriction of the neck, with the sensation of a ball, buzzing in the ears, and beatings in the temples; these two last constitute as you know the cephalic aura. These points, the excitation of which can give rise to an attack with singular facility, are, on the other hand, to make use of the terminology proposed by M. Pitres, only feeble *spasm-arrestors* [*spasmo-frénateurs*]; that is to say, even their intense and prolonged excitation, can but imperfectly arrest an attack in process of evolution.

In the *mental condition* of Rig— there is now, as formerly, always a dominant anxiety, fears, sadness. He cannot sleep in the dark; in the daytime he does not like to be alone; he is excessively sensitive and experiences great fright at the sight, or even recollection, of certain animals such as rats, mice, toads, which he sees, moreover, in his horrible nightmares, or in his frequent semi-conscious hallucinations [hallucinations hypnagogiques]. There is in him a certain restlessness of mind which betrays itself by the fact that he can with equal facility undertake or abandon five or six occupations almost at once. He is intelligent and relatively well informed. He is, moreover, of an amiable temperament and is totally devoid of vicious instincts.

The *attacks* may be either spontaneous or provoked. Whatever be the manner in which they are produced, they always commence with a burning sensation near the spasmogenic points, to which there succeed, first an epigastric pain, then a ball and sense of constriction in the throat, lastly, the cephalic aura consisting of buzzing in the ears and beating of the temples. At that moment the patient loses consciousness and the attack, properly so-called, begins. It is divided into four periods, quite distinct and separate. In the first, the patient experiences a few epileptiform convulsions. Then comes the period of the great movements of salutation, movements of extreme violence, during which his body makes from time to time the characteristic arc of a circle; at one time forwards (emprosthotonos), at another backwards (opisthotonos), the head and the feet touching the bed, and the body making a bridge. All this while the patient gives utterance to savage cries. Then comes the third stage, called the period of passionate attitudes, during which he utters words and cries in keeping with his gloomy delirium, and the terrifying visions which persecute him. Sometimes it is the forest, wolves, horrible animals; at others it is the cellar, the staircase, or the rolling barrel. At length he regains consciousness, recognises and names people around him, but the delirium and hallucinations persist yet awhile; he seeks around him and under the bed for the dark beasts which threaten him; he examines his arms, expecting to find there the bites of animals which he thinks he felt. Then he comes to himself, the attack is finished, but very often only to begin again a few seconds later, until, after three or four successive attacks, the patient regains his normal condition.

He has never bitten his tongue in the course of these fits, or passed urine in the bed.

For nearly a year has Rig— been submitted to a course of static electricity, which we are in the habit of giving in these cases, as you know, with good results; and at the same time we have given him all the tonics, all the restoratives imaginable. Nevertheless, the phenomena which have just been described, the stigmata, the attacks, persist much the same without appreciable change. On the whole they do not seem, after three years' duration, to have undergone the least alteration. However, we certainly have here, you will all agree, a case of hystero-epilepsy with mixed fits (epileptiform hysteria), as clearly characterised as possible; and it is quite certain that the stability of the stigmata, on which we have sufficiently insisted, should not, in the presence of the other symptoms, make us hesitate in our diagnosis for an instant.

In concluding this case, so perfectly typical, I will refer again to some peculiarities which a clinical analysis will enable you to recognise.

In the first place, I will particularly point out the hereditary neurosis so strongly marked in his family: hysteria in his father, very probably at least; his great uncle, and first cousin of his mother, epileptics; two daughters, one hysterical, the other hystero-epileptic. You will frequently meet, gentlemen, these hereditary conditions in an hysterical man, more accentuated perhaps than in an hysterical woman.

I would remind you, moreover, how in our patient the hysterical manifestations were developed in consequence, and on the occasion of an accident which threatened his life. The injury which then happened, a slight wound on the finger, was it sufficient to provoke the development of the nervous symptoms? It may be possible, but I should not like to affirm it. It is always necessary to bear in mind, that, along with the injury, there is a factor which most probably plays a much more important part in the genesis of these symptoms than the wound itself. I allude to the fright experienced by the patient at the moment of the accident, and which was betrayed shortly afterwards in the case before you, by a loss of consciousness followed by a sort of transitory paralysis of the lower extremities. This same psychic element is found, moreover, in some of the cases described by Messrs. Putnam, Walton, Page, Oppenheim, and Thomson, and in which this influence, often predominant, should not be lost sight of.

This same circumstance of the development of hysterical phenomena, following, and in consequence of, a "shock," with or without injury, but where emotion plays a great part, you will find again, gentlemen, in the other cases which will now be brought before you.

Case II.—The man named Gil—, 32 years old, a metal gilder, was admitted into the Salpêtrière in January, 1885. Nothing particular was discovered in his *hereditary antecedents*. His father, who was a violent man, died at sixty years of age from paralysis, which came on without any fit. His mother, who died of tuberculosis, was nervous, but she never had any attacks.

His *personal antecedents* are more interesting to study. At the age of ten he was a somnambulist. As a child he dreaded the darkness, and at night he was the subject of nocturnal hallucinations and nightmares. From an early age he indulged in sexual excesses; he has experienced from time to time a sort of irresistible impulse towards women, and he has been a masturbator. However, he is intelligent, is a clever workman, and easily learns; in his leisure hours he was a musician, played the violin and the accordion. He frequents the theatre, but he is nevertheless by disposition rather sad and taciturn, and he usually prefers solitude.

His occupation, in which mercury is employed, has never produced any symptoms which can be connected with mercurial poisoning. There are no signs of alcoholism; no syphilis.

His first attack occurred at the age of twenty without known cause. He was outside an omnibus when he felt the first warnings. He had time to descend and the convulsive attack took place in the street. After this, the attacks came on rathor frequently. He reckoned about four or five a month. It seems that on several occasions he passed urine unconsciously. The convulsive seizures were becoming much less frequent and only returned at long intervals, when in 1880 the patient was the victim of an assault in the street. He was stabbed with a knife *in the head* in the right parietal region. He fell down and lost consciousness, and was robbed and left for dead in the street. He was found and taken to La Charité, where he was placed in the wards of M. Gosselin, remaining for three or four days unconscious. A few days later, and erysipelas developed around the wound in the head produced by the knife. At the time when he was recovering an intense cephalalgia of a peculiar character commenced, which persists up to the present time.

For a long time after this accident he remained plunged in a sort of lethargy, from which he emerged only little by little and very incompletely; for since that time even at his best it has been impossible for him to work, or to occupy himself, or even to read, with any continuity; and soon he became melancholic. The attacks, moreover, which had become infrequent, now reappeared and were more intense and more numerous than formerly; for which reason in February, 1883, the patient presented himself at the Hôtel Dieu. He remained there up to March, 1884.

It was there that the complete left hemianæsthesia, which still exists, was first discovered. The attacks, which were then both frequent and severe, seem to have been regarded as epileptic [mal comitial], and treated for nearly thirteen months while he was in the wards by bromide of potassium in large doses, without the least amelioration. When the patient was admitted into the Salpêtrière (January, 1885) the following was his state:

His general condition, as far as concerns the nutrition, is fairly satisfactory. He eats well and is not anæmic. On the other hand, it is easy to discover a very marked mental depression. He is sad, taciturn, and mistrustful; he seems to avoid observation and does not mix with the other patients in the ward. He does not devote himself during the day to any occupation or any distraction. The left hemianæsthesia, which was already noted at the Hôtel Dieu, is complete, absolute as far as concerns common sensibility. The sensorial troubles of the same side (left) are also very well marked. On this side there is a notable diminution in the hearing; complete loss of smell and of taste; in the left eye complete achromatopsia was discovered by M. Parinaud, and a very pronounced retraction of the visual field for white light. Contrary to what is generally observed in cases of this kind the extent of the visual field and the notion of colours is absolutely normal on the right side. There is no alteration in the fundus of the eye either on the right or the left side.

He constantly complained of an intense headache of a dull, or rather of a constrictive, character, generally situated over the occiput, the summit of the head, the forehead and, especially, the temples, and it was more pronounced on the left than on the right side. It felt as though he carried a heavy helmet on his head which was too tight and compressed it. This permanent cephalalgia was notably increased a little before and after the attacks. It was specially increased when the patient attempted the slightest occupation, when he tried to read, for example, or to write a letter.

The attacks, which we have often witnessed in the wards, present the following characters. They may be either spontaneous or provoked, but in either case they do not differ in any essential particular. Three hysterogenic zones have been discovered; one on each side just beneath the right and left breast, and a third in the right iliac region; but pressure on the testicle or the cord on this side does not produce any abnormal sensation. When one presses lightly on the hysterogenic zones in the position above indicated, the patient immediately experiences all the symptoms of a cephalic aura, namely, beating of the temples, buzzings in the ears, vertigo, &c. And if one perseveres a little, an attack is surely produced. A few short epileptic spasms inaugurate the scene. They are soon followed by divers contortions and the great movements of salutation, interrupted from time to time by attitudes of *an arc of a circle;* and all the while the patient utters violent cries. Convulsive laughter, tears, or sobs terminate the attack. On coming round, Gil— has not the slightest recollection of what has taken place. His hysterogenic points are but very incompletely "spasm-arrestors" [spasmo-frénateurs]; for when pressure is made upon them during an attack, it ceases for an instant, but almost immediately resumes its course. Whether provoked or spontaneous, the attacks generally repeat themselves successively a certain number of times in such a way as to constitute a series. The rectal temperature under these circumstances has never been above 37·8° C. [99·5° Fahr.]

After this brief description you will recognise that the case of Gil— is very much like that of Rig— (Case I), from which it differs only in matters of unimportant detail. In both cases there are the same hysterical stigmata, the same melancholic tendency; the same attacks, with this sole difference that in Gil— the aura evolves with great rapidity, and that in his fits the passionate attitudes are wanting;—these are the only differences between the cases.

In some of his attacks Gil— has bitten his tongue and micturated involuntarily; facts which we have ourselves observed. We were at one time led to believe, from this, that it was a case of hystero-epilepsy with distinct crises; that is to say, true epilepsy at one time, hysteria major [grande hystérie] at another, appearing in the form of separate attacks. A more attentive examination has shown us that it is not so. All Gil—'s attacks have the characters of hysteria major [grande hystérie], and it is in the course of these attacks that he sometimes bites his tongue and sometimes passes his urine involuntarily. But biting of the tongue and involuntary emission of the urine are not by any means unique characters of the epiplectic fit [mal comitial]. These symptoms may be observed in hystero-epilepsy unassociated and uncomplicated in any way with epilepsy [mal comitial]. The occurrence is rare no doubt, but I have observed it, and published a certain number of undoubted examples.[1]

In concluding this case I wish to call your attention to the headache from which Gil— suffered so constantly but which invariably became worse whenever he attempted the least

[1] A few months later this patient died suddenly after having swallowed an enormous dose of chloral of which he had secretly possessed himself. The autopsy was absolutely negative, so far as concerns the nervous centres, and tends to confirm the diagnosis.

occupation. Combined with all the particulars that have been mentioned above, a cephalalgia of this nature does not belong to the description of hysteria; it is met with, however, as an almost necessary accompaniment of the neurasthenic neurosis [neurasthenia of Beard][1] of which it constitutes one of the prominent symptoms, and in which one also observes the mental depression that existed to so large an extent in our patient.

I particularly pointed out that in this patient the different symptoms occurred after a blow that he had received on the head. Now, gentlemen, the neurasthenic state, together with the collection of phenomena which Beard has assigned to it in his remarkable monograph, is one of the nervous affections which become developed most frequently in consequence of a shock, particularly in railway accidents. This statement is borne out by several of the cases reported by Mr. Page.[2]

I have myself met with two examples absolutely parallel to those published by this author, one of which relates to one of our colleagues in Paris. Hence we are justified in admitting I think that two perfectly distinct elements may exist in our patient Gil—. In the first place the neurasthenic state, which was an immediate and direct consequence of the injury he received three years ago. In the second place hystero-epilepsy with all the concomitant symptoms that characterise it. This latter condition had existed before the accident, though it was considerably aggravated afterwards, as you can see by referring to the details of the case.

We now come to the examination of the third patient, who belongs to the same group as those you have already seen.

Case III.—The man who is now coming in, named Gui—, is 27 years old and is a locksmith. On February 20th, 1884, he came under the care of my colleague, Dr. Luys. Concerning his antecedents he only knows that his father, who

[1] G. M. Beard, 'Die Nervenschwache (Neurasthenia),' 2e Aufgabe, Leipzig, 1883.

[2] H. Page, 'Injuries of the Spinal Cord and Nervous Shock, &c.,' pp. 170 and 172, London, 1885. See also L. Dana, "Concussion of the Spine, and its Relation to Neurasthenia and Hysteria" ('New York Medical Record,' Dec. 6, 1884).

died at the age of forty-eight, was an inveterate drunkard, and that his mother, who is still living, has not, so far as he is aware, suffered from nervous affections. He has had seven brothers and sisters; only one brother is living, who has never been ill and is not nervous.

About the age of twelve or thirteen Gui— became very cowardly, he was never able to remain alone in a room without experiencing a sentiment of fear, but in other respects he was neither irritable nor obstinate. At school he learned easily, and later on, when seventeen or eighteen years old, he proved to be apt and intelligent in his calling. Several times in the educational establishment for locksmiths he obtained medals. Unfortunately about this time he developed an inordinate liking for the other sex. He worked during the day like his comrades, but when the day was finished it often happened that he went to a ball and passed the rest of the night with girls. These debauches occurred several times a week, and consequently he was deprived of his necessary sleep. However, this mode of life did not seem to fatigue him very much, for on the morrow he returned to his work as usual, and performed his task with efficiency.

At the age of twenty-one (in 1879) during one of his nocturnal expeditions he received a blow from a knife which penetrated his left eye. He was taken immediately to the Hôtel Dieu, and placed in the wards of M. Panas, who soon afterwards enucleated the eye. On leaving the hospital Gui— was not long in returning to his old abandoned life.

At the commencement of the year 1882 it frequently happened that at the moment he closed his eyes to go to sleep he thought he saw a monster in human form coming towards him. He cried out in great fear, opened his eyes, and then the vision disappeared, but only to reappear as soon as he closed his eyelids. Then he fell into a condition of extreme anxiety, and not unfrequently he would remain thus the greater part of the night without being able to sleep.

These nocturnal hallucinations had existed about six months when, in July, 1882, he was the victim of a fresh accident, more formidable than the former one. Occupied in fixing a balcony on the third floor of a house, he, possibly a little intoxicated, fell into the street, alighting, as he affirms, on to his feet. He was unconscious for an hour. When he awoke he found himself again in the Hôtel Dieu, and again in the wards of M. Panas. It seems that they had reason to suspect the existence of a fracture of the skull. However, recovery took place in due course, and at the end of two months the patient returned home. Soon afterwards the terrifying hallucinations at night-time returned, and about this date convulsive attacks occurred for the first time. They were not at first as clearly characterised as they afterwards became. They consisted chiefly of attacks of giddiness, coming on suddenly, followed by rigidity, and then by clonic spasms of the limbs. There was not any loss of consciousness, nor were they very frequent.

Matters remained thus for nearly eighteen months. At the end of that time, the remedies given by the different doctors whom he consulted having produced no effect, Gui— decided to apply at the Salpêtrière, and was admitted into the wards of M. Luys. Soon after admission Gui— became the subject of frequent attacks of intestinal and gastric colic, followed by a feeling of constriction of the pharynx, and by vomiting which came on without effort. These symptoms did not yield to any medication, but ceased suddenly at the end of about six weeks. About that time the existence of a right hemianæsthesia was recognised, and also a particular trembling of the right hand, of which more will be said in a few minutes.

In January, 1885, owing to changes in the staff, the patients of M. Luys came into our wards, and it was then that I saw Gui— for the first time. He is, as you see, a well-built, vigorous young man; his general condition seems satisfactory enough, his mental condition does not show at the present time anything particularly abnormal. The nocturnal hallucinations have almost completely disappeared during the past year. Gui— is not sad, he converses freely with the other patients, and renders himself useful in the ward.

The hemianæsthesia on the right side is complete. Neither touching nor pricking are perceived on this side of the body at all. The organs of sense on the same side are also profoundly affected, hearing, smell, and taste in particular. As for the eyes, a methodical examination reveals very characteristic modifications; on the right side—you have not forgotten that he has lost the left eye—the visual field is extremely retracted, red only is perceived, and the circle of this colour is reduced almost to a point.

The trembling of the right hand which was just now mentioned is remarkable for the perfect regularity of its rhythm, as shown by the aid of a registering apparatus. It consists of oscillations numbering, on an average, about five per second. In this respect, consequently, it holds a position midway between the tremors of slow oscillations, such as paralysis agitans, for example, and the vibratile tremors such as the rapid oscillations of general paralysis and of Basedow's disease. It is not exaggerated by voluntary movement.[1] The patient is able to use his hand for eating and drinking, and he can even write passably well by firmly pressing with his left hand on his right wrist, an arrangement which causes the tremors to cease for an instant. The muscular sense is perfectly preserved in the whole of the right upper extremity.

The only hysterogenic zone discovered in Gui— is situated in the testicle and the course of the right spermatic cord reaching to the groin of the right side. The skin of the scrotum on this side is very sensitive, and when it is firmly pinched, exactly the same effects are produced as when one presses on the testicle itself or on the cord, that is to say, the development, or, on the other hand, the arrest of an attack.

These attacks, whether spontaneous or provoked by the artificial excitement of this hysterogenic zone, are always preceded by the sensation of a well-defined painful *aura* starting from the right testicle, mounting upwards into the epigastric and cardiac region, thence into the throat, where it produces a feeling of constriction, finally reaching the head, where it produces buzzings, chiefly in the right ear, and beatings, principally in the temple on the same side. Then the patient loses consciousness, and the epileptoid stage commences. The tremors of the right hand become much increased, and the eyes become convulsed upwards. The limbs stretch out, and the wrists flex and become twisted in

[1] 'Progrès Médicale,' 1885, No. 12.

position of exaggerated pronation. Next the arms cross one over the other in front of the abdomen owing to a convulsive

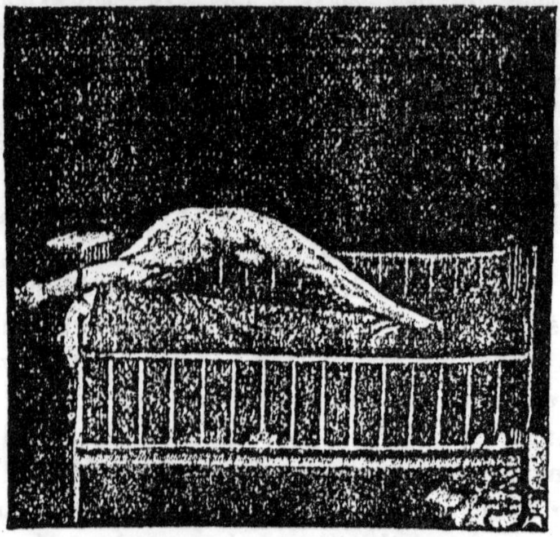

FIG. 49.—Arc of circle backwards.

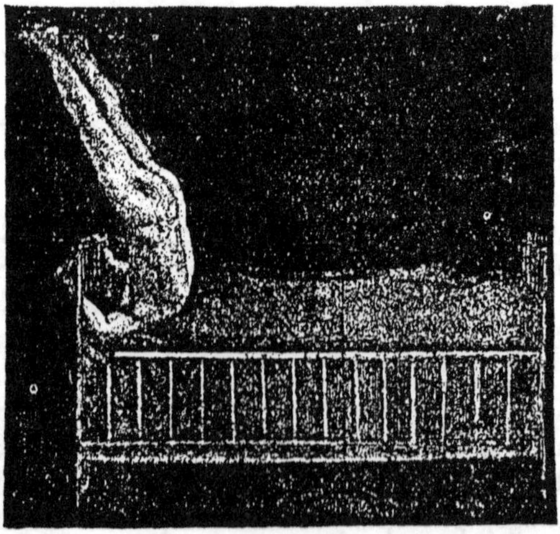

FIG. 50.—Illogical attitude.

contraction of the pectoral muscles. After this the period of contortions comes on, characterised by extremely violent movements of salutation accompanied by disorderly gestures. The patient breaks or tears everything on which he can lay his hands, and he assumes the strangest and most out-

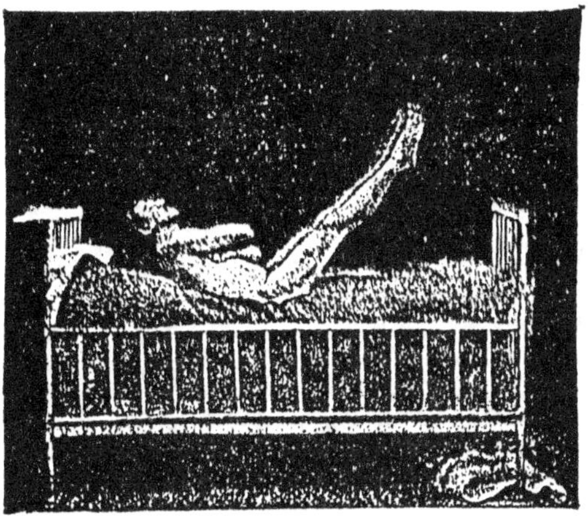

FIG. 51.—Arc of circle forwards.

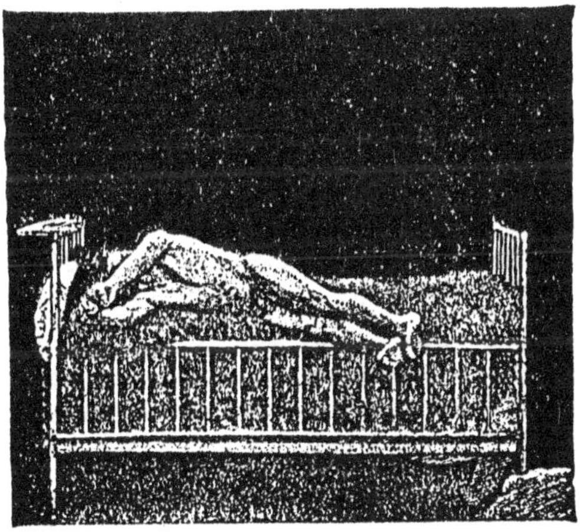

FIG. 52.—Lateral arc of circle (forwards).

rageous attitudes in a manner that fully justifies the denomination of *clownism*, which I have suggested as a designation for this part of the second period of the attack. From time

16

to time the contortions above described stop for a moment and give place to the characteristic attitude of an "arc of a circle." Sometimes it is opisthotonos, in which the loins

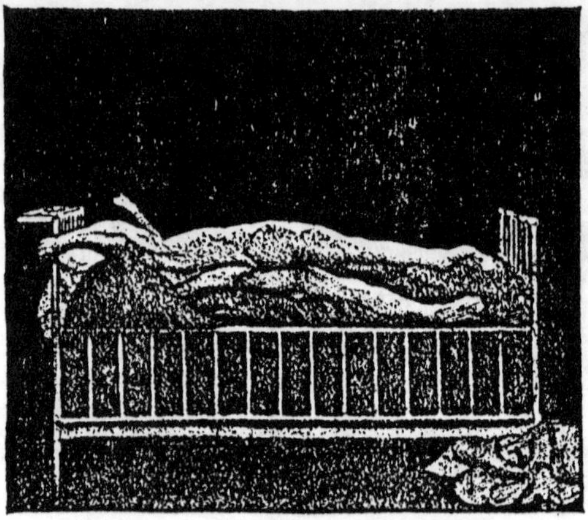

FIG. 53.—Lateral arc of circle (backwards).

are separated from the level of the bed by a distance of more than 50 centimetres [about 20 inches], the body only resting on the head and the heels. At other times the circle is made forwards with the arms crossed over the chest, the legs and the head raised in the air, the buttocks and loins alone resting on the bed. And at other times the body is bent into a lateral "arc of a circle," the patient resting only on the right or left side as the case may be. All this part of Gui—'s attack is very characteristic, and all its details are worthy of being recorded by the process of instantaneous photography. I am able to show you the pictures which have been thus obtained by M. Londe. You notice that in an artistic point of view they leave nothing to be desired, and for us they are most instructive. They show us, in fact, that in the regularity of the periods and the typical character of the different attitudes, Gui—'s attacks differ in absolutely nothing from those which we observe each day in hystero-epileptic patients of the female sex. And this perfect resemblance is worthy of all the more attention, in that Gui— has never been near the wards where the female subjects of such attacks are placed, so that the influence of contagious imitation cannot be said to be in operation.

The periods of hallucinations and passionate attitudes are generally wanting in Gui—. Sometimes, however, we have noticed that towards the end of an attack his physiognomy expresses fear or joy alternately, and that his hands extend into space as though he were searching for an imaginary being.

The conclusion of an attack in this patient is often followed by a sort of motor aphasia, which generally does not last more than eight or ten minutes, but which on one occasion persisted for nearly six days. When the patient wishes to speak, a few growling inarticulate sounds come from his mouth; he becomes impatient and agitated, but is able to make one understand by very expressive gestures. It has sometimes happened even that under these circumstances he is able to take a pen and write legibly a few correct phrases.

That is the conclusion of the history of this perfectly typical case. But we have not yet finished with hysteria in the male. We shall find the same features as marked as in the preceding cases, in three other patients that are now in the clinical wards [service de la clinique].

LECTURE XIX.

CONCERNING SIX CASES OF HYSTERIA IN THE MALE (*continued*).[1]

SUMMARY.—*Abnormal varieties of the hysterical attack in the male.—Account of a case in which the attacks assumed the characters of partial epilepsy.—Diagnosis of the case: importance of the hysterical stigmata.*

The convulsive attack may be wanting in hysteria in the male.—Description of a case of hysterical brachial monoplegia in a young man 19 *years old.—Difficulties of the diagnosis in this case.*

GENTLEMEN,—I hope to conclude to-day the subject which we were considering in the last lecture; adopting as heretofore the method of clinical demonstration.

In this method we are aided, for the material in our hands touching the subject of male hysteria is far from being scanty. Three new patients will be brought before you, and the principal details concerning them will be unfolded. I shall allow the facts to speak for themselves, only pointing out, by a few short commentaries, the teachings furnished by their cases.

CASE IV.—This case does not come quite under the category of those already referred to, inasmuch as it is that of a growing youth, and not a fully matured individual. But here, also, the disease presents the characters of permanence and tenacity which we have already encountered.

[1] Lecture edited by M. Georges Guinon, interne du Service.

Mar—, æt. 16, entered our wards on the 29th of April, 1884, that is to say, about a year ago. He was born and lived in the country up to the age of fourteen. In 1872 his mother had several hysterical attacks. His grandfather was a dissipated man, and of a very violent character. This is all that can be learned of his hereditary antecedents.

As to the young man himself, he is well-developed, though in infancy he suffered from some strumous manifestations, such as discharges from the ears, and glandular swellings in the mastoid region. He is intelligent, of a joyous disposition, and has never exhibited abnormal timidity; but he has been subject to paroxysms of anger in which he broke everything he could lay hands on. Two years ago he was placed as an apprentice to a baker in Paris. A short time afterwards he had congestion of the lungs, and the consequent enfeeblement of health was certainly not without its influence in developing the complications which supervened. Some time afterwards, while yet convalescent, he received a severe fright. He was, according to his own account, attacked in the street one evening by two young men. He fell, losing consciousness, and was in this state conveyed to the house of his employer. He showed no trace of any wound. From that time he remained during several days in a stupefied condition. He commenced to be subject to horrible nightmares, which torment him to the present time. He dreamt that he was being beaten, and he woke up crying out. About fifteen days later the hysterical attacks commenced. At first they occurred daily, and presented a series of from eight to ten, sometimes two series occurred in the same day; then they diminished in number and in intensity.

At the time of admission into the Salpêtrière the following conditions were noted:—The hysterical *stigmata* are very marked. They consist of an *anæsthesia in patches*, disseminated irregularly over the entire surface of the body, and in which there is complete insensibility to touch, to cold, and to pain. The senses of hearing, taste, and smell are blunted on the left side; and with regard to vision, a *diminution of its field* exists on both sides, but is more marked on the right. On this side the patient is unable to distinguish violet, while on the left he can distinguish all the colours.

But on both sides there exists a characteristic sign to which I have frequently called your attention, and which we have already observed in the first of our cases, the field of vision for red is more extended than that for blue, a condition as you know at variance with that which exists in the normal condition. There exists but one *hysterogenic point*, and that occupies the left iliac region. Even at the present time, notwithstanding that the disease has existed for two years, the attacks came on spontaneously, at short intervals, about every ten or twelve days. These attacks can be provoked very easily when a moderate pressure is exercised on the hysterogenic point. A more energetic pressure on this point arrests the attack.

The attack, whether spontaneous or provoked, is always preceded by an aura: iliac pain at the level of the hysterogenic point, a sensation as of a ball rising from the epigastrium up to the throat, buzzing sounds in the ears, and beating of the temples. Then the attack commences; the eyes are turned upwards in their socket, the arms become stiff and extended, and the patient, if standing, falls to the ground with complete loss of consciousness. The epileptoid phase is in general not very marked, and is short; but the period of great contortions which follows is excessively violent and of long duration. The patient utters cries, bites everything within his reach, tears the curtains, and performs movements of salutation, the body ultimately taking the characteristic form of an arc of a circle. The scene terminates by the phase of passionate attitudes, which is very marked in him, and differs somewhat according to the circumstances under which the attack has occurred. Thus, when the attack has been spontaneous, it may happen that the hallucinations are of a gay character; whereas if the crisis has been produced by excitation of one of the hysterogenic zones the delirium is always sombre or furious, and accompanied by indecent and reproachful speech. In general, many attacks succeed one another so as to constitute a series more or less numerous.

I must point out in this case the permanence and immobility of the hysterical symptoms, as is so often observed in the male. Thus, as you may have remarked in our young patient, notwithstanding that two years have now elapsed, the convulsive crises are now as frequent as ever, in spite of all our efforts; and the hysterical stigmata, anæsthetic, sensorial, and sensitive, have not altered since the day that he came under notice for the first time. There is nothing to make us to hope that they will soon be modified.

This is not the case usually with young persons, especially if the disease develops before the age of puberty. At that period of life, according to numerous observations which I have collected, the hysterical symptoms are, in general, more transitory, and no matter how pronounced they may be, they are most frequently amenable to appropriate treatment.[1]

Two days after this lecture was delivered, Professor Charcot admitted under his care a young Belgian named Fal—, 21 years of age, spare, tall, and with fair hair, who, as in the cases referred to, presented the classic characteristics of hystero-epilepsy with mixed crises. In the family history there was nothing noteworthy save a history of alcoholic indulgence in his father. In the history of his childhood, nocturnal terrors, frequent nightmares, and sometimes even in full daylight, visions of animals and horrible figures.

In November, 1884, Fal— had a bad attack of cholera. His convalescence was protracted, and for many weeks he remained feeble, subject to cramp in the inferior extremities, and abdominal pains. Three months after his recovery, being still in hospital, and convalescing, the sight of a dead body which was being carried frightened him, and almost immediately his first attack supervened. A subsequent fright, caused soon afterwards by a practical joke played on him by another patient in the same ward, seems to have determined the condition, for from that period Fal— did not cease to suffer from terrifying hallucinations, and the convulsions took place almost regularly every night. From the time of his entry into the Salpêtrière the following condition existed:—Scattered patches of cutaneous anæsthesia; a blunting of the senses of taste and smell on the left side; diminution of the field of vision limited to the right eye; very extended hysterogenic points in the form of hyperæsthesic area, occupying in front almost all the abdominal surface, and behind, the scapular regions, the buttocks, the popliteal space, and the soles of the feet, &c. The attack could easily be produced by moderate friction of the hyperæsthesic areæ. After the usual aura a marked epileptoid state followed. Equally characteristic was the period of the great movements, and the arc of a circle. Finally, succeeded the stage of passionate attitudes, during which the patient seemed to be a prey to a sombre or furious delirium. In this case, as in those we have considered, the hysteria supervened after an enfeeblement of body caused by a serious malady, and in consequence of a fright, and here likewise was observed all the genuine characteristics of hysteria as ordinarily observed in the female.

Apart from an anomaly in the form of attack, which I will advert to presently, the case I am about to submit to your consideration, that of a young man of 22, must be considered, like the preceding ones, as belonging to the type of hystero-epilepsy.

CASE V.—Ly—, a mason, æt. 22, entered the clinique of the Salpêtrière on the 24th of March, 1885. He was born in the country, in the neighbourhood of Paris. He is a young man of middle height, badly developed, and has a rather delicate appearance. His father—by trade a carter—is addicted to alcohol. His mother died of tuberculosis, and had had *hysterical attacks*. Further, in the family history we find a maternal grandmother also hysterical, who nevertheless attained to the age of eighty-two, and two *maternal aunts* the subjects of *hysteria*. Hence we have very important antecedents—four hysterical individuals and an inebriate in one family!

The personal antecedents are not less interesting. Our patient has always been of deficient intelligence. He was never able to learn at school, but otherwise he presented no striking mental peculiarity. He acknowledges to have drunk, for a long time, five or six little glasses of brandy per day, in addition to a considerable quantity of wine; but he states that he has abandoned this habit since he became an invalid. Three years ago he had erysipelas of the face, soon followed by an attack of acute articular rheumatism, not, however, of a severe nature, for he was only confined to bed for fifteen days. The same year he was engaged in efforts to rid himself of a tapeworm, from which he suffered, and for which purpose he took pomegranate bark, which had the desired effect. At first, fragments of the worm were voided, and then the whole. The sight of the tænia in his excreta so struck him, that for several days he suffered from slight nervous complications, such as colics, pains and tremblings of the limbs, &c.

A year ago, while working at his trade at Sceaux, he witnessed one of his comrades violently strike his son. Ly— desired to interpose, but his comrade turned furiously upon him, and while Ly— was fleeing hurled a stone at him. Fortunately, the stone did not strike him; but the fright experienced by Ly— was very severe. Immediately he was seized by trembling of the limbs, which persisted during the succeeding night, so that he was unable to sleep. The insomnia persisted during several days following. By night and day he was tormented by unpleasant ideas. He fancied every moment that he saw the tapeworm, or that he was again engaged in the strife with his comrade. Further, he suffered from pricking in the tongue, his appetite was gone, and he felt feeble and unable to work.

This condition lasted for fifteen days, when one evening towards six o'clock he experienced his first convulsive attack. All that day he had suffered from epigastric pain, the sensation of a *globus*, and from buzzing noises in the ear. At the moment when the attack commenced, he tells us that he felt his tongue retracted in his mouth towards the left side by a kind of involuntary and irresistible action. Then he lost consciousness, and when he came to himself he was told that his face was drawn towards the left, that his extremities were agitated by tremors, and that when the convulsions ceased he spoke in a loud voice without awakening.

During the months which followed, crises of a like nature were repeated about every eight or fifteen days, and during that long time he was obliged to abstain from all labour owing to his feebleness of body. These crises were considered to be epileptiform attacks of alcoholic origin, and for almost a year he was treated with bromide of potassium in large doses, without being benefited in the least thereby. During the day which followed his admission into the Salpêtrière, he was spontaneously seized with a series of five successive attacks which we were unable to witness.

On the following day, a systematic examination revealed the following conditions :—Generalised anæsthesia, disposed in disseminated areæ; considerable diminution of the field of vision on both sides, the field of the red being more extended than that of the blue; monocular diplopia. There exist two *spasmogenic* points, the one at the level of the right clavicle, the other below the false ribs of the right side. Moderate pressure exercised on the last point immediately determines an attack, which we are thus able to study in all its details.

The attack is preceded by the characteristic aura—epigastric constriction, a feeling of a ball in the throat, &c. At this moment, and even before the patient loses consciousness, his tongue becomes stiffened, and is retracted in his mouth towards the left side. It is found by aid of the finger that its point is carried behind the molars of that side. The mouth, half opened, is likewise deviated towards the left side. All the left side of the face shares in the deviation. The head itself is strongly drawn towards the left. The patient then becomes unconscious. The upper extremities are extended, first the right and then the left. The lower extremities remain flaccid, or at least they are very little stiffened. The movement of torsion towards the left, at first limited to the face, soon becomes general, and rolling over, the patient lies on his left side. Next, clonic convulsions replace the tonic spasm. The extremities are agitated by frequent vibrations, but of limited extent. The face is the seat of rapid tremblings, and then follows a stage of complete relaxation without stertor. But at this moment the patient seems tormented by horrible visions. He mentally sees again, without doubt, the scene of his quarrel with his comrade, and utters reproachful words: "Scoundrel . . . . , Prussian . . . . , struck with a stone, he is trying to kill me." The words are spoken in a perfectly distinct manner. Then, all of a sudden, he changes his attitude. Seated on his bed he is observed to pass his hand over one of his legs in such a manner as to disengage some reptile which encircles the limb, and during that time he mutters something about the worm. The scene at Sceaux comes back to him. "I will kill you . . . . , a gun-shot . . . . , you will see." After that period, signalised by delirium and corresponding passionate attitudes, the epileptoid stage is spontaneously produced, thus inaugurating a new attack which can in no wise be distinguished from the first, and which may be followed by many others. Pressure on the hysterogenic points interrupts the evolution of the different phases. On wakening, Ly— appears dazed and stupefied, and he states that he remembers nothing which has transpired.

All the attacks which we have witnessed, and there have been a considerable number, whether spontaneous or provoked, present exactly the same character. The different phases are always produced in the same order to the minutest details, the diverse incidents of the epileptoid phase, first commencing in the tongue and face, and then the various scenes of the delirious phase.

Here then, gentlemen, we have an attack of hystero-epilepsy, which in one respect forms a notable exception to the classic variety. In the first period, indeed, we observe the convulsive movements reproduce an almost perfect imitation of the symptoms of partial epilepsy; while the contortions, the grand movements, and the arc of the circle are wanting. But in the female this variety of the hystero-epileptic attack is known, and, though rare, I have set before you recently several perfectly authentic examples. This subject has, during the past year, been attentively studied by M. le Dr. Ballet, formerly my chef de clinique, now a hospital physician.[1] In comparing the cases narrated by Ballet, and that with which we are now concerned, you will be struck with the resemblance which exists between hystero-epilepsy in the male and that of the female, not only as regards the fundamental type, but also the aberrant forms.

Another anomaly, less rare and less unexpected, in hysteria of the female, is the absence of convulsive crises. You are aware that, according to the teaching of Briquet, about a fourth of hysterical females have no attacks. The disease in such cases, without losing anything of its individuality, is symptomatically represented only by the permanent stigmata, with sometimes several spasmodic or other manifestations, such as nervous cough, permanent contractures, certain arthralgias, forms of paralysis, and hæmorrhage from diverse sources, &c. Now, the attacks may also be absent in male hysteria. The case which I am about to submit to you offered a good example of this kind when the patient first presented himself before us. The disease has since become, as it were complete, for at the present time the attacks do exist. But during a long period of eleven months it was a latent case, and the interpretation of it was

[1] Ballet et Crespin, "Des attaques d'hystérie à forme d'epilépsie partielle," Arch. de Neurolgie,' 1884, Nos. 23 and 24.

sufficiently difficult, at least in certain respects, as you will be able to appreciate.

On March 10th last the young man before you presented himself to us with left brachial monoplegia. There was not the slightest trace of rigidity, the limb was perfectly flaccid. The paralysis, he informed us, dated from ten months previously, and had come on a few days after an injury to the front aspect of the left shoulder. There was no trace of paralysis, or even paresis, of the corresponding lower extremity nor the face. Nor were there any traces, in spite of the long-standing paralysis, of muscular atrophy; a circumstance which, combined with the absence of any modification in the electrical reaction in these muscles, led us to eliminate at once any causal effect—at least, any direct local effect—of the traumatism. We further noticed that the carotid regions were the seat of violent arterial throbbings.

Well-marked "Corrigan's pulse" and auscultation of the heart revealed the existence of a diastolic murmur at the base, and we ascertained that there was a history of an attack of acute articular rheumatism which had kept him in bed for five or six weeks. Hence, the idea naturally flashed upon us that this monoplegia depended on a focal cerebral lesion of the cortex, strictly limited to the motor zone in the brachial centre, and consequent on valvular affection of the heart. But a closer study of the case disabused us of this idea. Without doubt the monoplegia in question is due to a cortical cerebral lesion, principally localised in the motor zone of the arm, but it is not of the nature of a gross material alteration. The lesion is purely "dynamic," *sine materiâ*, of the nature, in short, of those whose existence we hypothetically suppose in order to explain the development and persistence of the different permanent symptoms of hysteria. That, at any rate, is the conclusion at which we shall arrive, I believe, from the detailed examination of our patient, upon which we are now about to enter.

CASE VI.—The patient, Pin—, aged 18, a mason by trade, entered the Salpêtrière on March 11th, 1885. His mother died at the age of forty-six in consequence of "rheumatism" (?); his father is an inebriate; one of his sisters, æt. 16, is subject to frequent nervous attacks. He is a well-built, muscular young man, apparently robust, but the functional exercise of the nervous system has always left much to be desired. From five to seven years old he was troubled with incontinence of urine. He has always shown a lack of intelligence, his memory is feeble, and he seems to have made but little progress at school. He was of a timid disposition, and the subject of nocturnal terrors. From a moral point of view he is of unstable equilibrium. From the time when he was nine years old he often left his father's house and slept under bridges and in the waiting-rooms of railway stations. His father apprenticed him to a greengrocer, then to a confectioner, and to other trades, but he always recommenced his escapades. One night he was arrested in company with a band of young vagabonds and shut up in La Roquette, where his father left him for a year.

About two years ago, at the age of sixteen, he was attacked with acute generalised articular rheumatism, preceded by facial erysipelas. It is very probable that the organic disease of the heart which now exists dates from this time.

Eighteen months afterwards, on May 24th, 1884, P—, then a mason's apprentice, fell from a height of about 2 metres (about 6½ feet), and remained for some minutes unconscious on the spot on which he fell. He was carried home, and then they discovered some contusions over the anterior surface of the shoulder, the keee, and the left ankle-joint—slight contusions which did not seriously interfere with the use of the affected parts.

For two days subsequently, matters remained in the same condition, but on the third day after the accident, May 27th, P— noticed that his left upper extremity had become feeble. He then consulted a doctor, who discovered a paresis of all the movements of the left arm, with anæsthesia of the limb.

On June 8th, that is, fifteen days after the fall and eleven days after the onset of the paresis, he entered the Hôtel Dieu. There he was examined with care, and the following conditions were discovered: Well-marked signs of aortic insufficiency. The parts which had been contused were not the seat of any pain, either spontaneous, or provoked by active or passive movements. There was incomplete paralysis of the left superior extremity. The patient was still able, though sometimes very incompletely, to flex the hand upon the forearm, and the latter upon the arm; but all movements of the shoulder were impossible. The paralysed member was completely flexible in all its articulations, and there was no rigidity. The condition of the face, and of the left lower extremity, was absolutely normal. So far as concerned the power of motion this was a case of monoplegia in the rigorous acceptation of the word. An examination of the sensibility furnished the following results. At this period there existed a general hemianalgesia of the left side; complete anæsthesia only in the upper extremity. There was also a retraction of the field of vision on both sides, but much more marked on the left. Finally, on the 25th of June, that is to say twenty-two days after the commencement, the paralysis had become absolutely complete.[1] The diagnosis was undetermined, and the treatment proved inefficacious. Faradization, many times applied on the left side, resulted only in rendering the anæsthesia of the trunk, the face, and inferior extremity less complete. The anæsthesia and paralysis persisted in the upper extremity. The condition of the field of vision was not modified when P— left the Hôtel Dieu.

It was on the 11th March, 1885, and consequently ten months after the accident, and nine months after the complete establishment of the monoplegia, that P— entered our wards at the Salpêtrière. We verified the conditions already referred to, and a more minute examination furnished the following results. The aortic insufficiency was very characteristic; there existed a souffle with the second beat at the base; violent arterial beating in the neck, visible to the eye; "Corrigan's pulse;" and capillary pulse perceptible on the forehead.

The motor paralysis of the left extremity is absolutely complete, it hangs flaccid and inert beside the body. There is no trace of voluntary movement, nor of contracture. The muscular masses have retained their normal volume and consistence; and their electric reactions, faradic and galvanic, are in no way modified. The tendon-reflexes of the elbow

[1] For all the information relative to his condition at the Hôtel Dieu we are indebted to Madlle. Klumpke, a pupil in the wards when P— was admitted.

and forearm are slightly augmented. Complete cutaneous anæsthesia to contact, cold, pricking, and the most intense faradization throughout the whole extent of the limb, hand, forearm, arm, and shoulder. In respect of the trunk the anæsthesia is limited by a circular line passing almost vertically beside the armpit and subclavicular space in front, and the external third of the scapular region behind. The insensibility extends in an equal degree to the deep-seated parts. The muscles and the nervous trunks themselves may be strongly faradized, the articular ligaments may be forcibly twisted, and diverse movements of the joints, torsion, &c., may be performed without the least consciousness on the part of the patient. The ideas attaching to the muscular sense have equally disappeared. The patient is unable to determine even approximately the attitude in which diverse segments of the limb may be placed, the position they occupy in space, or the direction and nature of the movements to which they have been subjected.

Apart from the left superior extremity, there does not exist on this side any modification of motor power, either in the face or the inferior extremity, but in these and over the left half of the trunk, the analgesia, discovered during the patient's stay in the Hôtel Dieu, still exists. An examination of the field of vision reveals a normal condition on the right side, while on the left it is considerably diminished; moreover, the circle of the red is outside that of the blue; and thus, since being in the Hôtel Dieu, an interesting change in the field of vision has occurred. Furthermore we discover by the usual methods that the senses of hearing, smell, and taste are much blunted on the left side.

We must now endeavour to determine the nature of this singular monoplegia supervening on the traumatism. The absence of atrophy and of any abnormal electric reactions in the muscles in a case of paralysis extending over ten months, repels, at first sight, the hypothesis of a lesion of the brachial plexus, while the absence of any atrophy alone, and the intensity of the perversion of sensibility, permits us to reject the idea that we have here to do with one of those cases of paralysis, so well investigated by Prof. Lefort and M. Valtat, which are caused by violence to an articulation.

A brachial monoplegia may, it is true, in exceptional cases supervene on certain lesions of the internal capsule, as has been demonstrated, among others, by Drs. Bennett and Campbell in 'Brain,'[1] but in such a case we do not certainly encounter the sensorial and sensitive hemianæsthesia, which is sometimes superadded to ordinary complete hemiplegia from lesion of the capsule.

The occurrence in the right hemisphere of a little hæmorrhagic point, or softening determined by embolism in consequence of an organic affection of the heart, a point which one can suppose limited strictly to the motor zone of the arm—such a lesion, I say, may account for the existence of left brachial monoplegia. But on this supposition the paralysis ought to supervene suddenly as on a "stroke," however limited the lesion, and not progressively. It would have been characterised almost certainly, some months after its commencement, by a certain degree of contraction, and by marked exaggeration of the tendon-reflexes. It certainly would not be accompanied by perversions of cutaneous and deep sensibility as pronounced as those we have observed in our patient.

We are obliged, then, to exclude in our diagnosis this last hypothesis, and likwise that of a spinal lesion which, as being inadmissible, we do not think even worthy of discussion. On the other hand, our attention has been vividly directed towards the significant hereditary antecedents of the patient, his psychical state and habits, the perversion of sensibility (extended—though unequally—over the whole of one side of the body), the diminution of the field of vision (so pronounced on the left side, and marked by the transposition of the red circle), and other sensorial troubles on the same side. All these constrain us, especially in the absence of any other reasonable hypothesis, to interpret the case as an example of hysteria. Further, the clinical characters of the monoplegia, its traumatic origin—and on that point I refer you to what I have already said—are in no way inconsistent with this view. Indeed, the limitation of motor paralysis to one limb, without involving at any time the corresponding side of the face; the absence of marked exaggeration of the

[1] 'Brain,' April, 1885, p. 78.

tendon-reflexes, of muscular atrophy, and of the ordinary electric reactions, the absolute stoutness of the member many months after the commencement of the disease; the cutaneous and deep anæsthesia, carried to a high degree in that member, and the total loss of notions pertaining to the muscular sense,—all these phenomena united in one case, as in that of our patient, amply sufficed to reveal the hysterical nature of the paralysis.

In consequence, the diagnosis "hysteria" was openly and resolutely adopted. Without doubt, the convulsive attack was an element wanting; but you do not ignore the fact that this is not inseparable from the nature of hysteria. Consequently the nature of the prognosis changed; we had not to deal with an affection arising from an organic cause, perhaps incurable; we were able to anticipate, despite the long duration of the disease, the occurrence, either spontaneously or under the influence of treatment, of some one of those sudden changes which are not rare in the history of hysterical paralyses, and of flaccid paralysis in particular. In any case we were able to prognosticate that sooner or later the patient would recover. A subsequent event soon justified our hopes, and amply confirmed our diagnosis.

On the 15th of March, four days after becoming our patient, we diligently searched, what had not been done up to this date, to find whether there existed in him any hysterogenetic zones. We found one situated under the left breast, another in each of the iliac regions, and a fourth on the right testicle. It was noticed that even a slight excitation of the sub-mammary zone easily determined the diverse phenomena of the aura—a sensation of constriction of the thorax, and then of the neck, beating in the temples, and buzzing sounds, especially in the left ear. But on insisting a little more P— was suddenly noticed to lose consciousness, to throw himself backwards, to stiffen his limbs, and then we witnessed *the first attack of hystero-epilepsy* which the patient ever experienced. This attack was absolutely classic; to the epileptoid phase immediately succeeded that of the greater movements. These were of an extreme violence; the patient, in the movements of salutation, went so far as almost to strike his face against his knees. Shortly afterwards he tore the sheets, the curtains of his bed, and turning his fury against himself, he bit his left arm. The phase of passionate attitudes immediately followed, and P— became a prey to a furious delirium; he became abusive, and cited imaginary persons to murder,—"Hold! Take your knife. . . . Quick. . . . Strike!" Ultimately he came to himself, and he affirmed that he had no remembrance of what had occurred. It is remarkable that during the whole of that first attack the *left superior extremity took no part in the convulsions;* it remained flaccid and perfectly inert. During the following days the attacks recurred spontaneously many times, always presenting the same characters as the provoked attack. In one of them, which took place during the night of the 17th March, the patient passed his urine in bed. Two other attacks followed on the 19th. On the 21st a fit occurred, *during which the left arm was agitated.* On awakening, the patient found to his great astonishment that he was able voluntarily to move the various segments of the limb, *of which he had not had the use for a single instant during the long period of close on ten months.* The motor paralysis was not completely cured, without doubt, for there remained a certain degree of paresis, but it was considerably improved. Only, the perversions of sensibility remained in the same degree as before.

This cure, gentlemen,—or, to speak more properly, this partial cure—after the diagnosis at which we arrived, ought not to be a matter of surprise to you. But, from our point of view, it had occurred prematurely. Indeed, it was evidently no longer possible to afford to you ocular demonstration of the characters in detail of that monoplegia, so worthy of study. The idea, therefore, occurred to me that, perhaps by acting on the mind of the patient, by *means of suggestion,* even in the waking state—we had learned previously that the subject was not hypnotisable—we might reproduce the paralysis, for a time at least. Thus it was that the following day, finding P— just coming out of an attack which had not modified the state of matters, I endeavoured to persuade him that he was paralysed anew. "You believe yourself cured," I said to him, with an accent of entire conviction, "it is an error; you are not able to raise your arm, nor to bend it, nor to move the fingers; see, you are unable to grasp my hand," &c. The experiment succeeded marvellously, for at the end of a few minutes discussion the monoplegia returned. I was not anxious on this account, it may be said in passing, for I know from long experience, that *what one has done, one can undo.* Unfortunately this did not persist for more than twenty-four hours. The following day a new attack supervened, in consequence of which the voluntary movements became definitely re-established. On this occasion all the attempts at suggestion which we made were found useless. To-day it only remains for me to apprise you of the modifications which, as far as voluntary movement is concerned, have taken place, in consequence of the fits, in a limb which was at one time completely paralysed.

The patient, you will notice, is able voluntarily to move all the parts of the limb. But these movements are not energetic; they do not overcome the least resistance which one opposes to them, and while in the right hand the dynamometric force is equivalent to 70, the left hand represents only 10. Hence, as I have already stated, if the motor paralysis is not so absolute as formerly, it still persists to a certain degree. Further, the troubles of sensibility remain as they were, affecting not only the weakened member, but all the left side of the body, and comprise the sensorial apparatus. The attacks continue frequently, from which you will understand that we have here simply amelioration, and for a complete cure much more remains to be done.

I shall have occasion to refer to some of the facts of this interesting case when we take up the subject of hysterical paralyses of traumatic origin, as I hope to do soon.[1] For the present, leaving aside the monoplegia, which constitutes but an episode in the history of our patient, I wish to point out to you once more, in conclusion, that, in the case of this man, as in the preceding cases, hysteria major [la grande hystérie] undoubtedly exists, endowed with all its characteristic attributes.

Gentlemen, in considering with you in these two lectures the six significant cases which chance has placed under our observation, I have been desirous of convincing you that

[1] *Vide* p. 284.

hysteria, even grave hysteria, is not so very rare a disease in the male, at any rate in France; that it may be found here and there in the ordinary clinical work, where only the prejudices of another age prevent its being recognised. I venture to hope that after the numerous proofs which have lately been accumulated, that notion is henceforth destined to occupy in your minds the place to which it is entitled.

LECTURE XX.

ON TWO CASES OF HYSTERICAL BRACHIAL MONOPLEGIA IN THE MALE, OF TRAUMATIC ORIGIN.—HYSTERO-TRAUMATIC MONOPLEGIA.[1]

SUMMARY.—*Case of Porcz—.—Antecedents, articular rheumatism.—Fall.—Monoplegia with anæsthesia of the arm and shoulder.—Examination of the patient; motor paralysis with flaccidity; loss of all kinds of sensibility having a peculiar delimitation; no trophic changes; no modification in the electric reactions of the paralysed muscles.*[2]*—Diagnosis; disturbance or contusion of the brachial plexus, characters of the symptoms observed in these cases, anæsthetic zone corresponds with the distribution of the affected nerves, trophic changes, modification of the electric reactions.*

GENTLEMEN,—To-day's lecture will be devoted to the clinical study of a case of right brachial monoplegia originating some months ago in a man, æt. 25, in consequence of a fall upon the shoulder, a form of monoplegia which presents serious difficulty in diagnosis. I do not wish to exaggerate these difficulties, and that you may be satisfied that they really exist you have but to recall the discussion on this case at the Société Médicale des Hôpitaux, when the patient was presented by M. Troisier at the meeting on 25th March last.

[1] Lecture edited by M. P. Marie, chef de clinique, et M. G. Guinon, interne du service. [The history of one of these cases, Pin—, is commenced on p. 252 *ante*.]

[2] Lecture delivered May 1st, 1885. At the meeting of the Société Médicale des Hôpitaux on July 24th last, Dr. Troisier again exhibited the patient Porcz—, the subject of this lecture (*vide* 'Gazette Hebdomadaire,' No. 31, 1885). At the same meeting Dr. Joffroy exhibited a patient from our wards, named Pin—, whose case was discussed in the preceding lecture, and to which I shall refer in the next.

You will then observe that the opinions expressed by our colleagues MM. Féréol, Déjerine, Rendu, and Joffroy, on the nature of the monoplegia, are very diverse, notwithstanding the very thorough investigation of the case.

M. Troisier has been good enough, and I am glad to express my obligations to him, to commit the patient to my charge. The history, I doubt not, will excite in you a lively interest.

You will not, I trust, be wearied by the minuteness of detail into which we shall enter in the analysis of this case, not one feature of which is wanting in its practical application. The patient is a man, æt. 25, named Porcz—a cab-driver, he became an inmate of our clinical wards on the 15th April last. The affection dates from over four months back, originating, as already remarked, in an accident, and it has not undergone any modification during that period. But before entering into further details, we will say a few words on the antecedents of this patient.

His mother died at the age of fifty-nine of disease of the liver; she was very nervous. Porcz— remembers that on many occasions when thwarted in anything she was wont to be affected with fits, in which she fell down and lost consciousness. His father was a great drinker of absinthe, but never had any nervous attacks. His sister is frequently the subject of nervous attacks, probably of an hysterical nature. There does not appear to be any insanity in the family.

Among the personal antecedents the following are disclosed:—In infancy, although not particularly nervous, our patient tells us that when left alone he always feared "robbers." At seven years of age he fell from a fifth storey on to an iron grating, whence he rebounded on to the pavement of a court. From this time his health has been notably enfeebled, and a short time afterwards the deviation in the vertebral column, which now exists, commenced. At the age of sixteen Porcz— entered as a "washer" with a carriage company, and shortly afterwards he contracted an attack of articular rheumatism, which confined him to bed for six weeks. From this period his right knee has been painful, and tumefied from time to time, and is at present the seat of *crepitus*. In consequence of this arthritis of rheumatic origin there is a certain amount of atrophy of the triceps extensor cruris (amyotrophy) of articular origin. This limb is notably more feeble than the corresponding one of the opposite side, and the patient limps a little on this side. This relative feebleness of the right limb dates, I repeat, from nearly ten years ago, but it has no connection with the present ailment.

This slight infirmity, and his miserable appearance, did not prevent Porcz— from following, since the age of eighteen, his employment, sometimes of an omnibus driver and sometimes a cabman.

Let us revert now to the monoplegia and its direct causes. On the 24th December, 1884, the horse which Porcz— was driving became restive, and our patient was pitched from his seat on to the pavement, falling upon his right side, the posterior part of the right shoulder receiving the first impulse. There was no loss of consciousness, no intense emotion. Porcz— was able to regain his feet, go to a chemist's, and mount the box. The right shoulder and arm were somewhat painful, but presented no bruising. The movements of the extremity were difficult, but possible, and Porcz— was able to drive his cab for five hours afterwards, holding the reins in his left hand. During the next five days the patient rested, and the pain and difficulty of movement seemed to diminish. He hoped soon to be able to resume his work, when, on the 30th of December, six days after the accident, and after a restless night, he found on awakening that the right superior extremity was flaccid, hanging motionless, and incapable of all movement, with the exception of the fingers of the hand, which he was still able to move a little. Practising friction, Porcz— noticed the insensibility of the shoulder, the arm, and the forearm, which we observe to-day. It is perfectly certain that neither at the time of the fall nor afterwards was there any trace of loss of consciousness, or any intellectual perversion, any sort of aphasia or embarrassment of speech, any deviation of the mouth or tongue, or any degree of paralysis in the right inferior extremity. We have therefore in this case to do with a brachial monoplegia plus anæsthesia, in the most rigorous acceptation of the term.

On the 8th of January, 1885, our patient presented himself at the Hôpital Tenon, under M. Troisier, who recognised, nine days after the commencement of the paralysis, all the features which we noted on receiving the patient. To-day, the 1st of May, four months after the commencement of the monoplegia, matters are in the same state. We find the patient exactly in the same state as he was four months ago when examined by M. Troisier, and also when he was presented a month ago to the Société Médicale des Hôpitaux.

Let us examine now with some attention this singular monoplegia, which has existed as you see it now during four months, despite the diverse forms of treatment employed.

A. *Motor functions.*—Porcz— is unable to perform any voluntary movement either with the elevator muscles of the shoulder or those of the shoulder itself, or the muscles of the arm or forearm. He is able to voluntarily move the fingers of the hand alone, and these movements are so feeble as not to be appreciable by the dynamometer.

Observe the absolute flaccidity of the limb. It lies along the trunk as an inert body, and falls heavily down after being raised. The patient is obliged to carry it in a sling to obviate the shocks and blows to which it would otherwise be exposed at each instant. There does not exist, as you perceive, the least trace of rigidity or contraction. This recalls the flaccidity of the monoplegia in *infantile spinal paralysis*. But here the tendon-reflexes at the elbow and the wrist are intact, perhaps even a little exaggerated, while you know it is quite otherwise in that form of spinal paralysis. Further, and this is an absolutely distinct characteristic, although the paralysis has existed for four months, there is no appreciable atrophy or diminished consistence of the paralysed muscles. Actual measurement of the right arm gives 23·5 c., of the left 24 c.; the right forearm 22.5 c., the left forearm 22 c.

B. There exists in the greater part of this limb, besides paralysis of movement, *profound perversions of sensibility*, Sensibility to contact, pain, and cold is completely and absolutely abolished, and this cutaneous anæsthesia, which exists exclusively in the parts of the extremity where there is motor paralysis, is marked off from the parts retaining their sensibility by lines presenting a singular disposition, especially as relating to the hand. Yet it is observable that it does not correspond with the anatomical distribution of the cutaneous nerves of the superior extremity, as you can see by looking at this diagram (Figs. 54 and 55, p. 268).

On the back of the hand the limit of anæsthesia is marked, so far as concerns the fingers, by a transverse line situated a few centimetres above the metacarpo-phalangeal articulations, while on the palmar aspect the limit is represented by a line parallel to the fold of the wrist, and about one centimetre below it.

Further, the *insensibility* is not limited to the skin, *it extends to the deeper parts;* and thus it is that faradization, no matter how energetic, either of the muscles or the trunks of the nerves, while provoking strong contractions, is not felt. Movements of torsion, or dragging, communicated to the shoulder, the elbow, or wrist, do not occasion any feeling whatever, no matter how violent they may be. But on the palmar surface and on the back of the hand, and over all the fingers, cutaneous and deep sensibility are preserved, at least in great part.

Further, in this extremity, the fingers always excepted, *the manifestations relating to what is called the muscular sense are in complete abeyance.* To appreciate this it is only necessary that Porcz— should be requested to shut his eyes and to find his forearm, held away from the body, and seize it by means of his left hand. At first he gropes in space, more or less remote from his object, and when he accidentally finds any part of the member, probably its upper end, he ranges with his hand over the whole arm until he arrives at the part at which he is requested to touch. When his eyes are shut, he does not know whether one bends his wrist, his elbow, or his shoulder. But, under like conditions he knows perfectly well when the same act is practised on his fingers, and which one is experimented upon. Porcz— has equally lost the notion of weight of objects placed in the palm of his hand. When he does not look he is unable to distinguish, without fingering them, a piece of 5 francs from one of 10 centimes, they both seem to him equally light.

To epitomise, we have, therefore, absolute motor paralysis of the muscles of the shoulder and of the arm and forearm;

complete loss of sensibility of the skin, of the muscles, of the nerves, tendons, and articular ligaments, &c.; complete absence of all notions relating to the muscular sense in all the parts which correspond to the motor paralysis; no rigidity in the parts deprived of movement, with preservation of the muscular outline, and slight exaggeration of the tendon-reflexes. These are the salient features hitherto disclosed.

But it behoves us to notice again the remarkable and significant fact that the muscles present no indications of trophic perversion, notwithstanding that the monoplegia has already existed for more than four months. You have satisfied yourselves that there is no wasting of the members; I would add that *the muscles, subjected to a rigorous examination, present no modification in respect of the electrical reactions either to faradism or galvanism.* There is not the slightest suspicion of the reaction of degeneration.

Finally, there is no lividity of the skin, and no œdema. There exists only, in the affected member, a slight diminution of the temperature. Thus, the axillary temperature of the two sides is 36·9°, that of the healthy member on the anterior aspect of the forearm 32·8°, while that of the paralysed member on the corresponding spot is only 32·4°, that is to say about four tenths of a degree lower.

Such are the phenomena disclosed to us by analysis of the condition of the paralysed member. There exist in our patient, beyond what relates to the monoplegia, several other interesting clinical facts; but they do not strike one at first sight, and we encounter them only after pursuing inquiry in a certain direction. I will reserve the noting of these peculiarities until, after the discussion, it becomes a question of definitely determining the diagnosis.

What, then, is the nature of this monoplegia which we have been studying so carefully, and of whose clinical characters we are now cognisant? Has it any connection with a lesion more or less pronounced of the peripheric nerves in consequence of a contusion or a shock to the brachial plexus caused by the fall on the shoulder? Does it relate to any spinal lesion? Or a focal cerebral lesion? Such are the questions which now have to be considered.

The first-named naturally presents itself at once to the mind. There are numerous examples of brachial monoplegia in consequence of a fall on the shoulder, and a certain number of the phenomena observed in our patient appear, at first sight, to admit of explanation on the hypothesis of shock or contusion of the brachial plexus. I am happy to be able to bring under your notice by the side of Porcz—, a patient in whom brachial monoplegia exists, and caused under circumstances similar to those which determined the brachial monoplegia in the case of Porcz—. It is true, we have not here to deal with a fall on the posterior part of the shoulder, as in Porcz—'s case, but with a violent shock to the same region caused by a blow from a large heavy beam. The traumatic conditions are analogous in both cases. Let us see what have been the consequences in our second case, of which the following is an abridged history.[1]

The patient Deb—, a vigorous, well-built navvy, æt. 31, had always enjoyed excellent health until, on the 3rd of April, 1884, that is to say, thirteen months ago, he received a blow on the posterior part of the left shoulder from the extremity of a beam, the violence of the shock being such as to throw him face forwards to the ground. He was at the same time struck on the posterior and the superior region of the cranium by an iron point carrying a block attached to the end of the beam, and a wound of some extent was the result. On receipt of the injury there was no immediate loss of consciousness, and during some time afterwards, for five or six minutes perhaps, the patient remained conscious. He recollects, at least, so he affirms, that at this moment he felt a sensation such as to lead him to believe that his superior extremity was entirely separated from the body. Then supervened a loss of consciousness which lasted during three hours. When Deb— came to himself, motor paralysis of the diverse segments of the member was as absolute as it is at this moment, the movements of elevation of the shoulder alone being preserved. With respect to sensibility, it seems to have been in the same condition as we find it now.

[1] Very recently the case of this patient has been given *in extenso* by Mdlle. Klumpke in her interesting work on "Paralyses of the Brachial Plexus" ('Revue de Médecine,' 10th July, 1885, 5th year, No. 7, p. 604).

From this time the patient has sojourned in various hospitals, where he had been subjected, unhappily for him without result, to various forms of treatment, and especially electricity. This treatment had to be interrupted from time to time, owing to the intense pain invariably caused by it, and could never, therefore, be followed out continuously.

I will first direct your attention to the derangements of sensibility. Sensibility of all kinds is absolutely abolished in the hand, including the fingers, the forearm, and part of the

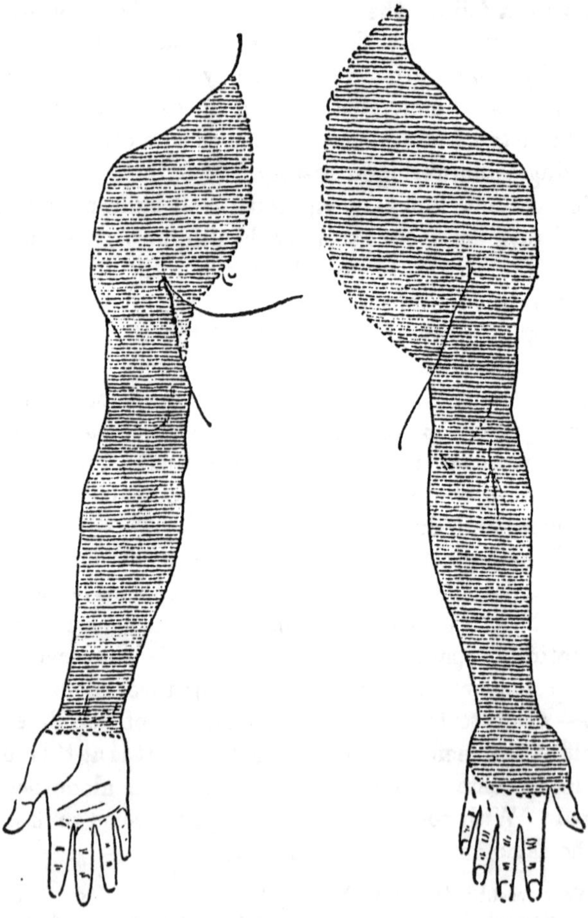

FIGS. 54 and 55.—Case of Porcz—.

arm ; in the same parts deep sensibility is likewise abolished, and likewise the ideas attaching to the muscular sense. Wherever the cutaneous anæsthesia exists it is as complete as we have seen it to be in the case of Porcz— ; only the mode of distribution is different in the two cases, for while in the case of Porcz— the zone of insensibility encircles all the shoulder, and even beyond, in that of Deb—, on the contrary, the area is much less limited, embracing neither the shoulder nor a considerable portion of the arm. Thus on the anterior and external aspect of the arm in the latter case the line of anæs-

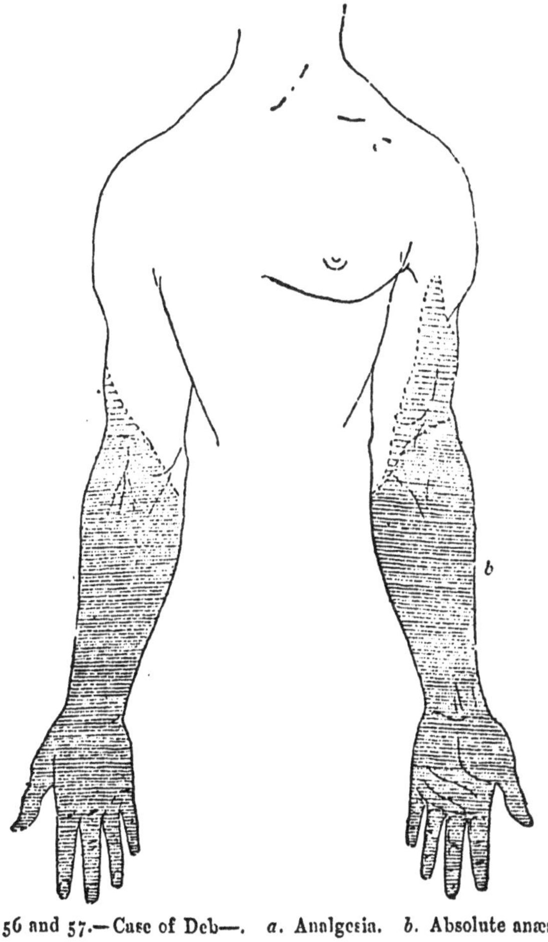

FIGS. 56 and 57.—Case of Deb—. *a*. Analgesia. *b*. Absolute anæsthesia.

thesia scarcely reaches the middle of the limb. On the external aspect it is higher. Behind it scarcely goes beyond the elbow, so that the posterior aspect of the arm is almost normal (Figs. 56 and 57).

I should like you to observe, gentlemen, that this disposition of the anæsthetic zone is exactly such as has been observed in cases where the brachial plexus has been severely injured, or even torn across completely, by injury or surgical division, cases of which have been recorded by Dr. Ross, of Manchester, in his important contribution to 'Brain.'[1]

You observe from an examination of the plates (Figs. 58 and 59) taken from Ross, and relating to a case of tearing of the brachial plexus, attended with motor and trophic derangements, both muscular and cutaneous, which have been determined by a rupture of all the branches of that plexus;[2] you notice, I say, that the disposition of the anæsthetic zone is exactly the same as that observed in our patient, Deb—.

Now, in the last-named case (Deb—), after noting the motor and trophic derangements to which we shall return directly, it must be conceded that there exists a grave and an extensive lesion of the whole plexus. This distribution of cutaneous anæsthesia appears to be the pathognomonic expression of deep and destructive organic lesions affecting all the motor and the sensory branches of the brachial plexus.

If, now, we revert to the case of Porcz— we notice that the distribution of the anæsthetic zone is totally different. It is much more extended upwards towards the trunk than in the case of Deb—. It involves the shoulder, and consequently, on the hypothesis of a contusion acting on the course of the nerves, not only the brachial but the cervical plexus also ought to be involved. Moreover, we know that in the case of Porcz— the zone of anæsthesia is limited below by the hand (Figs. 54 and 55). But the disposition of that line, marking the limit of anæsthesia, does not accord with the hypothesis of a lesion profoundly affecting all the sensi-

[1] "Distribution of anæsthesia in cases of disease of the branches and of the roots of the brachial plexus."—'Brain,' April, 1884, p. 70.

[2] With the exception of the communicating branch from the 4th nerve.

tive fibres of the brachial plexus. As we have already remarked, it is, on the palmar aspect of the hand, a straight line at right angles to the long axis of the limb, and parallel with the fold of flexion of the wrist-joint; and on the dorsal

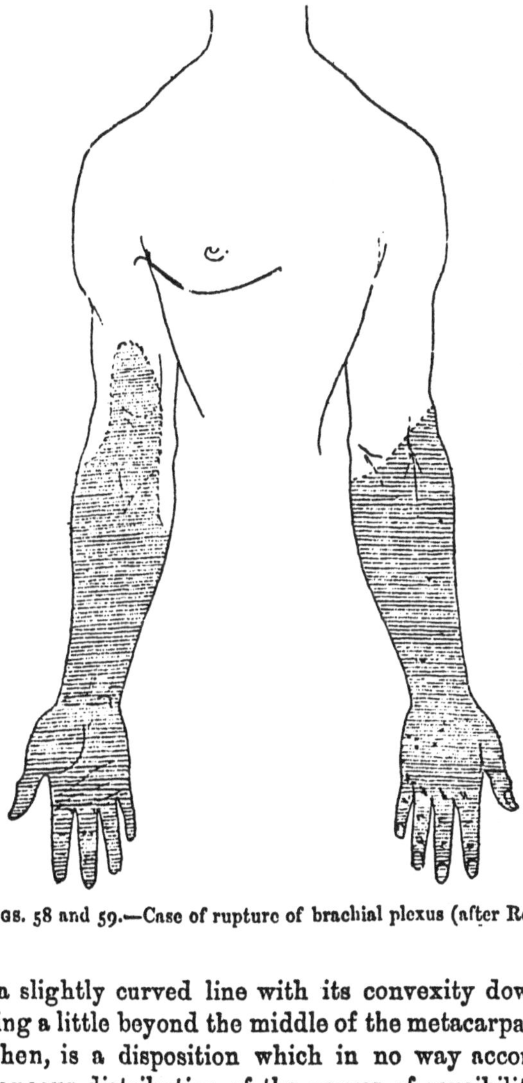

FIGS. 58 and 59.—Case of rupture of brachial plexus (after Ross).

aspect a slightly curved line with its convexity downwards, extending a little beyond the middle of the metacarpal region. Here, then, is a disposition which in no way accords with the cutaneous distribution of the nerves of sensibility in the lower portions of the hand (ulnar and radial for the dorsal aspect, median and ulnar for the palmar), and which, therefore, does not accord with the supposition of a deep and general lesion of the brachial plexus. The facts to which we have just referred do not better accord with the hypothesis of a slight contusion, or a simple "commotion" of the plexus, for numerous observations in those cases show, contrary to what obtains in our case, that under such circumstances perversions of sensibility are little marked, eminently transitory, or entirely wanting.

In the case of Deb—, which represents a typical example of a deep, old, and irreparable injury of the brachial plexus, we also discover trophic derangements, muscular and cutaneous, and certain other phenomena which, quite as much as the perversions of sensibility, contrast singularly with what we observe in Porcz—. Doubtless in both cases the paralysed member is flaccid and without traces of contraction or articular rigidity; but here is the difference, in Deb— the paralysed muscles are extremely atrophied. They present on electric examination the reaction of degeneration in its most aggravated form; the tendon-reflexes are abolished, the skin is cold, and its surface is marked by violet spots, especially towards the extremity of the limb, and the subcutaneous tissue is slightly œdematous.

There is nothing of the kind in the case of Porcz—. Here you see, notwithstanding the long continuance of the malady, the muscles have preserved their volume and consistence, they present no reaction of degeneration, the tendon-reflexes exist, and the colour of skin and the consistence of the integuments are normal. These, then, constitute the phenomena which do not permit of reconciliation with the theory of a serious and deep lesion of the brachial plexus, notwithstanding the existence of the malady for four months; and much might likewise be made of the remarkable fact of the non-participation of the fingers and of the hand in the motor paralysis and anæsthesia, so marked in all the other parts of the limb.

Thus, gentlemen, the brachial monoplegia which forms the subject of our present investigation, although occurring under conditions in which grave or trifling lesions of the brachial plexus by commotion or contusion might originate, does not really depend on a lesion of this nature. The seat of the disease has to be sought for elsewhere in the nerve centres. Have we therefore to do with a circumscribed organic cerebral or spinal lesion? It will, I think, be easy for me to indicate to you that this is not so.

LECTURE XXI.

ON TWO CASES OF HYSTERICAL BRACHIAL MONOPLEGIA IN THE MALE, DUE TO INJURY.—HYSTERO-TRAUMATIC MONOPLEGIA (*continued*).[1]

SUMMARY.—*Diagnosis continued.—Amyotrophies dependent on joint lesion; on spinal or focal cerebral lesions.—Symptoms pathognomonic of hysteria in this patient; right hemianæsthesia; monocular polyopia with macropsy; bilateral retraction of the field of vision.*

Case of Pin— :[2] *Flaccid monoplegia and loss of all kinds of sensibility in the left upper extremity following a fall. —Other hysterical symptoms; diminution of hearing, taste, and smell on one side; retraction of the field of vision with transposition of the red; monocular polyopia; anæsthesia of the back of the throat; hysterogenic areæ; hysterical attacks followed by an improvement in the paralysis of the arm.*

Psychic paralyses; their production by suggestion in hypnotism.—Different states of hypnotism considered in connection with the possibility of suggestion.

GENTLEMEN,—In our last lecture we had before us a remarkable case of brachial monoplegia in a man, æt. 25, supervening on a fall upon the shoulder, in which we were constrained to believe that the symptoms observed were not connected with a lesion of the nerves of the brachial plexus. This opinion we based upon the extent and dis-

[1] Lecture edited by M. Marie, chef de clinique, and M. Geo. Guinon, interne du service.

[2] Continued from p. 252.

position of the cutaneous and deep-seated anæsthesia, on the absence of trophic changes, and of Erb's reaction in the muscles of the paralysed limb. These same considerations also enable us to conclude at once that we have not to deal with an example of amyotrophic paralysis which is sometimes the result of traumatism affecting an articulation, and which has been specially investigated by MM. Lefort and Valtat.[1]

After eliminating these from the diagnosis it remains for us to examine the two following hypotheses. Does this monoplegia depend on a lesion localised in the spinal cord; or a circumscribed lesion in one of the cerebral hemispheres?

We shall not be long detained in discussing the first question to which we have more than once referred in the course of the preceding lecture. A destructive lesion strictly limited to a certain region of the anterior horn of the grey matter in the brachial enlargement of the right side, may it is true, as we see in cases of infantile spinal paralysis, produce a flaccid brachial monoplegia, without affecting in any respect the face or the leg of the same side, altogether corresponding in this respect to what is observed in our patient. But in such cases, not to speak of the sudden development, accompanied most frequently by a febrile condition of some days' duration, we certainly observe after a period of eight or ten days a very pronounced reaction of degeneration affecting all the muscles, and after four months manifest atrophy of those muscles. Further, the tendon reflexes are abolished from the commencement. And again, there would be no cutaneous anæsthesia or loss of the muscular sense. It is true that a concomitant lesion of the posterior cornua of the grey substance in corresponding regions of the spinal marrow, may cause, without doubt, more or less grave perversions of sensibility. But any such lesion exclusively involving one of the anterior horns and the region quite limited to the more posterior part of the posterior horn of the same side, has not yet been observed, so far as I know; and if that lesion instead of remaining limited, as we have already assumed, had invaded the median parts of the grey column, then the anæsthesia

[1] *Vide* Lecture II, p. 20, *ante*.

would affect not only the side corresponding to the lesion, but also the opposite side.

I will not further insist on that point, but we will consider a little more closely the hypothesis of a circumscribed cerebral lesion. In what region of the cerebral hemispheres ought any such lesion to be localised in order to produce the symptoms manifested in our patient? Could it be a lesion affecting the internal capsule? Such a lesion as one might suppose to be produced by the shock; and which would consist, I suppose, of a patch of hæmorrhagic or capillary apoplexy resulting from the commotion incidental to the fall. Such a condition would almost necessarily be accompanied by some apoplectic symptoms which have not certainly occurred in our patient. I would add that a pure brachial monoplegia, like the one before us, is almost unheard of in the history of lesions of the internal capsule.[1] It is further necessary to suppose a lesion strictly limited to the anterior parts of the capsule, and consequently perversions of sensibility would then be wanting. It is therefore higher in the hemisphere, that is to say, in the grey matter or the parts immediately subjacent to the *centrum ovale*, that we ought to search for the localisation of the supposed organic lesion.

A lesion sufficiently extensive and profound, localised in the middle third of the median convolutions (frontal and ascending parietal) necessarily results in a brachial monoplegia; that is now so well established that it is unnecessary to enlarge upon it. But it is necessary to remark that the existence of a *pure* monoplegia, without any participation of either the muscles supplied by the inferior facial, the tongue, or the inferior extremity of the same side, supervening on a cortical lesion, is undoubtedly very rare. We can scarcely collect a dozen such in a total of more than 250 cases observed by M. Pitres and myself, in our work relating to the question of cortical cerebral localisations.[2] But in the case

[1] *Vide* "A Case of Monoplegia due to Lesion of the Internal Capsule," by Drs. Bennett and Campbell, in 'Brain,' April, 1885, p. 78.

[2] Charcot et Pitres, "Etude Critique et Clinique de la doctrine des localisations motrices dans l'écorce des hémisphéres cérébraux de l'homme" ('Revue de Médecine,' 1883, Nos. 5, 6, 8, and 10).

of this patient, and this is a fact to be at once appreciated, it was clearly evident that at no stage of the malady, not even at the commencement, did the face, the tongue, or the inferior extremity present the slightest degree of paralysis or even paresis. From the outset, I repeat, the superior extremity alone has been affected.

I would remark that a cortical lesion sufficiently pronounced to provoke a paralysis of movement, as complete and as durable as is observed in the case of Porcz—, would necessarily determine a secondary descending cerebro-spinal degeneration, manifesting itself clinically by the existence of a certain degree of contraction in the paralysed member. But it is perfectly clear that in our case there is not the slightest evidence of any trace of such rigidity, rather, on the contrary, we observe that the motor paralysis is here remarkable by the softness and flaccidity of the parts, the diverse segments of the member opposing no resistance to the movements practised on them. Besides, although the tendon-reflexes are preserved in our patient, they are not notably exaggerated as would have been the case in a cortical lesion, with descending degeneration, four months after the appearance of the disease.

Finally, gentlemen, the perversions of sensibility, so strongly marked in the case of Porcz—, are not such as would be observed in a lesion of the cortex which one must suppose to be limited strictly to the middle third of the median convolutions. In a good number of cases of cortical lesion localised in one of the motor centres, the cutaneous sensibility and the muscular sense may, as you know, be absolutely intact. That is shown in many of the cases collected by my former chef de clinique, Dr. Ballet, in his inaugural dissertation,[1] and by a case published by Ferrier in 'Brain.'[2] It is true that MM. Exner, Petrina, Tripier, and more recently M. Starr[3] have collected a certain number of ob-

[1] G. Ballett, "Le faisceau sensitif et les troubles de la sensibilité dans les cas de lésions cérébrales" ('Archiv de Neurologie,' T. IV, 1882, et 'Thèse de Paris,' 1881, p. 67).

[2] 'Brain,' April, 1883. Ferrier's case relates to an example of crural monoplegia.

[3] Allen Starr, "Cortical Lesions of the Brain; a collection and analysis of the American cases of localised cerebral disease," pp. 48 and 49 (the 'American

servations relative to lesions limited to the median convolutions, in which, besides the motor paralysis, it was particularly noted that sensibility was affected in every manner (tactile sensibility, sensibility to pain, the muscular sense, &c.). But it appears established, notwithstanding, by these same observations, that, if the lesion is limited exactly to the motor centres without encroaching on the neighbouring regions of the parietal lobe, these various perversions of sensibility are always but little pronounced or eminently transitory. This contrasts signally, you observe, with what exists in our case, in which the diverse kinds of cutaneous and deep sensibility have been affected in a high degree and permanently during four months.

These considerations lead us to reject the idea that in this patient there exists a circumscribed cortical lesion, as we have already rejected the notion of a spinal lesion or a lesion of the peripheral nerves. With what then have we to deal? There is without doubt a lesion of the nervous centres, but where is it situated, and what is its nature? It is, I opine, in the grey matter of the cerebral hemisphere on the side opposite the paralysis, and more precisely in the motor zone of the arm. Further, taking into consideration the extent and intensity of the perversions of sensibility, we may believe, according to some recent works, that it is not strictly limited to the motor zone, and that it extends behind the median convolutions to the adjacent parts of the parietal lobe.[1] But certainly it is not of the nature of a circumscribed organic lesion of a destructive nature, as would have been the case in the diverse hypothesis we have passed in review. We have here unquestionably one of those lesions which escape our present means of anatomical investigation, and which, for want of a better term, we designate *dynamic* or *functional* lesions. And of this I shall now endeavour to offer you further proofs.

Journal of Medical Science,' 1884). "The Sensory Tract in the Central Nervous System," p. 78 (reprinted from the 'Journal of Nervous and Mental Diseases,' vol. vi, No. 3, July, 1884).

[1] Starr (loc. cit.); and Bechterew, "Ueber die Localisation der Hautsensibilität (Tast und Schmerzempfindungen) und des Muskelsinnes an der Oberfläche der Grosshirnhemisphären (Mendel's 'Neurol. Centr.-Blatt,' No. 18, 5th Sept., 1883).

As I have indicated, in demonstrating the symptoms observed in our patient, there are among them—and of a kind that are the most important—some which hitherto I have advisedly passed by in silence, intending to bring them into prominence at a proper time. That moment is now arrived. The symptoms in question do not strike the eye at first. In order to discover them it is necessary to direct the investigation on the lines of a certain hypothesis which the presence of these symptoms, if they really exist, would confirm and justify. You anticipate the hypothesis in question—is our patient hysterical? Is he the subject of sufficiently numerous and sufficiently accentuated hysterical stigmata to permit us to affirm that we have really to deal with the hysterical diathesis? In favour of this view the proofs abound. Here the motor paralysis, the anæsthesia and the other symptoms relate to hysteria. Such is my conclusion, confirmed on every point very explicitly by my colleague M. Joffroy, at a meeting of the Société Médicale des Hôpitaux.[1]

In the first place I would point out that in the case of Porcz— the perversions of cutaneous sensibility are not exactly confined to the right superior extremity. They are found though less pronounced, that is in the form of analgesia, over the whole extent of the same side, the face, the trunk, and lower extremity. We have here then, so far as relates to common sensibility, a generalised right hemianæsthesia, only much more pronounced on the extremity than elsewhere.

If, next, we examine the organs of sense, we find on this side valuable indications. The hearing is defective on the right side. The ticking of a watch, which on the left side is heard at a distance of 50 centimetres (20 inches) or more, is not heard on the right side beyond 20 centimetres (8 inches). Taste is completely lost on the right side. Then, observe the insensibility of the pharynx. The finger roughly introduced into the mouth as far as the epiglottis causes, in this patient, no reflex action. This phenomenon is, as you know, common in hysteria. Many observers, and particularly M. Chairou, have called attention to it in recent years. Having obtained these preliminary results, we naturally expect to find by an

[1] Séance du 27 Mars, 1885.

examination of the field of vision that characteristic retraction to which I have so often directed your attention. But, excepting on the first examination we have been deceived in our anticipations; we have now under observation a normal field of vision. I will show you how in this respect matters changed soon afterwards. However, investigation of the function of vision was not fruitless; it demonstrated, indeed, the existence of a phenomenon which, in the absence of others, acquires a great importance, and greatly contributes to identify hysteria in a case of diagnostic difficulty. I refer to the *Monocular polyopia of hysterical subjects*, a symptom which M. Parinaud[1] has investigated for some considerable time in the patients in my clinique, and which he was the first, I believe, to signalise.

Monocular polyopia (diplopia or triplopia) is, however, not exclusively peculiar to hysteria, but it generally occurs in that affection with special characteristics, by which, according to M. Parinaud it may be distinguished from other species of the same kind.

The crystalline lens, as you know, presents a segmentary structure, and may be said to be formed of three lenses. It will, therefore, be perceived that under certain conditions two or three images may be produced on the retina. This is a natural defect, as it were, more or less pronounced according to the individual, which in the healthy condition is corrected by the normal action of accommodation. It is easy to comprehend that when the physiological function of accommodation is affected, monocular polyopia results, and thus it may be noticed in the paralysis of accommodation produced by atropine, and in the contraction of accommodation determined by eserine. In the latter case it is generally not very pronounced, apparently owing to concomitant myosis. It is to the contraction of the muscle of Brucke,[2] in the absence of myosis, according to M. Parinaud, that the monocular polyopia of the hysterical ought to be ascribed. Without functional lesion of the apparatus of accommodation, mono-

[1] H. Perinaud, "De la Polyopie Minoculaire dans l'Hysteric," &c. (Extrait des 'Annales d'Oculistique,' Gand, Mai—Juin, 1878.)

[2] La contracture de muscle de l'accommodation dans l'hystérie a été étudiée par M. Galezowski ('Prog. Méd.,' T. VI, p. 39, 1878).

cular polyopia is seen in aged persons, in commencing cataract, and in certain cases of astigmatism, congenital, or due to keratitis.

But it will be easy to eliminate, in a given case, the causes of monocular polyopia above mentioned, viz. senile cataract, astigmatism from lesion of the cornea, or the effects of eserine or atropia, &c. Further, putting aside the absence of these causes, the polyopia of the hysterical appears, as I have said, to be characterised by special features. I refer to the *macrospy* and the *microspy* which, according to M. Parinaud, are peculiar to this condition, while they are not observed in the other cases. Place a pencil before Porcz—, held vertically at a distance of a few centimetres from one of his eyes, the other being shut, and he distinguishes but one image. But if the pencil is held further off he distinguishes two images. At eight or ten centimetres (three to four inches) from the eye they are distinctly separated the one from the other. Further, when the pencil is placed quite near the eye it appears unduly large, while, held at a distance of from fifteen to twenty centimetres (six to eight inches) it appears two or three times smaller than it really is, or than it would be seen normally. Such is the special monocular polyopia, which, associated with the sensorial and sensitive aberrations under consideration, constitute a significant feature in a case, especially where neither alcoholism, nor lead-poisoning, nor lesion of the internal capsule is operative. A second examination of the field of vision three days ago revealed a new feature. Five days ago the patient went out on an expedition, and returned very fatigued. Two days later perimetric examination disclosed concentric lessening of the field of vision, almost equally marked on both sides, though without transposition of the red circle.

It will not, after this, be necessary for me to enter into lengthy detail in order to show that the collection of symptoms which have been unfolded, so inexplicable on the hypothesis of an organic lesion of the brain, spinal cord, or peripheral nerves, admits of a very simple interpretation on the supposition of a dynamic hysterical lesion.

However, I should like to remark that the clinical characters of the monoplegia of Porcz— do not differ from those which distinguish undoubted cases of hysterical paralysis. Confirmation is afforded by reference to the most competent authorities on the subject. I would point out in the first place *the absence of any participation of the face* in the paralysis, a fact brought into prominence by Todd,[1] Althaus, Hasse,[2] and myself,[3] and by Weir Mitchell in his excellent book on the nervous diseases of females;[4] for my own part I have not yet found a well-marked exception to this rule. Secondly, the absence of any modification of electric reaction, of any atrophy of the muscles, notwithstanding that the paralysis has existed for several months; and the persistence of absolute flaccidity of the member without any marked change in the tendon reflexes; and also the absence of the muscular sense in a marked degree, such as is scarcely ever observed in paralysis of cerebral origin from other causes. Finally, I would point out to you the marked cutaneous and deep anæsthesia, its particular mode of distribution and limitation, which appeared singular at first sight no doubt, not having been carefully studied, and which does not correspond in any way to the distribution of the sensory nerves emanating from the brachial plexus.[5] I would not go the length of

[1] R. H. Todd, 'Clinical Lectures on Paralysis: Certain Diseases of the Brain, &c.,' London, 1856. "Again the extent of the paralysis in the limbs, and the total absence of it in the face and tongue, are certainly evidence in favour of its hysterical character, for although hysterical paralysis occurs in all parts of the trunk and extremities, it very rarely, if ever, attacks the face."—Loc. cit., p. 20.

[2] Hasse, 'Handbuch der Pathol., &c.,' II Auflag, Erlangen, 1869.

[3] Charcot, 'Leçons sur les Maladies du Système Nerveux,' T. I, 1st ed., p. 351. 12e leçon.—"Remarquez en premier lieu l'absence de paralysis faciale et de la déviation de la langue, lorsque celle-ci est tirée hors de la bouche. Vous savez que ces phenomènes existent au contraire toujours à un certain degré"—c'est presque toujours qu'il faut lire—"dans l'hemiplégie par lésion en foyer du cerveau."

[4] Weir Mitchell, 'Lectures on Diseases of the Nervous System, especially in Women,' 2nd ed., Philadelphia, 1885. "Unlike the hemiplasy of cerebral and organic cause, hysterical half-paralysis involves, more or less, all one side of the body, excepting the face; but in a few rare cases the neck is distinctly affected."—Loc. cit., p. 25.

[5] Compare Figs. 54, 55, 56, 57. That arrangement in geometrical segments limited by circular lines at right angles to the long axis of the member,

asserting that all hysterical paralyses necessarily present the whole of the characteristics enumerated, but I believe it may be affirmed that when these characters are found coexisting in a given case of paralysis its nature should not remain doubtful.

Such are the arguments, and they appear to me conclusive, by which I am constrained to affirm that, independently of hereditary circumstances, and the existence of stigmata, our patient must be considered to be hysterical; further that the monoplegia itself presents in him all the characteristic features of hysterical paralysis. In short, all the symptoms which we note in Porcz— reveal hysteria, and we find in his case nothing but what accords with hysteria.

Our diagnosis confirmed, there remains one concession which I am constrained to make, viz.: That this is not an absolutely complete case of hysteria, or, in a word, a classic case. But this renders it all the more interesting to the clinical observer, for if the hysterical nature of the affection is established by the foregoing, it should be remembered that it does not at first sight strike one as such, and that it is necessary to establish the diagnosis by minutely examining the clinical aspects of the case in their entirety. There is in reality something wanting in the picture, and that something, you all recognise, is the existence of hysterical attacks and of hystero-genic points. Evidently that circumstance need not seriously impede us, for the convulsive attack, as you know, is far from being a necessary characteristic of hysteria. According to M. Briquet it is wanting in a third of the cases of hysteria in the female, and, according to my experience, it may be absent in the male, and in equal proportion to the other sex.

To further establish the conclusions at which we have arrived, and to give them more weight, it may be useful to

really represents, at least for the limbs, the type of anæsthesia of cortical origin, by whatever cause produced. Only in hysteria that character will be, in general, much more accentuated and much more easy to recognise than in the case of an organic lesion, doubtless because in the former condition the dynamic lesion is much more extended, and may occupy the entirety of some circumscribed sensitive area of the cortex.—J. M. C.

compare with the present case that of another hysterical male whom I brought under your notice in the preceding lecture, and on whose case I dwelt at some length.[1] I refer to the patient Pin—, whom I again submit to your examination. Bearing in mind the principal features, you will recognise that his history is traced in some degree in that of Porcz—.

As with the latter, Pin— was affected with brachial monoplegia in consequence of a fall, only in his case the paralysis affected the left superior extremity and the anterior aspect of the shoulder, which was the one that had been struck. On the 11th March, at our first examination of him, the paralysis was absolute (as in Porcz—) the face never having been affected in any degree whatever. The paralysed member was pendent, flaccid, and without the slightest rigidity at the level of the joints; no amyotrophy nor modification of electric reaction, notwithstanding that the disease was of ten months' duration. Cutaneous and deep anæsthesia exists to the same degree in both Porcz— and Pin—, only it is more extended on the hands and fingers of the latter, but it is limited exactly in the same manner at the shoulder (compare Figs. 54, 55, p. 268, 60, and 61).

The loss of the muscular sense is equally pronounced in all the insensitive parts. These perversions of sensibility are not yet modified, and at this moment we can prove their existence in the two patients. You see how far the two cases resemble one another up to this point. Between them there is almost an identity. The details which follow will link them together still more closely.

In the discussion on the diagnosis in the case of Pin— we successively eliminated (as we have done in the case of Porcz—), the hypotheses of a lesion of the branches of the brachial plexus, any spinal lesion, or any organic lesion of the central hemispheres, which the presence of aortic insufficiency in his case might have rendered likely. And we arrived at the conclusion that the paralysis depended on a *dynamic* lesion localised in the grey substance of the brachial motor zone in the side opposite to that affected by the monoplegia. The existence of the hysterical diathesis further reveals itself in this patient by significant features; analgesia ex-

[1] *Vide* p. 251, *et seq.*

tending over the left side of the head, of the trunk, and the whole of the left inferior extremity; hearing, smell, and taste, tested by the usual processes, present a marked diminution on the left side. The field of vision presents a

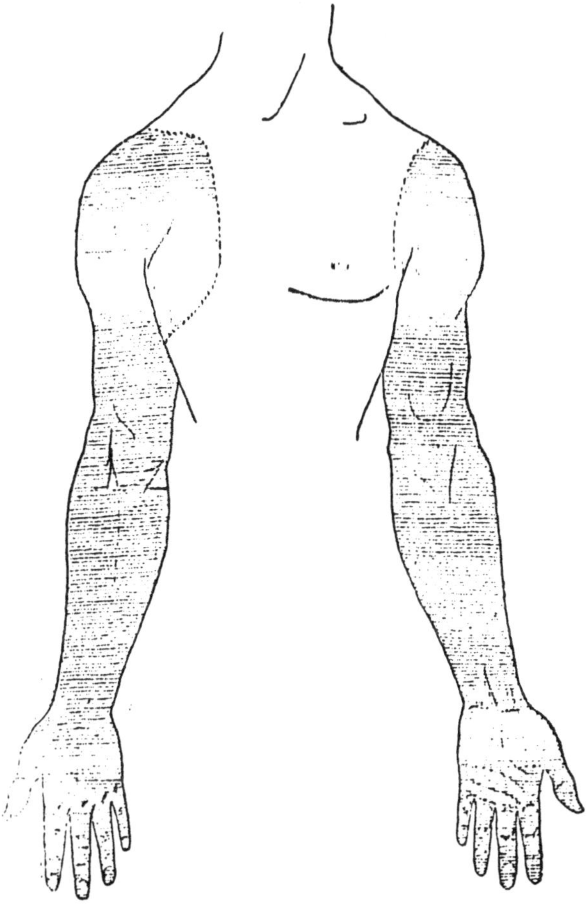

FIGS. 60 and 61.—Case of Pin—.

normal condition on the right side, but on the left there is a considerable diminution of its area;[1] further, on this side

[1] This case shows, with many others that I could cite, that although the concentric lessening of the field of vision in the hysterical exists more fre-

the red circle is wider than that of the blue (Figs. 62 and 63). To-day we find on the same side the presence of monocular polyopia, which has not been hitherto noticed. I would add that the finger introduced into the pharynx as far as the epiglottis does not cause any reflex action.

Finally, and this is the only feature in which the case of Pin— differs in a marked manner from that of Porcz—, there exists in the former several hyperæsthetic hysterogenic zones; one situated under the left breast, another in each of the iliac regions, and one on the right testicle.

On the 15th of March you will recollect that in consequence of a slight excitation of the submaxillary zone, Pin— was affected with a perfectly characteristic hystero-epileptic attack. This was the first that the patient had ever experienced. It was succeeded by many others of a like character. At the present time these attacks frequently occur spontaneously. After one of these attacks, on the 21st of March, an improvement in the motor power, which exists at the present time, was noticed in Pin—. He is able, as you see, to voluntarily move all the segments of the left superior extremity. But these movements are not very energetic, they do not resist the least opposing force. The dynamometric force on the right is represented by the figure 70, that on the left only by 10. Thus, if the motor power is not so complete as it once was, still there is much improvement. The derangements of sensibility remain, as they were at the commencement, not only in the impaired member, but over all the left side of the body and the organs of special sense. Consequently this is not a complete cure, but we have reason to hope that further improvement will occur, for clearly the prognosis is not so grave as paralysis arising from a destructive lesion in the grey substance of one of the cerebral hemispheres. Between the case of Pin— and that of

quently on both sides, this is not an absolute rule. This lessening may be limited to one side. The case of Gil—, in particular referred to in a former lecture (p. 232, *et seq.*), may be cited as an example. Apropos of this case, I may observe that the patient having unexpectedly died a few days ago (it appears he swallowed an enormous dose of chloral which he secretly procured) the post-mortem examination was absolutely negative as regards the nervous centres, a fact plainly confirming the diagnosis.—J. M. C.

Porcz— the presence of hysterogenic points in the former constitutes the sole difference; in all other respects they are identical. But it may be said that the case of Pin—, more

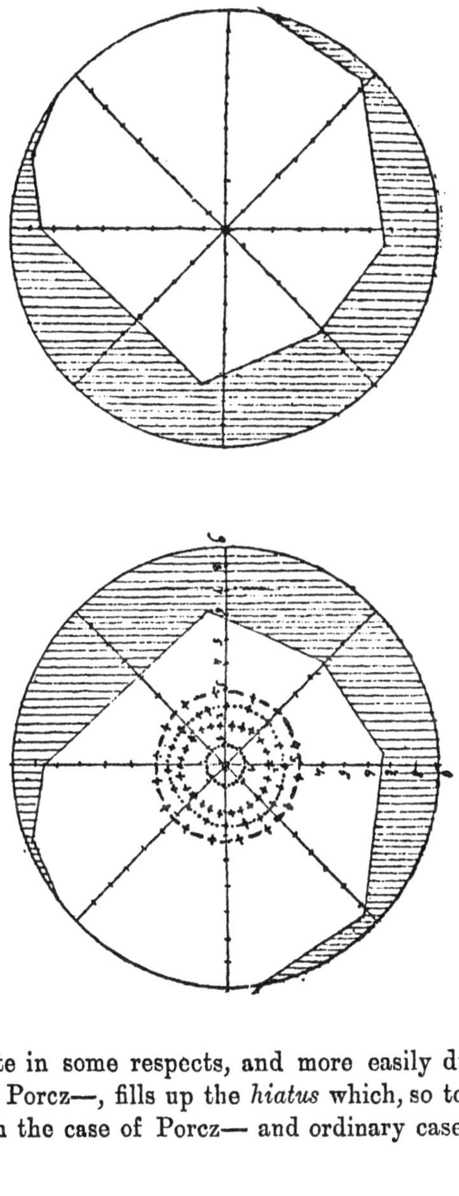

FIGS. 62 and 63.—Field of vision of Pin—.

.... green. + + + + blue. + . . + . . + . . + red. + — + — + — + white.

complete in some respects, and more easily diagnosed than that of Porcz—, fills up the *hiatus* which, so to speak, exists between the case of Porcz— and ordinary cases of hysteria.

It marks the transition, so that no part of the series is missing.

Here, then, are two examples of *hysterical brachial monoplegia of traumatic origin occurring in the male.*

I think that I have demonstrated that the brachial monoplegia supervening on an injury in the two men who formed the subjects of the preceding lectures, is of a hysterical nature.

The prognosis naturally follows from the diagnosis, and it is clear that it will be infinitely less grave in cases of this nature than in such as supervene on a destructive organic lesion. Without doubt, in our two patients, the paralysis, already of long standing, may persist, notwithstanding its hysterical nature, for months, or perhaps even years, especially if we do not intervene by means of appropriate therapeutic agents. Nevertheless the cure, we can safely affirm, will take place sooner or later, and our efforts ought to hasten the occurrence.

But how? According to what principles should the intervention take place? That is the question we have now to resolve. We may have recourse to the empirical measures which are resorted to in the treatment of hysteria—appropriate to rousing vital energies almost always depressed in such circumstances, such as the repeated application of æstheogenic means, and in particular static electricity, prolonged hydrotherapeutic appliances, &c. But these agents, which certainly ought not to be neglected, apply rather to the general condition, and, according to my experience, in so far as concerns the paralysis, their beneficial effects are long deferred. Certainly our interference will show itself with more effect if, instead of relying on empirical notions, it can be founded on a physiological basis; if, for example, we can recognise, at least in part, the mechanism of the production of traumatic hysterical paralysis.

This problem, bristling with difficulties of every kind, we must now proceed to face. I do not promise you, be it understood, a solution on all points, but in endeavouring to reach our aim we shall perhaps encounter glances at truths whose practical consequences ought not to be disdained. To arrive at the point to which I wish to lead you, I shall have to take a course apparently devious, and must return once more to a subject which has already occupied our attention.[1] I mean those remarkable paralyses which have been designated *psychical paralyses*, *paralyses depending on idea*, *paralyses by imagination* (*Paralyses durch Einbildung*). Now, observe, I do not say *imaginary paralyses*, for indeed these motor paralyses of psychical origin are as objectively real as those depending on an organic lesion; they simulate them, as you will soon see, by a number of identical clinical characters, which render their diagnosis very difficult.

Though they have been known for a long time, these paralyses were first investigated in a methodical and systematic manner in 1869 by Professor Russell Reynolds, in an excellent work treating of their etiology, their clinical characters, and their methods of treatment.[2] Their history still offers several obscure points. It is well known that in certain circumstances an *idea* may produce a paralysis, and conversely, that an *idea* may cause it to disappear; but between these two ultimate facts, many links remain obscure. Evidently this is a subject which would gain in clearness and precision if it could be submitted to experimental investigation.

Well, gentlemen, thanks to recent notions in relation to the science of hypnotic neurosis, it is possible to call in the aid of experiment in the study of cases of this kind. We know that in subjects in a state of hypnotic sleep it is possible—and this is a notorious fact now—to originate by the method of suggestion, or of intimation, an idea, or a coherent group of associated ideas, which possess the individual, and remain isolated, and manifest themselves by corresponding motor phenomena. If this be so, we know that if the idea suggested be one of paralysis, a real paralysis virtually ensues, and we see in such case that it will frequently manifest itself as accentuated as that arising from a destructive lesion of cerebral substance. These assertions I

[1] J. M. Charcot, 'Lezioni cliniche dell' anno scolastico, 1881-84; sulle malattie del sistema nervoso, redatte dal Dr. D. Miliotte.—Sulle paralis psichiche,' pp. 103—110, Milano, 1885.

[2] Russell Reynolds, "Remarks on Paralysis and other Disorders of Motion and Sensation dependent on Idea." Read to the Medical Section, Brit. Med. Assoc., Leeds, July, 1869; 'Brit. Med. Journ.,' Nov., 1869.

am about to try and justify by placing before you cases of paralysis produced by suggestion, and which we may consider as typical of psychical paralysis.

At the outset it is my duty to recall to your memory a certain number of facts with which our former studies have made you acquainted.[1] Bearing these facts in mind you will readily understand what follows. I would remind you that in the *lethargic* phase of what is called the *great hypnotism,* the mental inertia is so absolute that in general it is impossible to enter into relation with the hypnotised subject or to communicate any idea to him by any process whatever. But it is not thus in the other two phases of hypnotism. Thus in *catalepsy*—I speak here only of the true catalepsy, such I have described—certain phenomena of suggestion are easily obtained, and owing to their simplicity and their small tendency to become generalised, they are relatively easy of analysis. Here then, evidently, the study of hypnotic suggestions ought to commence. Here, as in the preceding phase, there is mental inertia, but it is less profound, less absolute; it has become possible, indeed, to produce a sort of partial waking in the organ of the psychic faculties. Thus, one can call into existence an idea, or a group of ideas connected together by previous associations. But this group set in action will remain strictly limited. There will be no propagation, no diffusion of the communicated movement; all the rest will remain asleep. Consequently the idea, or group of ideas suggested, are met with in a state of isolation, free from the control of that large collection of personal ideas long accumulated and organised, which constitute the conscience properly so-called, the *ego.* It is for this reason that the movements which exteriorly represent the acts of unconscious cerebration are distinguished by their automatic and purely mechanical character. Then it is truly that we see before us the *human machine* in all its simplicity, dreamt of by De la Mettrie.[2]

[1] J. M. Charcot, 'Essai d'une distinction nosographique des divers états nerveux compris sous le nom d'hypnotisme.' Note comm. à l'Académie des Sciences, 1883.—Id., 'Lezioni cliniche redatte dal Dr. Dom. Miliotti.—Sulle paralisi psichiche,' pp. 103—110, Milano, 1885.

[2] De la Mettrie, "L'homme machine," 'Œuvres philosophiques,' T. I,

In this cataleptic condition, in the greater number of individuals, the only means by which we can enter into relation with the person hypnotised is through the *muscular sense.* The gesture alone, or the attitude in which we put the subject, suggests to him the idea which we wish to transmit to him. By shutting, for example, his fists in an aggressive attitude, you observe the head carried backwards, and the forehead, the eyebrows, and the root of the nose become corrugated with a menacing expression. Or, again, if you place the tips of his stretched-out fingers on his mouth, then the lips relax, he smiles, and all the face assumes an expression of softness totally opposed to what it just manifested.

Having studied the influence of gesture on the physiognomy, we are also able, as M. Richer and myself have done,[1] to study the influence of physiognomy on gesture. But it is still to the muscular sense that the phenomena are due which are produced by the action of electricity on the diverse facial muscles, after the indications of Duchenne de Boulogne. If we determine, for instance, contraction of the *corrugator supercillii* (muscle of anger, D. de B.), you will observe the face suffused with anger, while the right arm is placed in an attitude of aggression, and the left in a position of defence. If, on the contrary, it is the zygomatic muscle (the muscle of laughter, D. de B.), which is excited, the expression of the physiognomy and the corresponding attitude are those pertaining to laughter. These phenomena, now indicated summarily, I have already brought under your cognisance.[2] But the feature to which I specially wish to call your attention at present is the way in which each impression thus originated by the intermediation of the muscular sense remains isolated without diffusion, and fixed,

Amsterdam, 1765; see also T. II, "L'homme plante. L'homme plus que machine."

[1] J. M. Charcot and P. Richer, "Note on certain facts of Cerebral Automatism, &c.: suggestion by the Muscular Sense," 'Journal of Nervous and Mental Diseases,' vol. x, No. 1, January, 1883; see also Bertrand, "Deux lois psycho-physiologiques," 'Revue Philosophique,' pp. 244, 245, No. 3, March, 1884.

[2] J. M. Charcot, 'Lezioni Cliniche,' loc. cit., p. 103.

so to speak, during all the time that the muscular action maintains the members in the expressive attitude artificially produced.

We now come to the third phase, the *somnambulic*, which is the only one that will engage our attention to-day. We have here to do solely with a state of obnubilation, mental torpor more or less accentuated. Here, again, without doubt, the awakening determined by suggestion remains partial, but the number of elements called into operation is less limited than in the preceding case, and frequently a diffusion occurs of the induced psychical phenomena sufficiently extensive to manifest a certain tendency to the reconstitution of the *ego*. Hence, it sometimes happens under these circumstances that the injunction, the suggestion, becomes the occasion of a certain amount of resistance on the part of the subject. In all cases this yields to a little insistance. Nevertheless, it does not always do so without a preliminary discussion. Let me add that the movements in connection with the ideas suggested are consequently often very complex; they have not, therefore, that character of mechanical precision which they present in the preceding form; on the contrary, they assume the likeness of voluntary acts, more or less premeditated, even to the extent of leading one astray.

Further, in the somnambulic stage all the senses are intact, and it may be said, indeed, that although the conscience is in abeyance, the sensibility to communicated impressions is exalted. It consequently becomes easier to enter in relation by diverse means with the hypnotised person. If he be urged to look at some object, the simple view of that object will arouse in that patient a certain number of ideas associated with the nature of the object, and those ideas will manifest themselves objectively in the form of corresponding acts. If, by significant gestures, an object or an animal is figured in space, that animal or that imaginary object will appear to the eyes of the hypnotised person as real, and will call into action a corresponding series of ideas and movements. And again, in a manner still more perfect, suggestion can be effected by the aid of speech, either alone, or better, combined with gestures.

This is enough, gentlemen, to remind you in a general

way of the chief characters of hypnotic suggestion in the somnambulic period, and how unlimited our power is in this domain, for really we can vary our action almost without end. Hence you will not be surprised to find that, in suggesting to a somnambulistic subject the idea of a morbid state, for example motor paralysis of the extremities, the paralysis becomes objectively manifest, and thus lends itself to our clinical investigation.

I would remark, and this is a point interesting in the highest degree, that that paralysis which we can make by the aid of suggestion, we are able at will to modify both in degree and character up to a certain point, and to unmake it equally well by suggestion. One can therefore anticipate that the study of paralysis thus artificially produced may one day be employed to elucidate the whole group of psychical paralysis.

After these preliminary remarks we may proceed to the demonstration of facts. The hysterical girl, Greuz—, who is now before you, presents on the left side the usual complete hemianæsthesia; on the right side there is no appreciable perversion of sensibility. We shall be able, then, on this side, easily to observe any perversion of sensibility which may occur during the evolution of the perversions of motor power which we are about to provoke. I may inform you in passing that this girl has been subjected only four or five times to the influence of hypnotism, so that in her case there is wanting the influence of training [entraînement], produced in subjects frequently hypnotised. Further, I can assure you that the phenomena which you notice to-day are exactly the same as in our first experiment.

Greuz— is put into a somnambulic state by means of slight pressure exercised on the eyeballs for a few seconds. The peculiar rigidity of the members which you observe produced by light touches over their surface, or even by movements performed at a distance (somnambulic contracture), is of a somatic nature which, as you know, enables us to appreciate when the sleep is well established. Then, in order to determine the production of the phenomena which we have purposed studying, I proceed by affirming in a loud voice,

"Your right hand is paralysed," saying to the patient in a tone of conviction, "You cannot move any part of it, it hangs by your side." The patient demurs to some extent.[1] "But no," she replies, "you are mistaken. My hand is not in the least paralysed, you see I move it." And really she does move it, though very feebly. Then I insist, and always with an accent of authority. I repeat a certain number of times my first affirmation. You notice that after a few minutes' discussion the paralysis is definitely established. Now we have really produced a brachial monoplegia whose clinical characters we must minutely study, for perhaps this monoplegia is allied to that referred to in our last lectures in the case of two hysterical men, Porcz— and Pin—. This we intend to do.

The motor paralysis which we produce in Greuz— by hypnotic suggestion is, as you can see for yourselves, absolute and complete. The right upper extremity in its entirety is flaccid and hangs by the side. There is no trace of rigidity in any of the joints. It falls heavily down after being raised for a second. The patient is unable to move the arm in any manner, nor can she flex the wrist or the fingers. Hence in this limb all active movement is abolished, as also all resistance to passive movements. No muscle, I repeat, manifests the slightest contraction, no matter what efforts are made by the patient at our solicitation.

Moreover, the sensibility, recently normal, has now completely disappeared in the whole extent of the limb. You can prove that the anæsthesia has even invaded the region of the shoulder and a portion of the right side of the chest. It not only affects the skin, but the deeper structures, viz. the muscles, the trunks of the nerves, the ligaments, &c. Thus, as you see, the most violent torsion of the joints may be practised without feeling, and faradization of the nerve trunks to such an extent as to cause violent contraction of the muscles can be effected without determining the slightest facial expression of pain or of any sensation whatever. The tendon-reflexes of the wrist and elbow-joint are very notably enfeebled.

[1] Other subjects submit to the suggestion without protest; there are numerous individual varieties in this respect.

Lastly, as far as regards the muscular sense, the former existence of which I took care you should recognise, you see that it is now completely wanting. The patient, when a screen is placed before her eyes, is unable to find with the left hand any spot whatever indicated on the right, and she has no notion whatever of the movements which we impart to the various articulations of the limb.

In short, we have here to deal with a complete monoplegic paralysis characterised by absolute flaccidity of all the parts, cutaneous and deep anæsthesia occupying the whole extent of the limb and extending even beyond, enfeeblement of the tendon-reflexes, and total loss of the muscular sense. These clinical characters, you will at once recognise, are exactly those disclosed in our patient Pin— when he entered our wards, and which now exist in the case of Porcz—, with this *sole difference,* evidently of a secondary order, that in the latter *motion and sensibility are preserved* in the fingers.

LECTURE XXII.

ON TWO CASES OF HYSTERICAL BRACHIAL MONOPLEGIA IN THE MALE (*continued*).[1]

SUMMARY.—*Production of a monoplegia of the whole upper extremity in a hysterical subject by* suggestion; *its disappearance effected by the employment of similar means.—Production of paralysis of the different segments successively in the upper extremity of the same patient (shoulder, elbow, wrist, fingers).—The sensation and tendon-reflexes disappear simultaneously in the parts attacked with paralysis.—Monoplegia can be artificially determined in a hypnotic by a blow on the shoulder (traumatic suggestion).—Repetition of the same phenomena in an hysterical subject awake, but in a natural and permanent condition of hypnotism.*

Remarks on the treatment of two men affected with brachial monoplegia; hydrotherapy; static electricity; special exercise.—Mode of action of this last agent; psychic motor images.—Good results of treatment.

GENTLEMEN,—We are now furnished with incontestable and very valuable information. But we are enabled to push the analysis still further. Thus, instead of paralysing the whole member by one stroke, we can paralyse it partially, segment by segment, and by these successive operations we can more thoroughly investigate the essence of the phenomena.

In order to do this we must in the first place, if you will allow me to use the expression, "deparalyse" our patient. It suffices for this that we destroy the effects of the initial

[1] Lecture edited by MM. P. Marie, chef de clinique, and Geo. Guinon, interne du service.

suggestion by the intermediation of a new suggestion of an opposite nature. I therefore assure Greuz— that her arm has ceased to be paralysed, that she can move the limb as well as ever. You notice that after a few minutes' discussion the member assumes all its normal functions in respect not only of its mobility, but all forms of sensibility.

And then proceeding successively to paralyse segments of the member, in the first place I suggest the idea to the patient that she is unable to move the *shoulder-joint*, and forthwith she is in reality unable to move it in any direction, while she freely moves all the other joints, viz. the elbow, the wrist, and the fingers. Moreover, in every part where voluntary movement is abolished, and there only, observe that there is not only cutaneous but deep insensibility; thus, in the region of the shoulder, pricking, faradic excitation, &c., are not felt; movements of torsion and extension, however violent, at the scapulo-humeral articulation occasion no pain. All the impressions derived from the muscular sense relative to passive movements of this articulation are likewise completely wanting.

It will not be without interest to consider briefly the extent and limits of that anæsthesia (Figs. 64 and 65, A). The insensible portion represents a sort of plate moulded over the shoulder, similar to the sixteenth century piece of armour designed to protect that region. Superiorly the line which limits the anæsthesia commences at the level of the base of the neck; it extends anteriorly almost to the external border of the sternum, involving the superior third of the breast, and is directed obliquely towards the axilla, affecting its entire extent, and prolonged for four or five fingers' breadth along the axillary portion of the thoracic region. Behind (A′) it takes almost a vertical direction from the base of the neck to about three or four fingers' breadth above the angle of the scapula. In the transverse direction it extends to within four or five fingers' breadth of the spinous processes. The arm is almost entirely encased, to continue the metaphor, in an anæsthetic armulet.

I wish particularly to call your attention to the singular manner in which the anæsthesia is limited below. You observe that the line determined by successive prickings is very distinctly circular. It forms a line at right angles to the axis of the limb, about two inches above the flexure of the elbow in front, and passing behind just above the superior extremity of the olecranon process.[1]

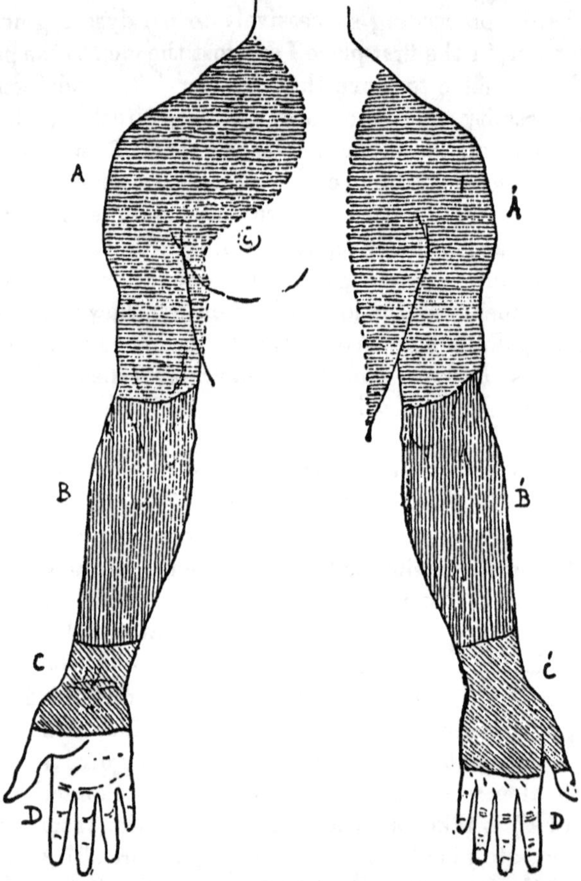

Figs. 64 and 65.—Case of Greuz—.

Such is the anæsthetic region corresponding to the isolated paralysis of the shoulder. We shall now see that this condition is capable of being modified by the same procedure of suggestion which we have just employed; and we now deter-

[1] *Vide* note 5, p. 282.

mine paralysis of the movements of the *elbow*. As soon as the motor paralysis of this joint becomes complete you will observe that the zone of anæsthesia extends lower down and involves not only the shoulder and the arm, but the elbow

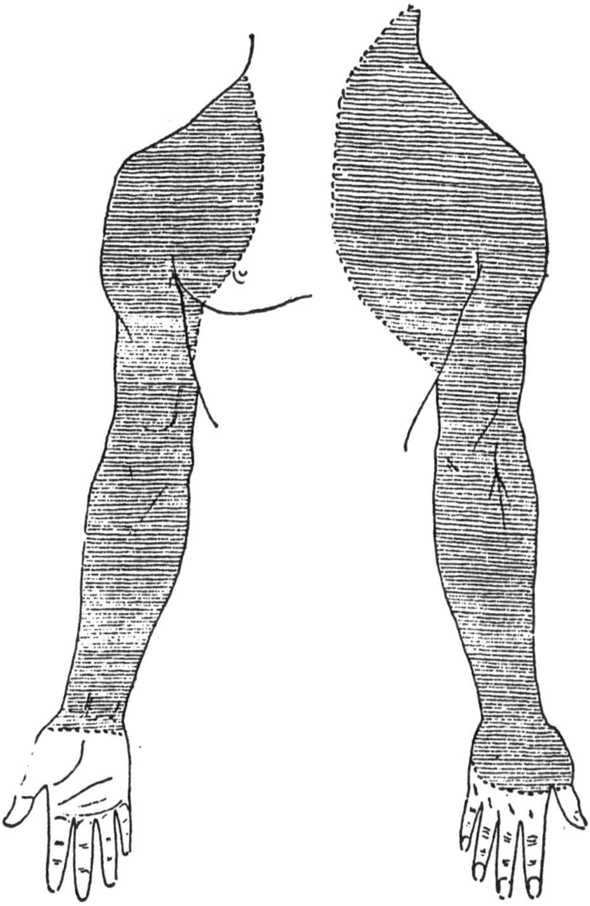

FIGS. 66 and 67.—Case of Porcz—.

and the forearm. Its inferior limit is formed by a circular horizontal line, situated about two inches above the wrist-joint, and forming a plane at right angles to the long axis of the extremity (Figs. 64 and 65, B, B′).

Let us pass now to another segment, that of the *wrist.* Here again, in consequence of a new suggestion analogous to the preceding, the paralysis creeps onward and the patient is now unable to move her shoulder, her elbow-joint, and her

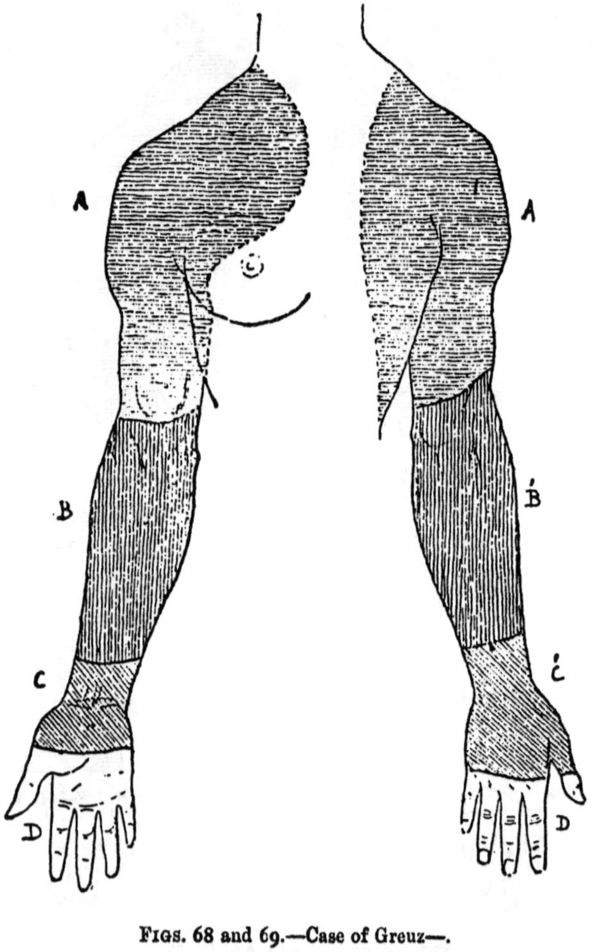

FIGS. 68 and 69.—Case of Greuz—.

wrist, she is only able to move the fingers of her hand. In consequence, the inferior limit of the anæsthetic zone is again displaced (Figs. 64 and 65, C, C′). You can satisfy yourselves now that it is limited anteriorly by a horizontal line across the hand in a transverse direction almost on the level of the metacarpo-phalangeal articulation of the thumb ; behind, the limit extends lower down than in front, and is situated only a few millimetres above the line formed by the heads of the

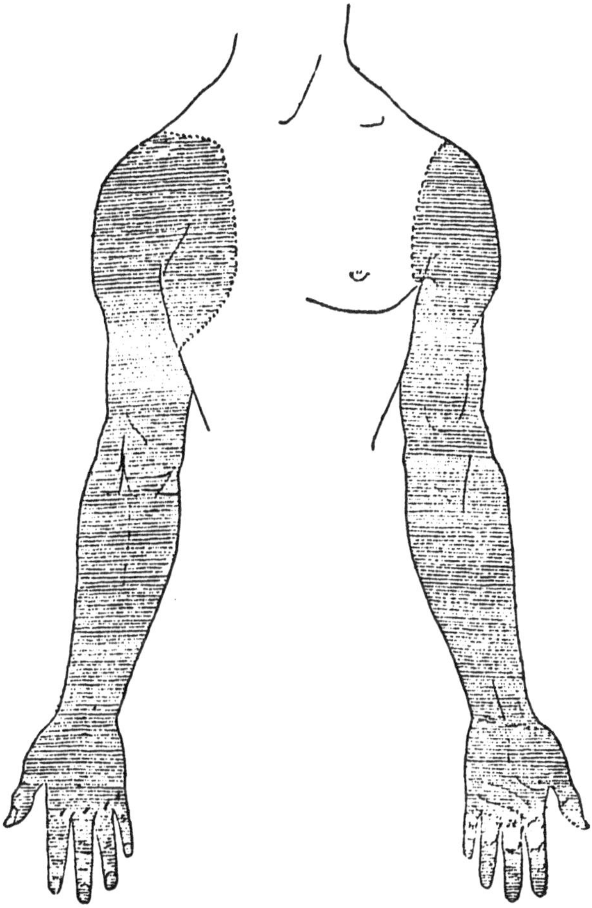

FIGS. 70 and 71.—Case of Pin—.

metacarpal bones, and on the back of the thumb at the level of the articulation uniting its two phalanges.

But, gentlemen, you have doubtless remarked that the paralysis which we have now determined in Greuz— by a series of successive suggestions, reproduces in its minutest details the clinical characters presented by the monoplegia of our patient Porcz—. Indeed, in the two cases it is actually the same segments of the superior extremity, the shoulder, the elbow, and the wrist that are affected with motor paralysis, the movements of the fingers remaining intact. And equally in the two cases, wherever the paralysis of movement exists there is cutaneous and deep anæsthesia, and loss of the muscular sense; whereas the fingers, where the motor power remains, present no perversion of sensibility. Truly, the imitation which we have obtained is perfect; it extends, I repeat, to the minutest details. You can convince yourselves of this by the aid of these figures which I submit to you, and by comparison of the anæsthetic territory in our hypnotised subject, and in our patient Porcz—. You observe that these territories have the same extent, present the same configuration; I might say that they are *superposable* (Figs. 64 and 65, and Figs. 66 and 67).

That is no doubt remarkable; but we can go further, and complete in Greuz— the monoplegia by determining, by suggestion, motor paralysis in the fingers, which, as you will observe, is immediately followed by a loss of all kinds of sensibility in the parts. And now we have a paralysis artificially produced invading all the parts, and involving perversion of sensibility as well as perversion of movement which are exactly identical with the monoplegia observed in our second case, that of the patient Pin— (Figs. 70 and 71). *We have been able, then, to obtain artificially in our hypnotised patient by means of suggestion, a perfect imitation of the monoplegia caused in our two other patients by a process apparently very different, the action of traumatism.*

Not to lose sight of the principal object in view in this series of lectures, I will return in a moment to the important results which we have realised. At present I desire to demonstrate a few more facts relating to the hypnotic suggestion, in order to fix in your minds those which we have already gathered, and to convince you moreover that these facts are not accidental (forming an appendage to a subject unique of its kind), but that they may on the contrary be reproduced with absolutely the same features in a certain number of cases.

In the first place I will proceed to "*unmake*" the artificial paralysis of Greuz—; operating segment by segment, as I recently did in producing it, only now I proceed inversely, that is to say, beginning with the hand, taking in turn the wrist, the elbow, and the shoulder successively. At each step of the operation you can prove once more that the mode of distribution of the anæsthesia corresponds to each segment of the motor paralysis.

In another hysterical subject named Mesl— I am about to repeat all the phenomena that have been produced in Greuz—. Mesl— is hemianæsthetic on the right side, it is therefore on the left superior extremity that I am obliged to operate. The results which follow, as you observe, are exactly the counterpart of those described in the case of Greuz—. An identical result has been obtained in the case of other hemianæsthetic "hysterics" whom we recently investigated in our wards, and whose cases I might present to you did time permit.

In subjects of this kind the paralysis of the non-anæsthetic member, determined by suggestion, is always accompanied by anæsthesia, cutaneous and deep, loss of the muscular sense, and finally the diminution or abolition of the tendon-reflexes in the segments of the member affected with motor paralysis.[1]

However, I would further remark that we are able even in hemianæsthetic "hysterics," to obtain motor paralysis without any perversion of sensibility. It suffices to accomplish this, as I have many times seen, to persuade the subject at the moment when the suggestion is made, that movement *alone* will be lost, and that the sensibility will remain intact. I do not wish to generalise too hastily with reference to experiments not yet very numerous, but I am bound to mention that hitherto I have not observed any variation in the hemianæsthetic "hysterics" to whom I suggested *purely* and *simply* the motor paralysis of the member, *without saying anything of sensibility*. I am not considering at present the cases of non-anæsthetic "hysterics."[2]

[1] This fact is not constant; the tendon-reflexes are sometimes manifestly exaggerated.

[2] Compare also Appendix II.

That will suffice for the present on this subject, and I must now revert to the principal object of to-day's investigation. You perceive that the monoplegia of our two male patients Porcz— and Pin—, and the condition designedly produced in the hysterical patients are, so far as relates to clinical features, not only comparable to one another, but really perfectly identical; motor paralysis with flaccidity of the parts, cutaneous and deep insensibility, the delimitation of the anæsthesia by circular planes at right angles to the long axis of the limb,[1] the loss or impairment of tendon-reflexes, and the abolition of all notions of the muscular sense. The syndrome is, in the two cases, absolutely identical.

There is, however, a difference on one point which at first sight appears very essential, namely, the mode of production of the paralysis. In the case of our two male patients you have not forgotten that the cause was traumatic, a *blow* more or less violent on the shoulder; while in the case of our hypnotised females it was *suggestion by speech* which occasioned the paralysis. This difference, apparently so essential, can be made to disappear. For, as a matter of fact, we can cause in our "hysterics," re-hypnotised, all the paralytic phenomena first obtained, *not now by means of a verbal injunction, but through an agency analogous to that which occasioned the monoplegia both in the case of Pin— and Porcz—, viz. a shock applied on the posterior part of the shoulder*, by sharply, yet not very forcibly, striking this region with the palm of the hand. The result is, you see, not long in appearing. Immediately the patient starts, emits a cry, and being interrogated as to what she feels, she states that she experiences in the whole extent of the extremity a sensation of enervation, of weight and feebleness; it seems, she says, as if *the member struck did not belong to her, that it had become strange to her*. And then we find that the paralysis is really established. It attains its maximum at the very outset, and presents all the clinical features with which you are familiar.

In this way the resemblance between the two kinds of cases which we are comparing is strikingly complete even in its causal bearings. Without doubt in our two male

[1] See note 5, p. 282.

patients—in the case of the coachman when he fell from the cab, and the mason when he fell from the window—the material shock was much more energetic; but this simply amounts to a question of quantity, not to a generic difference, of such a nature that it may be attributed to the varying degree of impressionability of the subjects. Without doubt the two men were not at the moment of their fall in a hypnotic sleep, nor subsequently, when the paralysis was definitely established. But in this respect it may be inquired whether the mental condition occasioned by the emotion, by the Nervous Shock experienced at the moment of the accident and for some time after, is not equivalent in a certain measure, in subjects predisposed as Porcz— and Pin— were, to the cerebral condition which is determined in "hysterics" by hypnotism.[1] Upon the assumption of this hypothesis, the peculiar sensation felt by our hysterical females in the member submitted to shock, and which we may suppose to have been produced in the same degree and with the same characters in our two male patients by a fall on the shoulder, that sensation, I say, may be considered as having originated, in the former as in the latter, the idea of motor paralysis of the member. But because of the annihilation of the *ego* produced by the hypnotism in the one case, and, as one may suppose, by the nervous shock in the other, that idea once installed in the brain takes sole possession and acquires sufficient domination to realise itself objectively in the form of paralysis. The sensation, in question, therefore, in both the cases plays the part of a veritable *suggestion*.[2]

[1] It is very probable that, by a mechanism of this nature, most of the various nervous affections become developed which are frequently so obstinate (although not connected with any organic lesion), and which our English and American colleagues have studied under the names of "Railway Spine" and "Railway Brain." The same mechanism was alluded to when I was directing your attention (in a preceding lecture, p. 221 *et seq.*) to the influence exercised by material shocks, in those predisposed, in the production of hysterical manifestations even in the male.

[2] So far as concerns the sensations produced by the shock, our two male patients are unable to enlighten us. The one, Pin—, in falling instantly lost consciousness; the other, Porcz—, asserts that he was conscious. Neither the one nor the other knows exactly how the affected member felt at the moment of the accident, nor for some days afterwards. We know that on

I give you, gentlemen, that explanation for what it is worth, and without attaching to it more importance than it merits. However, I believe it worthy of being more closely examined, and tested by more numerous observations. And in the meantime I may be allowed to mention additional evidence which seems to me to plead in its favour.

There are subjects, and perhaps they are more numerous than one thinks, in whom most of the manifestations of hypnotism, both psychic and somatic, may be encountered in the waking state, without the necessary intervention of hypnotic practices. It appears that the hypnotic condition which in the case of others is an artificial state, may be for those singular beings an ordinary one, their normal condition. These individuals *sleep*, if you will allow the term, while they appear perfectly awake. They comport themselves in ordinary life as in a dream, treating as parallel the objective reality and the dream imposed on them, at least they make hardly any difference between the two.

I submit for your examination, as an example, a subject of this kind. I refer to a hystero-epileptic patient well known to you through former investigations, the woman Hab—.[1] For many years this patient has been affected with general anæsthesia of a permanent and complete nature, and with Attacks which from every point of view correspond to the classical type. You notice that, although no hypnotic manœuvre has been resorted to, and hence she is presumably in a waking state, we can obtain contraction by pressure exercised on the muscles, on the tendons, or the nerve-trunks (lethargic contraction); and cataleptic immobility of the extremities placed in the most diverse positions; and likewise, by means of light stroking or movements at a distance, somnambulic contraction. All these somatic phenomena occur in this subject commingled as it were at the same moment, without distinction into periods, contrary to what obtains in *great hypnotism*. But from the psychical point of

being awakened, no matter how slight the hypnotism may have been, hypnotised subjects retain no consciousness of what took place during that state.

[1] J. M. Charcot, 'Lezioni Cliniche, &c.,' redatte dal Dr. Miliotti, Lez. 20, p. 159, "Dello Stato di malo Istero-Epileptico."

view they are evidently the features of the somnambulic state which predominate. Well, if proceeding by *verbal suggestion* we affirm to this patient, not asleep, I repeat, that her right arm is paralysed, that she is not able to move it voluntarily, we see that immediately flaccid monoplegia is effectively produced, endowed with all the characteristics with which we are familiar; after which the simple affirmation that she is able to move her arm, just paralysed, suffices to re-establish voluntary movement. Finally, and this is a point specially interesting at present, by the operation of that kind of *traumatic suggestion* to which I referred a short time ago, and which consists in the application of a blow sharply applied to the shoulder, you notice that immediately the member becomes paralysed anew. This time the identity between the monoplegia artificially produced and the monoplegia originating in the cases of Porcz— and Pin— as the result of traumatism can hardly be contested, as it appears to me. Not only from the symptomalogical, but from the pathological point of view, the similarity is as perfect as it can be, for neither in the one case nor the other is there the intervention of the hypnotic practices—everything happens in the *state of waking*. The demonstration, if I mistake not, is sufficiently convincing, and I do not believe that in any experimental physiologico-pathological research whatever is it often possible to reproduce artificially with more fidelity an affection which it is desired to study and investigate.

These considerations, gentlemen, have not a purely speculative import; they have already furnished us with certain practical deductions which, especially from the therapeutic point of view are, as you will see, of some utility.

Our two patients, Porcz— and Pin—, have been subjected for some days to a regular treatment, on which I will say a few words. The treatment consists of two elements. On the one hand, it is in a sense indirect, in that it relates either to the general state or to the hysterical diathesis. Twice a day Pin— receives a general cold douche; Porcz— not being able to sustain the douche, takes a sulphur bath three times a week. Every other day both are treated with static electricity. This agent is useful, as you know, to modify perversions of sensibility. Experience has for a long time taught us that, as a consequence of an electro-static bath, sensibility, in most cases of hysterical anæsthesia, reappears, at first for a time, for some hours perhaps, then according as the baths are repeated, for a longer period, for several days, for example; and finally by the continuation of treatment it becomes re-established in a definite manner. Further, at the same time that a more or less durable return of the sensibility takes place, the other hysterical phenomena, the attacks, for example, are favorably modified, or disappear.[1]

But I wish specially to call your attention to the second part of our treatment; it is based on that idea which we have just been discussing, viz. that in our two patients the paralysis may have been caused by a mechanism analogous to that which in the "hypnotics" determined paralysis by suggestion. The various attempts at hypnotization which we made in these two men, and which, if they had succeeded, would have singularly lightened our task, being unsuccessful, we were constrained to adopt the following means. In the first place we acted, and continue to act every day on their minds as much as possible, affirming in a positive manner a fact of which we are ourselves perfectly convinced—that their paralysis, in spite of its long duration, is not incurable, and that, on the contrary, it will certainly be cured by means of appropriate treatment, at the end possibly of some weeks, if they would only be good enough to aid us.[2] In

[1] J. M. Charcot, "De l'Emploi de l'Électricité Statique en Médecine." Conférence faite à l'Hospice de la Salpêtrière, le 26 Dec., 1880. 'Revue de Médecine,' 1881, T. I, p. 147.

[2] The influence of mental impression on movement, says Maudsley ('Le corps et l'esprit,' p. 269), is shown in the sudden cure of imaginary (?) paralysis by energetic injunction. In these cases the idea of movement, the belief that it will take place, is, in the inner conscience, the movement itself. It is the active nervous current which, directed on the appropriate nerves, really causes external movement.—The idea of a particular movement, says Müller, determines a nervous current towards the affected muscles, and produces their contraction. We know that a sudden injunction sometimes determines the cure of a psychical paralysis of long standing, and which may have resisted the most varied therapeutic agencies. Thus, for example, a patient is forcibly made to leave her bed, in which she may have long remained motionless from a paraplegia of this kind; and being placed on

the second place the affected members were submitted to methodical exercise. We availed ourselves of the voluntary movements which still subsisted, though in a feeble degree, in the two patients, and we endeavoured to progressively augment the energy of these by a very simple method. A dynamometer was placed in the hand of each of them, and they were exhorted to squeeze it with all their power, and to progressively increase the figure indicated by the needle of the instrument. This exercise was regularly repeated every hour of the day for three or four days. These attempts must not be too prolonged, nor too frequently repeated. We have noticed that when the exercise is excessive, or too frequently repeated, the maximum figure reached by the needle declines. It is necessary then to have patience; an excess of zeal would, I am convinced, result in fatigue, and thus retard the expected result.

Here we act *psychically*. It is well known, unless I am mistaken, that the production of an image, or of a mental representation, no matter how summary or rudimentary it may be of the movement to be executed, is an indispensable preliminary condition to the execution of that movement.[1]

her feet, she is told to "walk," and forthwith she walks. Here we have an example of a "miraculous" cure which explains many others. There is nothing better established than these facts, to which I have frequently borne testimony ('Leçons sur les Maladies du Système Nerveux,' T. I, 3e édit., p. 356, et suiv.:—P. Janet, 'Revue Politique et Litteraire,' No. du 2 Août, 1884, p. 131). Nevertheless, we cannot be too guarded, even with the very best intentions, against assuming the part of a miracle-worker, for even in a case of psychical paralysis of an undoubted nature injunction is a remedy, the mechanism of which we know little. Failure would compromise the authority of the operator, and subject him to ridicule. "Never prophesy unless you are sure," say the English. To proceed by a slow and progressive method of mental training will always be more prudent, and often more efficacious.—J. M. C.

[1] *Synonyms:* Idea or conception of the kind of movement to execute, (James Mill); Ideal recall of the movement to be executed (Bain); Motor intuition (Maudsley); Locomotor faculty (W. Hamilton); Mental representation of the movement to be executed (Spencer); Sentiment of innervation (Wundt, Meynert). See also James Mill; Bain, 'Senses and Intellect,' p. 411; Spencer, 'Psychology,' vol. i, and 'First Principles,' pp. 216 and 497; H. Jackson, "Clinical and Physiological Researches on the Nervous System" (reprints from the 'Lancet,' 1873, p. 216); Ribot, 'Philosophie Anglaise,' p. 280; Maudsley, 'Physiology of Mind,' p. 250; Wundt, 'Physiolog.,'

But it is probable that, in the case of our two male patients, the conditions which normally preside over the representation of the mental image have been so seriously affected as to render its formation impossible, or at least very difficult, in consequence of an inhibitory action exercised over the cortical motor centres by the fixed idea of motor weakness. It is to that circumstance that the objective realisation of the paralysis is greatly due.[1] If this be so, we can readily conceive that the repetition of the dynamometric exercise would tend to revive in the centres the motor representation, which is a necessary preliminary to the voluntary movement; and that, as we have seen, these movements tend to become more and more energetic, according as they are repeated. Frictions, massage, passive movements of the paralysed limb and those determined by faradization, all such means, I say, act in the same sense, and may be employed at the commencement of the treatment when the motor paralysis is complete.

Be this as it may as to theory, the treatment we have adopted, although in operation but for three or four days, has already given encouraging results.

Thus in the case of Porcz— the dynamometric indication has increased in that short space of time in a remarkable manner. The instrument indicated but 15 K at the commencement of the treatment, and you notice to-day that the figure 40 K is attained. I should like you to remark, in passing, the depressing influence that the closing of the eyes exercises in the case of Pin— as to the force developed. The figure obtained when his eyes are shut is always 8 K. or 10 K. below that obtained when, the eyes being open, he receives a visual image of the movement accomplished. Hence, to profit by the dynamogenic influence of the visual on the motor centre, we advise our patients to attentively regard the hand during operations with the dynamometer.[2]

p. 447; Ferrier, 'Functions of the Brain,' chap. xi; C. Bastian, 'Brain the Organ of the Mind,' vol. ii, pp. 165, 171—176, 196, and Appendix, p. 278; Stricker, 'Studien ueber de Sprachvorstellungen,' Wien, 1883; Ribot, 'Revue philosoph.,' No. 8, Août, 1883, p. 188; Herzen, 'The Journal of Mental Science,' April, 1884, p. 44.

[1] See Appendix II at end of this volume.

[2] On the dynamogenic influence of sensorial and sensitive excitations, see

Analogous results have been obtained in the case of Porcz—, notwithstanding that in him motor power was more affected than in Pin—, voluntary movement being entirely abolished in the shoulder, the elbow, and the wrist, and very

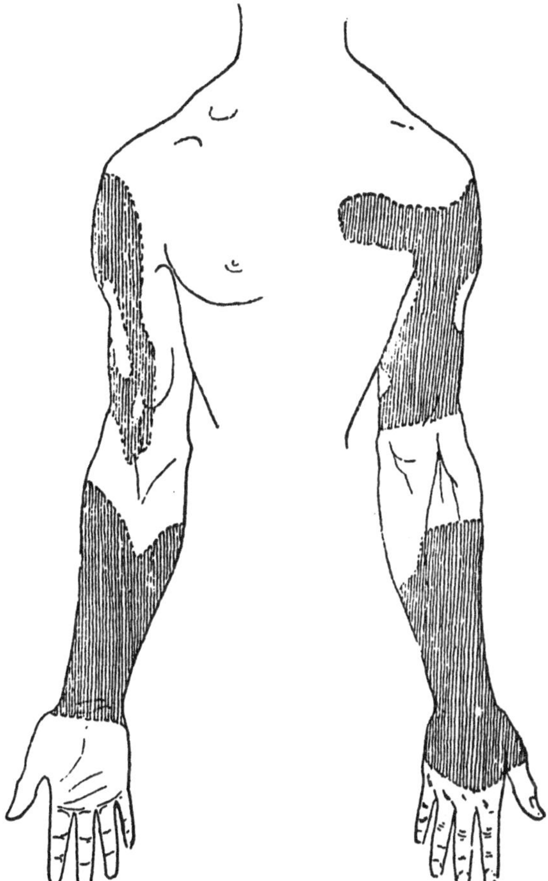

FIGS. 72 and 73.—Case of Porcz—, July 7th.

feeble in the fingers. So far as concerns the large articulations, the paralysis remains the same when the muscular

M. Féré's researches ('Bulletin de la Société de Biologie,' Avril, Mai, Juin, Juillet, 1885; 'Brain,' July, 1885; 'Revue Philosophique,' Octobre, 1885).

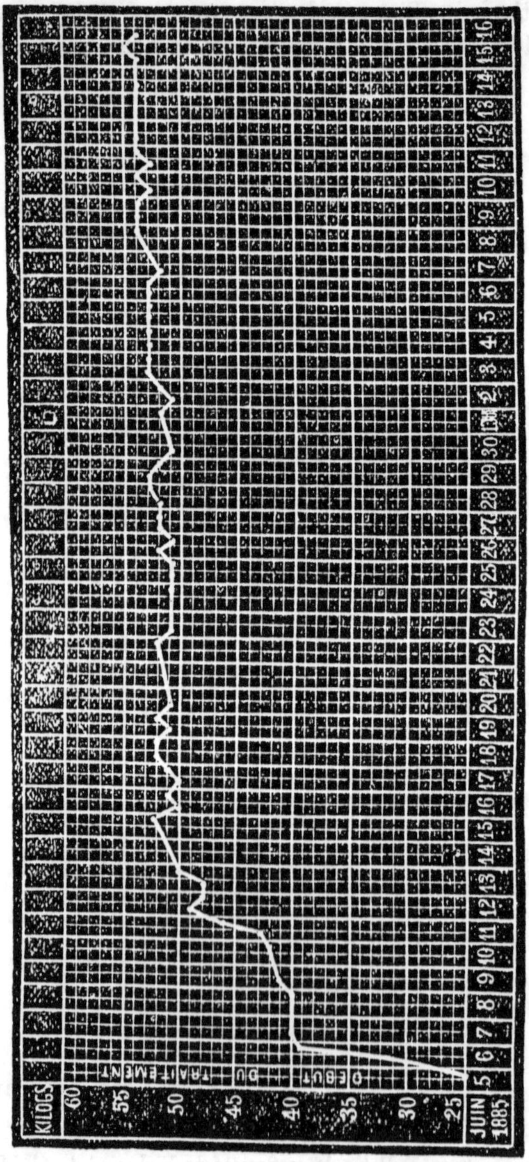

Fig. 74.—Case of Pin—, June 5th to July 16th.

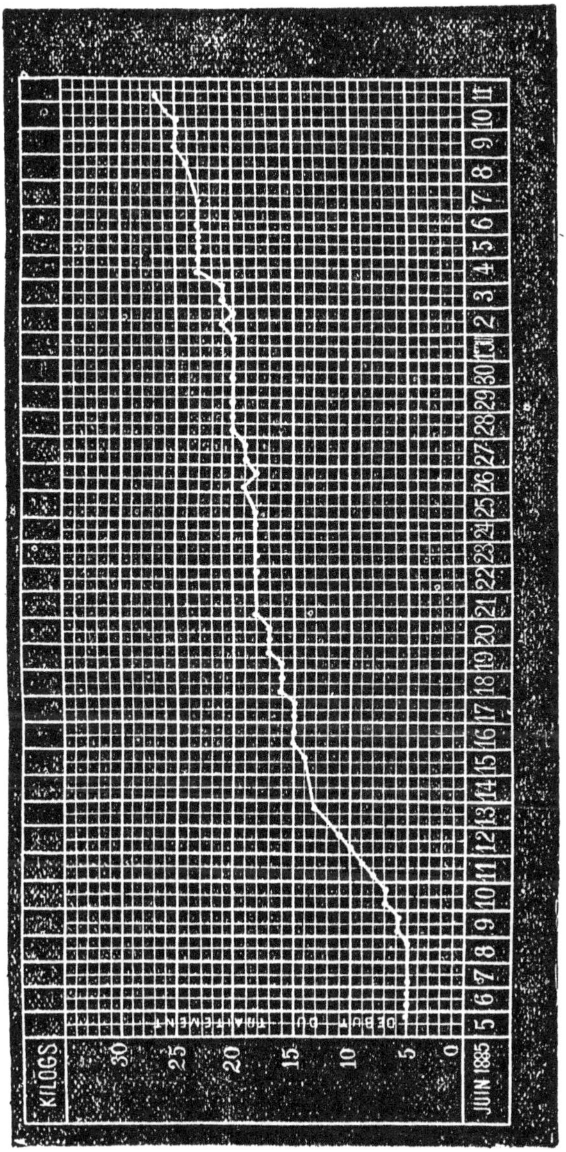

FIG. 75.—Case of Porcz—, from June 5th to July 11th.

groups which move those joints are called into action separately.

But the patient having several times repeated in our presence the dynamometric exercise, we have observed that on each occasion the muscles which move the large articulations have a tendency to contract at the same time. When the patient presses the dynamometer, these muscles appear under the skin in marked relief. At this moment you can observe that the wrist becomes flexed when the fingers press the instrument, and how it presents a marked resistance to passive movements of flexion or extension.

These results, however imperfect they may be, are meanwhile of such a nature as to encourage us in following this course. I make bold to hope that in a few days—say fifteen, or perhaps a month—we shall have made substantial progress.

This lecture was delivered on May 29, 1885. And subsequently when speaking incidentally of the two patients under treatment, M. Charcot continued as follows:

I am happy to be able to show you such progress as has been made in our two hysterical male patients during the past eight days, in consequence of the treatment adopted. In the case of Pin—, though matters move slowly, the progress is very real. Thus, eight days ago the maximum dynamometric figure was 40 K; to-day it is 53 K. And at the same time as the dynamometric force is augmented, cutaneous sensibility is restored, to a limited extent it is true, at the level of the shoulder.

In the case of Porcz—, during the past week the needle of the dynamometer did not indicate beyond 5 K. This week we have gained somewhat, for on one occasion the figure 13 K has been attained. Besides, cutaneous sensibility is reappearing in the armpit and at the flexure of the elbow. At the same time the patient appears to appreciate the notion of position of the member where the parts have become sensitive. You see therefore that our anticipations seem likely to be realised. It will not be without interest to follow closely the changes which will doubtless occur in our patients, under the influence of more prolonged treatment.

These modifications we have followed step by step. Each day the results of pressure exercised on the dynamometer are registered hour by hour; and the progress realised in the sensibility is noted daily. From the latter point of view the condition is now almost stationary in the case of Pin—, and to-day, the 16th of July, there exist only two small areæ of sensibility on the posterior aspect of the arm. On the other hand favorable results have been realised in respect of mobility. In order to realise the progress better, the figures obtained by the dynamometer, are daily noted in the morning and in the evening (Fig. 74), so as to form a chart.

It will be observed that during the first week of treatment (commencing on the 5th of June), the increase of force was rapid and considerable, when the figure increased from 25 K to 49 K. In the course of the following fifteen days the average oscillation was between 50 K and 52 K. Eight days subsequently it attained to 53 K, and finally from the 3rd till the 17th July it attained to the average figure of between 54 K and 55 K.

We know that in the case of Porcz—, the cutaneous anæsthesia was absolute at the commencement of the treatment (5th June) over the whole extent of the member, the hand excepted (*vide* Figs. 66 and 67, p. 299). Eight or ten days subsequently it began to reappear at the flexure of the elbow and in the armpit. On the 7th of July the condition was as follows (Figs. 72 and 73, p. 311). Sensibility had reappeared over a good portion of the region of the shoulder, before and behind; and over the inner half of the anterior aspect of the arm patches of sensibility are disseminated here and there on the portions of the arm and shoulder still anæsthetic. Sensibility is again re-established at the elbow, before and behind, extending upwards about 10 or 12 centimetres. It is remarkable to observe that in respect of the hand the limit of anæsthesia does not vary one line. We find in the arm, more especially behind, and in the forearm, the tendency peculiar to such cases—viz. the limitation of the anæsthetic patches by a circular line at right angles to the long axis of the member.[1] On the shoulder and on the anterior portion

[1] See note 5, p. 282

of the arm the borders of these patches are, on the contrary, irregular or jagged.

As to the restoration of movement, the results obtained in this patient are not less remarkable (Fig. 75). On the 5th of June the dynamometer gave only 5 K; at the end of a week the figure was 11 K; it was 17 K in two weeks, and fifteen days later 21 K. On the 11th July the patient suddenly left the hospital. During the week preceding his departure the average figure was 27 K.

It is thus rendered probable that if the treatment had been continued a complete return of the sensibility of the limb, and of movement, would soon have been obtained. Despite this, it is proper to remark that the cure was not perfect when (July 11th, 1885) we lost sight of the patient, for the hysterical stigmata—the monocular polyopia, the diminution of the field of vision, the right hemianalgesia, &c.,—were in no sense modified.[1]

In the case of Pin— it is the same. In spite of the very important amelioration produced in the movements of the left superior extremity, the diverse perversions of sensibility, and the hystero-epileptic attacks, persist almost to the same extent as when he first came under observation.[2]

[1] In the early part of February, 1886, Porcz—, who was then in the surgical wards, had a dispute with another patient about a game of dominoes. The emotion which he experienced was so great that the movements of the paralysed limb returned immediately; but it was not the same with the loss of sensibility, which remains up to the present time (February 20, 1886).

[2] *Vide* Appendix I, at end of this volume.

LECTURE XXIII.

ON A CASE OF HYSTERICAL HIP DISEASE IN A MAN, RESULTING FROM INJURY.

SUMMARY.—*Works of Brodie and other authors on hysterical affections of the joints.—Characters of hysterical joint disease.—Attitude of the limb; special features of the pain.—Case of Charv—; initial injury of the left inferior extremity; attitude of the patient; shape of the buttock and gluteal fold. Considerable clinical analogies with true organic hip disease.—Distinctive features: Brodie's sign; hemianæsthesia; pharyngeal anæsthesia, &c.—Necessity of examination under chloroform.*

GENTLEMEN,—The lecture of to-day will be devoted to proving that the vigorous young man before you is the subject of hysteria, and that the pain in the hip of which he has complained for nearly three years—an affection which supervened after an injury, and which has rendered it impossible for him to carry on his work—reveals hysteria, and that consequently we have to deal with a malady *sine materia* which is capable of being cured, not a severe organic malady which will necessarily result in an incurable infirmity.

In committing myself to this theory, which I hope to be able to prove beyond doubt, I must confess that the appearance of the patient, which is so far from what is regarded in the present day as the classical type of an hysterical subject, is apt to mislead some of those amongst you newly arrived, who will probably think that I have undertaken an imprudent wager, or committed myself to a paradoxical opinion in order to give myself the vain satisfaction of revealing some dialectic expedient.

But I am convinced that among my hearers those who did me the honour of following these lectures last session will be more reserved before passing judgment, and will, I hope, wait with more confidence until the end of the demonstration. These will remember that hysteria may exist even in a robust adult man, in an artisan, neither of delicate nor nervous organisation, and without intellectual culture; and they will also remember that it may occur on the very first occasion in the form of a purely local manifestation, such as, for example, a paralysis or contracture of the limb. In the patient I am going to show you to-day we have in fact neither paralysis nor contracture, but an affection, at least this is my view of the case, described for the first time by Brodie in 1837, under the name of "hysterical affection of the joints."[1]

It is an affection but little known even yet I believe, although since Brodie's time it has formed the subject of important works in England,[2] in France,[3] in Germany,[4] and in Italy.[5]

It will be useful by way of introduction, and to render our

[1] 'Lectures illustrative of certain Local Nervous Affections,' London, 1837, Lecture II, "Various Forms of Local Hysterical Affection," p. 35, *et seq.* The lectures of Sir Benjamin Brodie have been translated into the French by Dr. Aigre ('Libraire du Progrès Médical,' 1880).

[2] W. Coulson, "Hysterical Affections of the Hip-joint," 'London Journal of Medicine,' vol. iii, 1851, p. 631. Barwell, 'A Treatise on Diseases of the Joints,' 1st edit., 1861, 2nd edit., 1881, "On Hysterical Pseudo-disease or Mock Disease of the Joints." F. C. Skey, 'Hysteria: Local or Surgical Forms of Hysteria; Hysterical Affection of Joints,' 3rd lecture, London, 1867. Sir James Paget, 'Leçons de clinique chirurgicale,' trad. du Dr. L. H. Petit, 3ième leçon, "Affections neuromimetiques des articulations," p. 274, Paris, 1877. See also among American authors—S. Weir Mitchell, 'Lectures on Diseases of the Nervous System,' Philadelphia, 1885, 2nd edition, p. 218, "Hysterical Joints."

[3] M. A. C. Roberts, 'Conférences de clinique chirurgicale,' recueilles par le Dr. Doumic, chap. xvi, "Coxalgie hystérique," p. 450. Verneuil, 'Bull. de la Société de Chirurgie de Paris,' 1865-66. Giraldès, 'Leç. sur les mal. chir. des enfants,' p. 610.

[4] E. Esmarch, 'Ueber Gelenkneurosen,' Kiel und Hadersleben, 1872. O. Berger, "Zur Lehre von den Gelenkneuralgien," 'Berl. klin. Woch.,' 1873, p. 255. M. Meyer, "Ueber Gelenkneurosen," 'Berl. klin. Woch.,' 1874, p. 310.

[5] Angelo Minich, 'Della coscialgia nervosa,' Venezia, 1873.

clinical analysis more easy, in the first place to recapitulate briefly the chief features of the classical description of Brodie. Subsequent authors have added some interesting details, but they have not, as it seems to me, altered anything essential.

We have to deal, according to Brodie, with a painful affection, a neuralgia, a hyperæsthesia, so to speak, of the extremities of the articular nerves, which may find its seat in diverse joints, and simulate so as to render the diagnosis extremely difficult, a serious organic lesion of the articulation. The diagnosis of this affection is especially difficult when it affects the hip-joint; a non-organic coxalgia may be so easily mistaken for a serious organic arthritis, scrofulous or other, and *vice versâ*. The absence of material lesion in the former is, however, sufficiently demonstrated (1) by the progress of the malady, which terminates in a complete cure, and often very rapidly; (2) by a certain number of autopsies.

Yes, although it may surprise you in an affection which is undoubtedly benign, there exist a certain number of these, though they are most frequently autopsies made during life, *veritable biopsies*. In fact, by a singular coincidence, the patients attacked with this affection clamour loudly for active surgical intervention, and thus you will readily understand that, when these patients, attacked with a *mania opperativa passiva*, as Textor says, find themselves unfortunately in the presence of surgeons affected with an analogous, though this time active, madness, *mania opperativa activa* (of Stromeyer), the most fantastic operations may result from this unlucky collision. Amputations have been done. Brodie quotes several instances, and Coulson also. One mentioned by the last author is particularly interesting. The patient was a young girl who had suffered for three years from an affection of the knee; the leg remained flexed upon the thigh, the pain became unbearable; every surgeon had refused to intervene, but finally one was found who consented to operate. Amputation was performed, and an examination of the knee-joint revealed a normal articulation with the synovial membrane absolutely healthy, presenting all the delicacy and transparency of a physiological condition; the bones were a trifle light, offering but little resistance to the saw, the cartilages a trifle thin, such as is commonly seen in limbs that have remained a long time immovable.[1]

I might mention several other examples of the same kind, but I think you will perceive that there undoubtedly exist *painful non-organic affections of the joints* capable of simulating articular affections due to grave lesions, and so leading by an error of diagnosis to the most serious consequences.

But what are the signs that enable one to recognise an arthralgia *sine materia*, and distinguish it from an organic arthropathy? The diagnosis is particularly difficult when, as in our patient, the hip-joint is involved. The following are the principal characters ascribed to these arthralgiæ by authors, who, however, as I just said, have scarcely been able to do more than reproduce the description of Brodie.

1. The extremity of the affected side seems shortened on account of the muscular contraction raising the pelvis on the corresponding side.

2. The thigh is in respect to the pelvis in an absolutely fixed condition in such a way that every movement imparted to the thigh is immediately communicated to the pelvis. Here again it is due to the muscular contraction.

As you know, gentlemen, these two characters are not peculiar to hysterical arthralgia, for both are invariably found in organic coxalgia, at any rate in what is commonly known as the third stage.[2] But the following characters will enable us doubtless to distinguish the two affections:

3. The pain presents special characters. It is undoubtedly situated in the hip and the knee, and is exacerbated by percussion of the hip, the knee, or the heel. But then, and this is what Brodie has so well pointed out, it is not exactly limited to the joint itself, it extends to the skin corresponding to the joint, and stretches upwards over Poupart's ligament, spreading over the lower abdomen and even occupying the buttock. It is therefore a superficial pain situated, so to speak, in the skin in such a way that pinching that part of the external integument which covers the joint is often much more painful than severe deep pressure in the same region. At night the patients suffering from organic

[1] Coulson, loc. cit., p. 631.

[2] Barwell, loc. cit.

coxalgia are not infrequently awakened by starting pains in the hip; those suffering from hysterical coxalgia, on the other hand, though they may be kept awake by the pain, when once asleep they are not roused by it.

4. The mode of development of the affection and its course of evolution furnish us with very important particulars. In the hysterical disease it may supervene quite suddenly, and disappear in the same way, very often after a moral impression. Or, again, the subject has convulsive attacks, and it may be after one of such that the coxalgia makes its appearance, &c.

Finally, Brodie adds that, over the affected parts of the limb the temperature is not elevated, and that, whatever be the duration of the affection, no kind of atrophy comes on. We shall see presently that, although the first of these statements is true, the second is not always so.

There are, gentlemen, it is no use to hide the fact, many delicate shades of difference. Further, in difficult cases it may be necessary to have recourse, as we have been able to do for the last thirty years, to the employment of chloroform, so as to determine whether or not the joint is the seat of a material lesion. However, it is necessary to mention, as Prof. Verneuil has shown, that in recent organic coxalgiæ an examination by means of chloroform does not always exclude every suspicion of a material lesion, and thus one cannot assign to this means—at least in the stage referred to—an absolute diagnostic value.

You see, gentlemen, I hold that the diagnosis between hysterical and organic coxalgia presents many serious difficulties; and, as a matter of fact, in nearly all cases where I have been consulted I have seen both physicians and surgeons considerably embarrassed.

After these preliminaries let us return to the patient, of whom I affirm that the coxalgia from which he has suffered for nearly three years is of a purely hysterical nature.

He is a man of forty-five years of age named Ch—, the father of seven children. His antecedents, either hereditary or personal, present nothing worthy of being noted. He served for seven years as a Zouave, but during that time he was never ill. He has never experienced at any time of his life either nervous attacks or rheumatic manifestations. He has exercised his calling as a sawyer, and has worked with a straight saw in the service of one of our great railway companies. On May 13th, 1883, he was the victim of an accident: the connecting-rod of a steam engine situated below the place where he worked struck the plank violently under his feet, and he was projected into the air, so he tells us, to the height of two or three metres [six to nine feet]. He did not lose consciousness, but he experienced immediately a sharp pain, accompanied by a numbness in the limb, so that it seemed, he said, at the same time both *painful and absent.* He was able, however, to make a few steps; they carried him home; he remained two months in bed, and at first he says the limb was swollen. At the end of that time he commenced to walk with crutches, then he managed to get on with only a stick. For more than a year his condition has remained as you see it now.

If we examine the patient first of all *lying down* this is what we find. There exists a notable shortening of the left inferior extremity which corresponds exactly with that which is observed in organic hip disease in the third stage. The joint is rigid, the thigh being fixed to the pelvis in an almost immovable position. The patient complains of a spontaneous pain in the groin, the hip, and the knee, which pain is increased when one presses out these regions, when one moves the limb, or when one percusses the great trochanter or the heel; and, moreover, I should like you particularly to notice that the whole of the left limb, thigh and leg, is a little less voluminous than the right,—the circumference is less by about a centimetre.

Now, when the patient *stands up*, if you look at him from the front (Fig. 76, A) you will see that he stands resting on the healthy side, holding his stick in his right hand; the left foot does not rest on the ground, or only on tip-toe. The left leg is extended, and is carried a little in front of the right. This position, as my colleague Prof. Lannelongue—to whom I showed a good photograph of the patient standing—said the other day, is the typical attitude of hip-joint disease when the patient is able to stand upright.

If now we examine the patient from behind (Fig. 76, B), we notice in the first place the contrast that exists between the two buttocks. The right buttock is rounded, and presents the little fossa behind the trochanter resulting from the contraction of the gluteus maximus, but the left seems larger, flatter, and more flaccid. These characters are to be found in or-

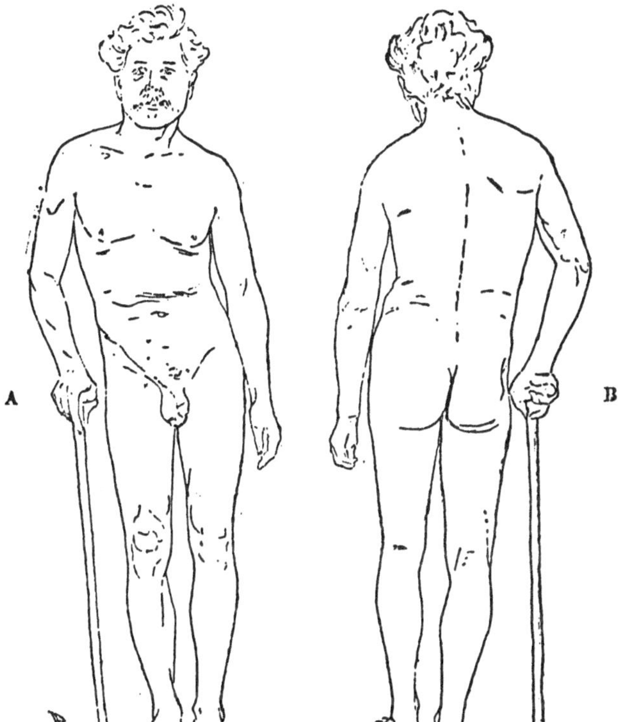

FIG. 76.

ganic coxalgia, and have been pointed out by certain authors[1] as possessing much clinical importance.

As a matter of fact, this contrast between the two buttocks depends entirely upon the attitude of the patient. We are assured of this by placing beside our patient a healthy indi-

[1] Barwell, for example, loc. cit.

vidual who is accustomed to pose for painters, and whom we have instructed to imitate as much as possible (after careful study) the attitude of the patient. The results of this comparative study are well realised in the drawing that I place before you, which has been made from a photograph (Fig. 77).

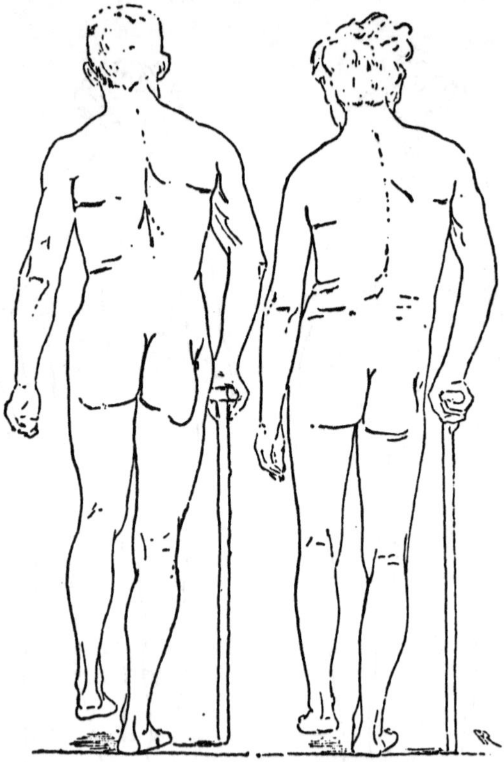

FIG. 77.

It may be noted that the gluteal fold is higher and larger on the left than on the right, and that the right is double, whereas the left is single. The intergluteal fold is inclined upwards from the left towards the right, from the affected to the healthy side. There exists a fairly marked spinal curvature, with its concavity towards the left. These different deformities depend in an evident fashion on the abnormal position in which the hip is maintained, and especially on its elevation on the affected side. I should like you to remark in the last place that this inequality of volume of the two thighs and of the two legs is more easily seen in the upright position.

It is doubtless not necessary to dwell on the halting gait of our patient, you will recognise that it does not essentially differ from that presented by individuals who are the subjects of old-standing organic coxalgia.

In brief, gentlemen, you see that we do not find at first sight anything contrary to the idea of a serious organic articular affection which has terminated without abscess in ankylosis of the joint.

But is there true ankylosis? A thorough exploration under chloroform at the present time, that is to say three years after the onset of the affection, would enable us to reply to this question in a very definite way, and I shall return to this point directly.

But, I should like you in the first place to examine the patient from another point of view. Let us accept the hypothesis that he is the subject of a coxalgia *sine materia,* and see if the symptoms that he presents correspond to Brodie's description.

And, firstly, if we consider the general condition of this man we find that although he has been ill for two and a half years he has not become enfeebled; no wasting, no anæmia, never any fever, and all that time he has had an excellent appetite. This preservation of the general health is scarcely in accord with the idea of a grave organic articular affection lasting for many months, even if it had made a most favorable progress.

In the next place you will notice that the *rigidity* of the limb occupies not only the hip, but also the knee, and even the ankle. Now, these are not the symptoms which belong to common coxalgia, any more than the relative coldness and purple colouration of the parts which are so marked in the knee and leg of this patient.

Again, let us examine the character of the pain which we have already noted in passing. This pain, which is intense, though intermittent, is greatly increased as we have said by percussion over the trochanter or the heel, and consequently by every attempt made to move the joint. But it also has this peculiarity, that it is diffuse and spreads upwards over Poupart's ligament, radiating over the lower abdomen, almost as far as the left breast, and extends also down to the buttock. Moreover, when the skin at the level of the groin, or even over the anterior part of the knee, is raised and slightly squeezed between the fingers it produces an acute pain quite out of proportion with the degree of force exercised in the pinch. I should like to insist on the value of this hyperæsthesia of the skin in the neighbourhood of the hip. It has been discovered by most authors who have written on hysterical coxalgia; but it is worthy of being designated by the name of *Brodie's sign* because it is to this celebrated English surgeon that we owe the value of the sign from a diagnostic point of view.

I should add that, having remarked the signs of extreme anxiety presented by Ch— after these excitations of the skin in the groin and the knee, the wrinkling of the face, the swelling of the veins in the neck and the temples, &c., we interrogated him as to what he experienced at that moment; and the description which he gave us of his sensations corresponds exactly with the description of an ordinary hysterical aura, namely, epigastric constriction, cardiac palpitations, constriction of the throat, buzzing in the ears on the left side, and beatings in the temple on the same side. The same results occurred after percussion over the great trochanter or on the heel, or after any attempt at movement imparted to the hip. Thus you see, gentlemen, that although the hysterical attack does not exist in our patient, one can at least provoke in him the phenomena of an aura by an excitation of veritable hysterogenic zones, some of which occupy the skin covering the hip- and knee-joints, and the others, situated more deeply, appear to be seated either in the synovial membrane or the capsule of the joint.

The discovery of the facts just mentioned have naturally induced us to suppose that a more attentive examination of this man, conducted in a certain direction, would enable us, perhaps, to discover other symptoms in him capable of rendering the existence of the hysterical diathesis still more evident and tangible. In this expectation we have not been disappointed. A methodical exploration of the different modes of sensibility has revealed that over almost the entire half of the left side of the body—a few areæ existing unaffected —there is complete anæsthesia both to pricking and for temperature (Fig. 78). In the movements of certain joints

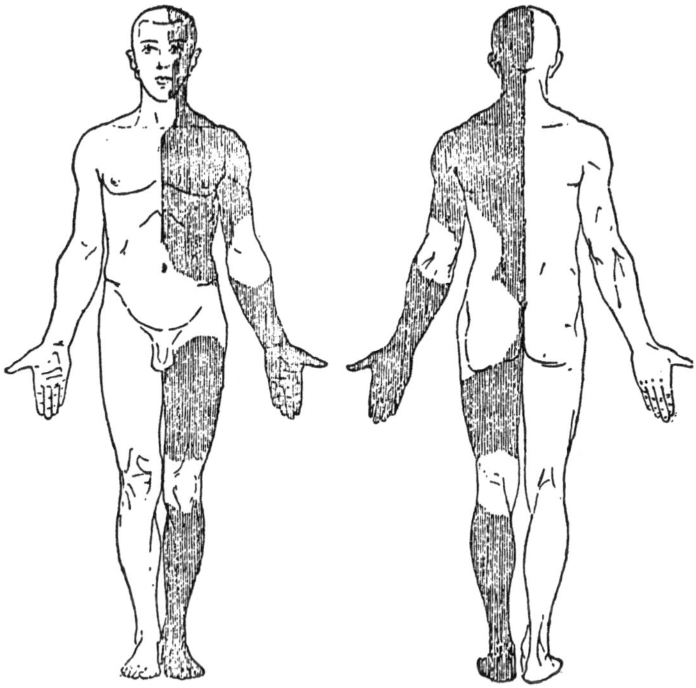

FIG. 78.

(feet, hands, wrists, shoulders) the notions of muscular sense are lost, whereas in others (the elbow, for example) they are preserved. The special senses, taste, smell, hearing, are notably affected on the left side, and on the same side the visual field is considerably retracted, although the right eye is not similarly affected. It may be added, and here is a very significant character, that the pharynx can be tickled and irritated in any way you like without producing the least trace of reflex action.

All that has been said leads us to the conclusions:— Firstly, that our patient is an "hysteric"; secondly, that the articular affection from which he suffers presents a large number of the characters which belong to hysterical coxalgia, and that none of them necessarily indicate the existence of a profound lesion of the joint. The wasting of the limb itself does not correspond to the muscular atrophy with flaccidity which is to be found in organic coxalgia, and it may be satisfactorily explained by the relative functional inactivity during two and a half years. Everything, therefore, may be of an hysterical nature in this patient whether it refers to the general or local condition. The traumatic origin of the symptoms are not, far from it, opposed to this interpretation, for we know from our former studies that in men, more perhaps than in women, an injury may have the effect of developing an hysterical diathesis which has up to that time remained latent.

Nevertheless, I should be the first to allow that even in the presence of the arguments which we have accumulated, doubts may still exist as to the diagnosis. It is not easy, in fact, in presence of a loss of power so pronounced, and extending over years, to altogether dispose of the idea of an organic hip-joint disease. It may be asked amongst other things whether the hysterical symptoms although pronounced have not supervened at a given moment, and become grafted, as it were, on to an organic coxalgia, which would thus have called into existence the manifestation of the neurosis. It is evident that the administration of chloroform would alone dispose of all doubts. Naturally we were anxious to employ this method of differentiation, but up to the present time the patient has obstinately refused to allow it to be employed. But I do not despair of persuading him to listen to reason, and of his deciding one day to lend himself to a method of examination which cannot but be to his own advantage.

However, gentlemen, in the absence of an examination made by ourselves we can avail ourselves of the result of an exploration which was made scarcely five months ago by an eminent surgeon. The results of that exploration have been communicated to us by a colleague who assisted, and who states that during the administration of the anæsthetic the joint was discovered to be perfectly mobile, exempt from any rigidity and from all adhesions.

The conclusions drawn from that examination were the following:—First, that there did not exist in this patient any trace of an organic affection of the joint. Secondly, that this individual very probably was one who simulated.

From the facts we have made out it is difficult for us to endorse the second of these conclusions.

Most certainly there is no organic disease of the hip-joint in this patient, that is well-established. He is the subject of an hysterical coxalgia *sine materia,* as you may call it. But however *dynamic* it may be, the disease is perfectly legitimate, perfectly real, and nothing, absolutely nothing, authorises us to tax this man with simulation.

You will readily understand, gentlemen, that as soon as it is established, as we have affirmed here, that we have to do with an hysterical coxalgia, the prognosis is much less serious than it would have been on the hypothesis of an organic affection. Without doubt, an hysterical coxalgia may be very chronic, may last for months or even years—and this case offers us an unfortunate example of this kind—but the cure must always necessarily follow some day sooner or later.

But what should we do in order to hasten this favorable termination? That is a question which to be properly dealt with requires a somewhat lengthy exposition, and must be dealt with in the next lecture.

LECTURE XXIV.

ON A CASE OF HYSTERICAL HIP-DISEASE IN A MAN, RESULTING FROM INJURY (*continued*).

SUMMARY.—*Results of an examination under chloroform.—Symptoms then presented by the patient.—Mixed or hystero-organic hip-disease—Hip-disease artificially produced in two women presenting the phenomena of great hypnotism.—Different proceedings employed to produce this coxalgia.—Characters of artificial hysterical coxalgia.—Nervous shock.—Traumatic suggestion.—Method of treating hysterical coxalgia; massage, its good but transitory results; influence of the psychical state.—Probable recovery.*

GENTLEMEN,—I bring before you once more the patient whom I have already presented to you in the last lecture, as offering a remarkable illustration of an affection that is now known by the name of *hysterical coxalgia.*

You have not forgotten the numerous and weighty arguments by the aid of which this diagnosis was established, but nevertheless it is possible that certain scruples may still remain in your minds; and, as a matter of fact, in the absence of the administration of chloroform to the patient, we have not been able to assure ourselves of the integrity of the joint.

Well, gentlemen, these doubts are now removed. The patient, who, under the influence of I know not what fear, refused to submit to chloroform, now realises his own interests better and submitted himself to examination last Friday.

These are the results of our exploration. At the end of six or seven minutes, after a very brief period of excitement (contrary to what we had reason to fear in this respect from what we know of the effects of chloroformization in hysterical subjects), sleep became profound. The muscles became perfectly flaccid, those of the affected limb being the last to succumb, and the skin became insensible to pinching, even in the most hyperæsthetic places. One was able to impart to the leg and the thigh most extensive movements without being arrested by the least resistance. Percussion of the great trochanter or of the heel was without result, and we were unable to discover the least crackling during the execution of these movements either by the hand or even with the stethoscope. The conclusion, therefore, to which we are driven is, that the joint is perfectly free from adhesions, that the articular and osseous surfaces present none of those deformities or lesions which would most certainly exist in a coxalgia of such old standing as this, if it had been really of an organic nature.

I should like to mention the interesting symptoms presented by the patient as he was coming round. The stiffness commenced to reappear to a certain extent in the affected muscles before any painful manifestation was evident in the joint. The sensibility in the skin had already partly reappeared and the patient was beginning to reply to questions before the sensibility of the deep parts (percussion of the trochanter or the heel) had become at all marked, showing that the deep hyperæsthesia was the last to return. But when he had completely come to, that is to say at the end of twenty or twenty-five minutes, the deformity, the pain, and the limping returned absolutely to the same condition as before chloroform was administered.

Thus, our diagnosis is amply confirmed. But we are not so sure about the line of treatment which should be adopted. It is to this side of the question that we must now turn our attention. But before coming to the question of therapeutics I think it may be useful to draw your attention to another point touching the diagnosis of hysterical coxalgia. The reason I was so desirous of giving chloroform to our patient was that I thought it quite possible we might be in the presence of some such combination as the following: (1) Organic lesions of scrofulous coxalgia; with (2) Dynamic lesions of hysterical coxalgia. Our patient most certainly is hysterical, and clearly presents the symptoms of hysterical coxalgia, but it might have so happened that these symptoms served only to mask a true hip-disease. We might thus have a mixed form, a *hystero-organic form*, if you like to call it so.

This mixed form; does it really exist in clinical experience? Yes, most certainly; and perhaps it is more frequent than we think, although authors do not touch upon it, as far as I am aware. In view of the importance of the facts perhaps I may be allowed to say a few words upon the subject. Thanks to the kindness of my colleagues, Messrs. Lannelongue and Joffroy, I am able to narrate to you three cases in which this combination occurred under circumstances which rendered it very difficult to avoid error. In these three cases the first impression was that the affection was hysterical, but a more attentive examination demonstrated that the hysterical phenomena masked an organic lesion of the hip which had been overlooked for a time.

[1] Here is a summary account of the three cases:—

First case (communicated by Prof. Lannelongue).—A boy, 11 years old, whose mother had had numerous hysterical attacks. The limb on the affected side was *contracted not only at the hip- but also at the knee- and ankle-joints.* It was not possible to touch this limb without the child being seized with a nervous attack [attaque de nerfs]. Under chloroform the existence of loud articular cracklings was revealed. There was a shortening of two centimetres [about three quarters of an inch], due to the head of the femur over-riding the cotyloid cavity. Later on symptomatic abscesses occurred.

Second case (communicated by Prof. Lannelongue).—A little girl of 13. Her father was the subject of infantile paralysis; her mother had hysterical seizures up to the age of thirty. When seven years old the patient had painful contracture of the right foot; at nine, nervous attacks, and again at ten; when eleven she suffered from pain in the right hip with limping. *There occurred a complete remission which made them think that it was a purely nervous affection and they consequently allowed the child to walk.* A return came on and the child was submitted to chloroform. Then cracklings were discovered and a very great difficulty in bending the joint, consequent on the deformity of the bone. A deep-seated swelling caused them to suspect an abscess.

Third case (communicated by Dr. Joffroy).—Mdlle. X—, of St. Petersburg, 18 years old. No hereditary antecedents. From six to fourteen she had numerous nervous attacks which seemed to be of an hysterical nature, somewhat like partial epilepsy. When six years old she had *transient coxalgic* symptoms. When eighteen years old *the same symptoms reappeared on several occasions.* At the age of eighteen the same symptoms reappeared five months before the patient came under notice. Severe pain in the hip and knee; apparent short-

In reference to this combination of organic lesion with hysterical symptoms I should like to observe in passing, that you must not believe that slight material disorders of the organism necessarily exclude hysterical phenomena. It may so happen without doubt, but if it be so in a few cases, in other cases which are perhaps more numerous the hysterical stigmata persist during the evolution of more or less serious organic lesions. This was what occurred in the course of a case that we have recently had in our wards of acute articular rheumatism complicated with endo- and pericarditis, followed by death.

I need not insist further upon this point; enough has been said, I think, to show you that when an organic affection becomes developed in an hysterical subject, the symptoms relative to each of the two affections combine in such a way as to constitute a pathological hybrid, whose clinical history should be recognised by the physician.

And now to come back to our patient. He is, as has been shown, the subject of "hip disease" of an undoubted hysterical nature, without any admixture, without any organic lesion. We may therefore affirm that he will probably recover sooner or later; but when will the cure be effected, and what means must one employ to arrive at that result?

I should like in the first place to examine the theory, the pathological explanation, of these cases, hoping that by the way we may meet indications which will enable us to found our therapeutic intervention on a rational basis. We have a means at hand—a means that I have already made use of under similar circumstances. I refer to the artificial pro-

ening; the patient walked with the aid of crutches, resting the point of the foot with difficulty on the ground; no hysterical stigmata. However, in view of the opinion of the doctors whom she had formerly consulted, the singular walk of the patient, and particularly the remissions, followed by the reappearances, which had occurred for nearly ten years, they inclined towards the diagnosis of hysterical coxalgia, though with reservation. The employment of tepid douches at first produced a decided amelioration; a fresh remission was thus produced and the patient became able to walk with very little pain. However, in the meantime, chloroformization having been performed, it was discovered "that complete relaxation of the hip was impossible, and that the movements imparted to the joint determined characteristic cracklings, leaving no doubt as to the existence of very advanced osseous lesions."

duction of the symptoms of hysterical coxalgia, and it is by the aid of this that one may hope to more readily recognise the conditions and the mechanism which preside over the development of the disease.

In this investigation we do not avail ourselves of any animal, however elevated it might be in the scale of natural history, but of man himself placed under the mental conditions special to the hypnotic state.

The two patients that are now brought before you are women, the subjects of inveterate hysteria, who reveal all the well-marked features of great hypnotism. They present, as you see, in a waking state all the features of hysterical coxalgia,—pain, limping, &c., details into which I need not further enter. But what I want you to realise specially is that the affection has been produced by us purposely, artificially, during the hypnotic state.

Naturally in these patients matters have not been pushed too far, but even when kept within the bounds of prudence it is sufficient for us to discover in them all the features of the affection described by Brodie, albeit under a benign form.

In one of these women it was produced during a somnambulic state by a moderate torsion of the thigh on the pelvis. She immediately complained of pain in the hip, and also—please to note this well—in the *knee*, although this latter had not been submitted to the slightest tension.

In the other patient it was enough to affirm to her when she was in a state of hypnotism, that she had just had an attack during which she had received a blow upon the hip. The animated recital of the supposed incident, and the picture of the severe pains that would follow, produced the desired result. Here again, strange to say, although we had only spoken of a blow upon the hip the patient complained at the same time of a pain in the hip-joint and also in the *knee*. And whereas the patient was formerly anæsthetic on this side, it will now be seen that the skin over the hip and over the knee is very sensitive. I should like you to remark that our patients after being aroused from the hypnotic state are absolutely ignorant of our intervention, and both of them firmly believe that they have hurt their hips during an attack.

You have not forgotten, gentlemen, the two men Porcz— and Pin—, whom I showed you recently for the second time, and in whom an hysterical paralysis of the corresponding arm was developed after an injury to the shoulder. I demonstrated to you moreover that this paralysis could be produced segment by segment in subjects under hypnotism, either by means of verbal suggestion, or by the traumatic action of a blow on the shoulder, which constituted, as one might say, a veritable *traumatic suggestion.*

My opinion is that this hypnotic condition, during which "suggestion" produces these effects, is assimilable in more points than one to the state which in England has been called by the name of *nervous shock* in opposition to *traumatic shock*, with which it may often be combined, but from which it may also remain distinct. This nervous shock is produced by some strong emotion, a fright, a feeling of terror determined by an accident, especially when this accident menaces life, such as may be seen, for example, in railway collisions. On these occasions a peculiar mental condition is often developed, recently studied with care by Mr. Page, which is very intimately connected, in my judgment, with the hypnotic state.[1] In both of these conditions, in fact, the *mental spontaneity*, the *will*, or the *judgment*, is more or less suppressed or obscured, and suggestions become easy. And thus the slightest traumatic action for instance, directed to a member may become the occasion of a paralysis, of a contracture, or an arthralgia. It is in this way that one so often sees after railway accidents cases of monoplegia, paraplegia, or hemiplegia, simulating organic lesions although they are no other than dynamic or psychical paralyses, very analogous, to say the least, to hysterical paralyses.

[1] "We are . . . . disposed to believe that the primary seat of functional disturbance lies in the brain itself, and that, as in the hypnotic state, ... there is a temporary arrest in the function of that part of the sensorium which presides over and controls the movements and sensations of the periphery" (Page, 'Injuries of the Spine and Nervous Shock,' p. 207, 2nd ed., London, 1885). See also Wilks, "On Hysteria and Arrest of Cerebral Action," 'Guy's Hosp. Rep.,' vol. xxii, p. 35; and Tuke, 'Influence of the Mind upon the Body,' p. 99. We may, I think, write in French indifferently *Shock* or Choc—Shock, synon.: Fr., choc; Germ., shok. See R. Quain, 'Dict. of Medicine,' London, 1882, art. *Shock*.

I regret that I am unable to dwell longer on the connection which I have indicated between the mental state produced by nervous shock, and that which characterises the somnambulic period of hypnotism; but I think enough has been said to attract your attention to this point and to induce you to make it the subject of your meditations.

With reference to the man Ch— suffering from hysterical coxalgia, you will have perfectly understood, gentlemen, that in my opinion the coxalgia of this patient must be interpreted according to the theory applied in our lectures last session to cases of hysterical monoplegia of traumatic origin.[1]

You have, in fact, observed the pain and also the paralysis suggested in the hypnotic state whether by the means of oral suggestion or by a slight traumatism. And this pain the observer is able at will to localise to one or other part of the limb.

Thus, just as there are psychical paralyses produced by what has been called in former lectures *traumatic suggestion*, so also there are spasmodic coxalgiæ due to the same mechanism. Our patient is an illustration of this. The injury from which he suffered produced in him a nervous shock and a corresponding mental condition. Without doubt his hip has incurred a concussion, perhaps even a contusion more or less pronounced. But this local action has not determined serious organic lesions, and the pain which has been experienced has only become developed, exaggerated, and definitely established as a permanent "arthralgia" by reason of the psychical state produced by nervous shock.

Such, gentlemen, is the theory which I propose. If I have dwelt a little on this point it is that the treatment follows as it were naturally from the consideration thereof. We have here a psychical affection, it is therefore by a mental treatment that we must hope to modify it. But how shall this be accomplished? We know from the observations of different authors that psychical arthralgiæ, whether of traumatic or other origin, sometimes recover quite suddenly after some strong emotion: a religious ceremony, for example, or anything which strongly appeals to the imagination. Unfortunately,

[1] Pp. 304 and 305.

neither of these means are available for us. We have attempted to assume a position of authority, to persuade the patient at the moment when he was coming out of the chloroform narcosis, at a time when the pain and limping were lessened, that he was cured; but I must confess that we have not been very successful. May we count on the influence of a simulated operation, following the advice of Hancock and Barwell? I am afraid not. Moreover, you understand that when one employs means of this kind one should be sure of success, for to fail under these circumstances would be to run the risk of losing our patient's confidence. As for the employment of hypnotic practices, which would perhaps furnish us with powerful means of action, this man will not hear of it.

For the last twelve days our patient has been submitted to a very simple treatment, consisting of massage. Up to the present time this treatment has not been followed by very definite results. Nevertheless I should like you to see the application of it so as to enable you to realise the immediate consequences of these manipulations, which are repeated on him each day.

You have not forgotten, gentlemen, that Ch— is absolutely hemianæsthetic on the left side, excepting certain areas where the skin is not only sensitive but hyperæsthetic. These hyperæsthetic zones are found especially in the region of the elbow in the upper extremity, and over the hip and the knee in the lower extremity; in these regions pinching of the skin produces pain and all the phenomena of an aura. Moreover, this hyperæsthesia is not limited to the skin that covers the joint, but involves also the deeper parts (ligaments and synovial membrane); percussion of the heel or of the great trochanter are also followed by severe pain, and so also are movements communicated to the lower extremity. I would remind you also that this articular pain is attended by contracture of the muscles which move the knee, the hip, and even the pelvis; and that the tilting of the pelvis thus produced is the cause of the apparent shortening of the left leg.

Having decided to try the effects of massage on our patient, I asked Dr. Gautier, who for several years has devoted himself in a scientific way to the employment of this agent, to be so good as to lend us his assistance, which he has very kindly given us.

We have left the conduct of this treatment entirely in his hands and he will demonstrate to you the mode of operation which he employs. You will see that the manipulation consists in the first place of a simple *stroking* [*effleurage*] of the hand over the left buttock of the patient; little by little the hand is pressed more firmly, and then it becomes a true deep massage. A week ago the patient supported these manipulations very badly, but now he bears them much better; at the end of four or five minutes you notice that he ceases to feel the hand that rubs, then he experiences a heaviness in the whole limb; and soon he states that he has "ceased to have a leg," in other words, the whole of the lower extremity has become completely insensitive; the hyperæsthesic zones over the knee and hip have disappeared, and one can pinch the skin with impunity. And moreover, the anæsthesia has extended to the deeper parts, for one can strike the heel or the great trochanter without producing the least pain. Finally, and this is still more interesting, the contracture has disappeared, and one can move all the joints of the left lower limb in every direction, even with some roughness, without encountering the least resistance and without the patient showing signs of the slightest pain. And now you see again that we can, as we have already done during the chloroform sleep, demonstrate that the joints are entirely free and mobile, that they are not the seat of the least crackling, in a word that the synovial membranes of the articular surfaces are absolutely healthy; and finally, that all notions relating to muscular sense are completely abolished. Thus, gentlemen, we have, properly speaking, transformed a coxalgia with contracture, into a flaccid hysterical paralysis which corresponds precisely with the most perfect type of that complaint.

How long will these flaccid paralytic symptoms persist? Probably from about an hour to an hour and a half. Then what will happen? The pain will reappear in the limb, it will rapidly reach the degree of intensity which it formerly had, and then the contracture and the apparent shortening of the limb will reappear. It is therefore a very transient amelioration that we have effected up to the present time by these applications of massage. But it is a fact that I want to point out, that for two or three days the return of the pains and the contracture has not been quite complete, and the patient himself recognises that as the applications increase in number the coxalgic symptoms improve, and in this way we hope to arrive some day at the desired result.

We are counting also on another circumstance that I will narrate to you when the patient has gone out. . . . .

The circumstance is the following. The affection from which this man suffers was, as I told you, contracted in the service of a railway company; and this company is now paying him every day very nearly the same amount that he earned by working. If this subsidy should happen to stop it would be for him, incapable as he is now of earning his living, and for his seven children, a very great misfortune. Thus he is in a condition of perpetual inquietude on this point, of mental depression which is of itself enough to perpetuate his malady, which is undoubtedly of psychical or, if you like it better, of mental origin. Now, I have reason to believe that the administration of the railway company has resolved to make Ch— a pension on which he will be able to count for the future; consequently, the mental condition of the patient will be, I hope, considerably improved when he no longer has this spectre of misfortune perpetually before his eyes. That state of mental depression in which he has continually lived will rapidly disappear. It will become more easy to persuade him that his malady is not incurable, that he can and must be cured, and that he himself can, if he sincerely wishes it, materially help towards that end. Thus, the practices of massage also aiding, all will go well—at least, I hope so.

Before finishing I should like, gentlemen, to draw your attention a little more particularly to the results obtained in this patient by massage. Undoubtedly, you will hesitate to believe that a simple massage is able to produce effects so pronounced in every case. Without doubt we know that it can in the long run ameliorate and even cure articular pains, &c., but to determine even temporarily a veritable motor and sensitive paralysis of a limb, that is what seems so unusual.

On what then do the singular results obtained in this patient depend? I think it may be affirmed that they are due to the nature of the subject, to the *material* with which we are dealing. It is because it is applied to a hysterical subject that massage has produced in this man such marked results. Perhaps one might say that in this case massage represents a sort of local hypnotism. I may mention in support of this notion that analogous practices applied to two hysterical hemianæsthesic women in my wards have given rise to similar results. In less than five minutes we produced in them, on the sensitive side, an anæsthesia of the skin, then of the deeper parts, and finally a complete but transitory motor paralysis of the limb, with the loss of muscular sense. Here again then, is an additional argument in favour of the existence of the hysterical neurosis in our patient; but I believe that I have sufficiently convinced you on this point and I do not wish to insist any more.

I have expounded to you the means that we are now employing in order to arrive at the desired end: will our efforts be crowned with success? Without being too confident I am in hopes that it will be so and that I may have the pleasure of showing you in a few weeks, or perhaps in a few months, the patient, whom we have just studied together with so much care, cured of the affection from which he has suffered for nearly three years.[1]

[1] The patient left us and abandoned all treatment. We saw him again six months later and the affection was not perceptibly modified.

LECTURE XXV.

THE CASE OF SPASMODIC CONTRACTURE OF THE UPPER EXTREMITY OCCURRING IN A MAN AFTER THE APPLICATION OF A SPLINT.[1]

SUMMARY.—*Development of a brachial monoplegia having all the characters of so-called hystero-traumatic monoplegia, due to a blow from a heavy body falling on the limb.—Fracture of the forearm.—Nervous shock; what it is that constitutes "local shock;" the part it plays in the production of hystero-traumatic paralysis.—Application of the splint; monoplegia with flaccidity becomes transformed into monoplegia with contracture which presents all the characters of hysterical contracture.—The tendency to spasmodic contracture is a frequent occurrence in hysteria in either sex.—The most certain means of producing it is the application of a ligature around the limb.—The artificial production of contractures constitutes a veritable stigma of the hysterical state.—Amelioration of the patient after the different kinds of treatment; although the hand still preserves a certain degree of deformity which does not yield to the action of chloroform and which appears to be due to the formation of fibrous tissue.*

GENTLEMEN,—The patient who forms the subject of our lecture to-day is, as you see, a man of robust appearance. He presents another example of those hystero-traumatic affections to which we have been particularly devoting our attention during this and last year. One cannot, I think, collect too many facts in connection with this subject. It

[1] Lecture edited by Dr. Babinski.

has hitherto been insufficiently explored, and if I am not deceived, it promises for the future an ample harvest of results which possess great practical interest.

This man has, as you see, a contracture of the left upper extremity, which for several months has deprived the limb of all movement. The contracture became developed at a time when the limb was enveloped in a plaster splint, the application of which had become necessary owing to a fracture of the bones of the forearm; a fracture determined by a blow from a heavy body—that is to say, half an ox weighing about 300 kilogrammes [about forty-three stone]—on this part of the body.

Well, gentlemen, we propose to demonstrate that this contracture, which is a more or less direct consequence of the injury, is of an hysterical nature. We shall seek afterwards to interpret the mechanism involved in its development.

Here, in a few words, is the clinical history of this patient. He is a man, 30 years of age, named Dum—, born in Dordogne, and only having lived in Paris for the last five years. There is nothing particular to point out in his hereditary or personal antecedents. He is a young man without any education, and he lived quite in the country up to the age of twenty-five. He has looked after sheep, attended fairs, and slaughtered animals for butchers. Since being in Paris he has worked for different butchers in the town and at slaughter-houses. He assures us that he has never drunk to excess. He has, it would seem, like most of his comrades, followed the repugnant practice of drinking every day several glasses of blood: "I like blood better than wine," says he, "it gives more force."

The accident which particularly concerns us happened under the following circumstances. About four and a half months ago—the patient cannot be precise about the date—he was engaged with one of his comrades at the Central Market in unhooking half the carcass of an ox of considerable weight; the hook broke and the patient was knocked over, falling with his left arm underneath the carcass. He assures us that he did not completely lose consciousness at the moment, but he remembers that he was stunned, and that for several instants he did not know where he was nor what took place. They were obliged to carry him to a chemist's shop near by.

It is probable that the *nervous shock* which he experienced then was considerable, for even now there seems to exist in him a certain degree of amnesia relating principally to matters connected with the accident, but also to those of more recent date. There does not appear to be in this respect any simulation or dissimulation. As we have said, he is unable to indicate exactly the date of the accident; and further, when he is asked to tell us the place where he now lives he hesitates; but almost immediately draws from his pocket a paper on which his address is written, and we have ascertained that the information it contains is correct. We have, therefore no good reason for doubting the veracity of his account.

Returning to the circumstances of the accident, he states that at the moment when it happened he heard the sound of a crack which seemed to him to come from the left arm, but he says that at that moment he did not experience any pain, either on the day of the fall, nor on the following days. Not only did he experience no pain in the arm at that moment but he declares "that he was unable to feel the limb at all," that "it seemed like dead," or again as though it were absent "from the shoulder to the end of the fingers." "In place of an arm," he adds, "it seemed to me that this side carried a weight of forty pounds."

The limb moreover appears to have been absolutely flaccid. It was able to be moved in all directions although no voluntary movement was possible.

From this account it appears that in all probability the phenomena which occurred in this man's arm, at the time it was injured, consisted of a superficial and deep anæsthesia and absolute motor paralysis without muscular rigidity; and that consequently the symptoms were very similar to those that we have minutely studied in the preceding lectures, in male subjects attacked with hystero-traumatic monoplegia.[1]

You will, moreover, remember how we were able to produce this same kind of paralysis in several hypnotised sub-

[1] Lectures XX, XXI, and XXII.

jects during the somnambulic period by a blow with the fist of moderate intensity on the upper part of the limb. The sensations of weight, of absence of the limb, and finally the weakness which occurred after a blow on the limb in these cases (as in those where the phenomena are produced independent of hypnotism), would be the point of departure of the "suggestion," which has the effect of developing the paralysis (already initiated, as it were, by the circumstance of contusion), and of completing it and establishing it in a definite fashion. You will remember that such was the theory, as I proposed it to you, in order to interpret facts of this nature.[1]

I am not sorry, gentlemen, to have the opportunity of pointing out that these sensitive and motor troubles, to which I have called your attention and which occur in limbs subjected to a contusion, do not belong, far from it, to hysterical subjects alone. In such subjects without doubt they occur under the influence of shocks to all appearance very slight, and they easily acquire a considerable development, out of all proportion to the intensity of the injury. But they are also to be found, quite apart from hysteria, in any individual following a contusion, provided it be of a sufficient intensity. Thus it is that under the influence of a shock produced, for example, on the forearm by the penetration of a rifle-ball, the whole of the limb may become paralysed and insensitive for a longer or a shorter time. A simple blow without wound may even suffice to determine phenomena of the same sort.[2] One may affirm, I think, in general terms that the lighter the contusion and the less neuropathic the subject, the less hysterical he is if one may put it so, then the slighter, more circumscribed, and more transient are the paretic and sensorial symptoms consequent on the blow.

M. Billroth relates[3] that having inadvertently received a blow on the back of the hand, it became insensitive, and at the same time the voluntary movement was for the moment lost in the fingers, but that the duration of these phenomena did not exceed three minutes. M. Gussenbauer relates facts

[1] See specially in Lecture XXII.

[2] O. Berger, 'Berlin. Klin. Wochensch.,' p. 234, 1871.

[3] See G. H. Grœningen, 'Ueber den Shock,' Wiesbaden, 1885, p. 78, *et seq.*

of the same kind. This collection of phenomena, this syndroma [syndrôme], to which I am just now calling your attention has been described by certain authors under the name of local shock (*localer shok*, Fischer; *localer wundschreck*, Bardeleben; *localer oder peripherer shok, local shock*, Grœningen, &c.).

Under these circumstances there occurs a cutaneous and deep anæsthesia, with more or less accentuated motor paralysis for a certain distance above and below the place where the blow occurred, sometimes throughout the extent of the limb; consequently we have to do, not with a lesion of any single nerve, but very probably with the result of a participation of the nervous centres in a reflex manner.

One can, I think, without forcing the analogy too much, imagine that there is here, as it were, a sketch, a rudiment, or germ, of the hystero-traumatic paralysis, and one can understand that in a subject psychically predisposed, this rudimentary paralysis, provoked by the shock, becomes realised and developed to the full extent by reason of a mental elaboration, by a process of auto-suggestion, the mechanism of which I have attempted to explain to you in the preceding lectures.[1]

This *local shock*,[2] relatively benign, must not be confounded with *local stupor*,[3] which has been recently described by Professor Verneuil in one of his clinical lectures. In this condition following a blow, which is always severe, there is a suspension of the circulation, of the calorification, and of the innervation (motor and sensory paralysis), with a threatening of gangrene. All these symptoms in such a case, according to Professor Verneuil, would be accounted for by a compression of the arterial and nerve trunks by a deep-seated effusion. Free incision, allowing the blood to flow away, suffices in fact, to cause all the symptoms to disappear.

However, to return to our patient, the phenomena of *local shock* in his case seem to have been very accentuated, because not only did the fracture occur without pain, but, further,

[1] Lectures XX, XXI, and XXII.

[2] Concerning the orthography of the word *shock* see p. 335, foot-note 1.

[3] See 'L'Union Médicale,' 1886.

the limb seems to have been affected with complete anæsthesia throughout its entire length, at the same time that it was deprived of all voluntary movement. There existed at that time without doubt a flaccid monoplegia analogous on all points to those that we have recently studied in several hysterical subjects, resulting from injury. In reference to the flaccidity you will see directly that at the present time it is not a flaccid paralysis, but a spasmodic contracture; and this is just the point that we shall reserve for special discussion in the sequel, but in the first place it will be well to examine the incidents which occurred shortly after the accident.

Two days after the accident the patient decided to go and consult a surgeon at the hospital of San Antoine. The wrist, hand, and fingers had become very swollen, all voluntary movement was lost, though passive movement was possible, and there did not exist any trace of stiffness in the affected limb, though it was still, as at the beginning, completely insensitive.

During a period of fifteen days the forearm was kept in a hollow splint, and covered with carbolised compresses and poultices. Then it was decided to apply a plaster apparatus, which he kept on for forty-five days.

At the end of this time the splint was taken off, and it was discovered that the upper extremity was contracted. The elbow and the fingers were in a state of flexion exactly as you see them at the present time (Fig. 79).

Chloroform was administered, and then they were able to recognise that there was no articular lesion, no trace of fibrous retraction, and that it consisted of a true spasmodic contracture.

Profiting by the resolution produced under chloroform, they attempted to modify the position of the hand, and to straighten the fingers. For this purpose a small straight splint was applied along the palm of the hand, and maintained in position by a bandage. But this contrivance was constantly becoming disturbed owing to the invincible flexion of the fingers; they were obliged to take it off at the end of two days, and the hand left to itself resumed its former attitude.

Since this epoch a great number of doctors have been consulted, but no fresh means have been adopted. Quite recently my colleague M. Périer, the surgeon of the Lariboisière Hospital, who was consulted amongst others, had the goodness to send the patient to me (16th May, 1886), he being under the impression that the case was more interesting to the physician than to the surgeon.

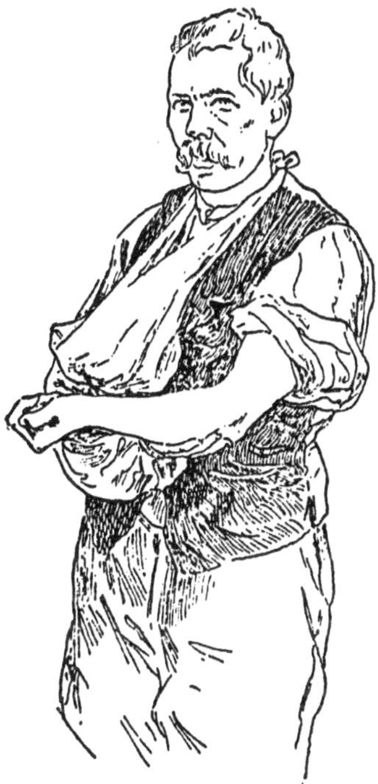

Fig. 79.

You can now see for yourselves that in this patient the left upper extremity, habitually carried in a sling, is flexed to an obtuse angle at the elbow-joint (Fig. 79). The forearm is maintained in a state of supination, and the fingers flexed on the palm of the hand, showing a marked tendency to overlap each other. The thumb is bent towards the axis of the hand, and its nail has produced a deep impression on the skin of the external surface of the index finger (Figs. 80 and 81).

The voluntary movement is almost completely lost in the different segments of the limb, and even passive movement is, by reason of the rigidity of the different joints, extremely limited. At the elbow and at the wrist the tendon reflexes are obviously exaggerated, and a trepidation of the fingers and the whole hand is very easily produced when attempts are made to straighten them.

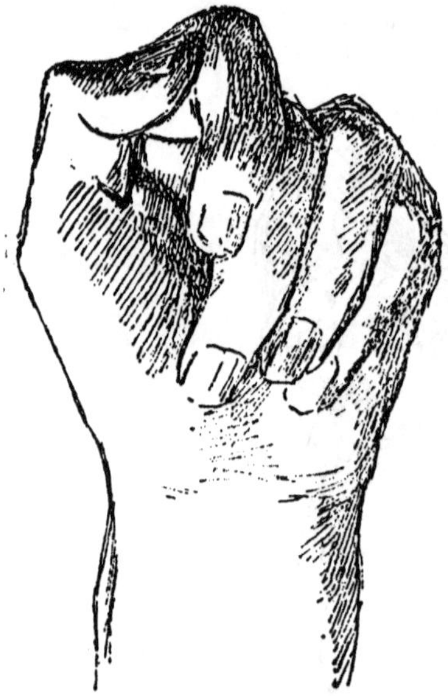

FIG. 80.

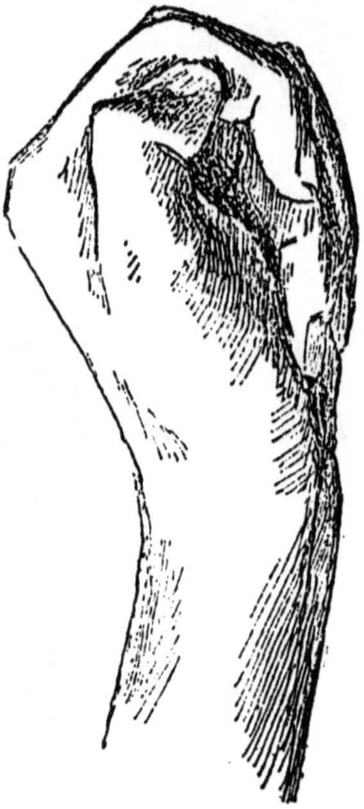

FIG. 81.

There is a certain degree of wasting, of atrophy of the limb, but the electrical reactions are normal. There is not the slightest trace of the reaction of degeneration.

We have here evidently a spasmodic contracture of neuromuscular origin.

It is easy to show that the deformity and the loss of power of the limb are not in this case the result of one of the complications of another sort, such as may occur after prolonged rest of the parts, or of a too forcible compression of them by means of a bandage.

Prolonged rest of a joint may produce, as you know, in certain cases and in certain subjects, a growing together of the synovial surfaces, a sort of arthritis sometimes followed by fibrous ankylosis (Teissier and Bonnet, Hueter, &c.). This arthritis is very similar, it may be noted in passing, to those which M. Bouchard and I have formerly studied in limbs which have been for a long time rendered immobile as a consequence of hemiplegia of cerebral origin. But the disappearance, beyond dispute, of all rigidity in the present case, when the subject is placed under the influence of chloroform, suffices to show that it is not this pathological condition with which we have to deal.

The same test enables us to state at once that it is not a matting together of the synovial sheaths or the tendons, nor yet a hyperplasia, with retraction, of the subcutaneous areolar tissue. A compression of a nerve-trunk would be able, no doubt, to produce a paralysis of a muscular group—of the extensors, for example—and consequently a paralytic contracture determined by the predominating action of the non-paralysed antagonistic muscles, but in such a case it would be easy on the one hand to exaggerate the flexion and on the other to overcome to a certain degree the predominating action of the flexors. But it is exactly the contrary that is here observed. The action of the extensors is quite as difficult to overcome as that of the flexors, and this is, as you know, precisely one of the characters of spasmodic contracture.

Of late years Professor Volkmann, in the first place, and after him M. Leser,[1] have described a particular kind of contracture which is observed in cases of fracture, especially in the upper extremities, which follows and is due to the too-forcible application of a bandage. This contracture seems to be due to the ischæmia produced in a limb by the excessive compression of a bandage; and it might be assimilated, according to the authors above recited, to the rigidity which shows

[1] R. Volkmann, "Die ischaemischen Muskellähmungen und Contracturen," 'Ctbl. f. Chir.,' 1881, No. 51, 'Ctbl. f. die med. Wiss.,' 1882, p. 445; E. Leser, "Untersuch. ueber ischaemische Muskelcontracturen und Muskellähmungen," Hallesche Habilitationsschrift, Leipzig, 1884; 'Centr. für Klin. Med.,' 1885, No. 17, p. 282, and 'Samm. klin. Vortraege,' No. 77.

itself in ischæmic parts in the experiments of Stenon, or again in man after ligature of the principal artery of a limb. You will understand this from the details I have given you in a lecture that was devoted this year to the study of intermittent limping produced in man by arterial obliteration.[1]

The contracture, or better, the rigidity of the limbs which appears under such conditions, may perhaps be considered as representing, so to speak, an early stage of cadaveric rigidity supervening in a living subject, and which, if the experiment is sufficiently prolonged, inevitably terminates at length in mortification of the limb. Now this, if I am not deceived, is the mechanism invoked by M. Volkmann and M. Leser to explain the development of the rigidity in the cases they have observed. According to them the phenemenon of cadaveric rigidity with coagulation of the myosine[2] occurs under these circumstances in some of the muscular fasciculi which are submitted to a high degree of ischæmia; while in the muscular fasciculi less completely involved there supervenes a condition consisting of a sort of alimentative myositis, followed first of all by a reabsorption of the coagulated myosine, then by muscular sclerosis, and lastly it terminates in a definite shortening of the muscle. M. Leser, in the experiments which he has made on animals, believes that he has obtained results which enable him to confirm on every point the theory proposed by M. Volkmann. But this is not the time to enter into a critical examination of these works. I will confine myself simply to pointing out that chief amongst the clinical characters which distinguish the contraction of M. Volkmann must be placed, according to him, the existence of profound modifications in the electrical reactions of the retracted muscles; and beyond doubt another equally important character is the impossibility of obtaining the resolution of the rigidity of the limb by the intervention of chloroform administered to its fullest extent.

Now you will remember that in Dum— the results of electri-

[1] Charcot, 'Della claudicazione intermittente, &c.,' Lez. raccolte dal Dr. G. Melotti di Bologna ('Gaz. degli Ospitali,' No. 73, p. 581, 1884).

[2] The recent researches of Brown-Séquard throw considerable doubt on the theory of the "coagulation of the myosine" as a cause of cadaveric rigidity ('Académie des Sciences,' Octobre, 1886).

zation and those of chloroformization are absolutely opposed to this pathological condition, and it is rendered abundantly evident that between the condition of contracture described by M. Volkmann and that which we have before us no kind of similitude can be established.

This is enough, I think, to enable one to affirm that the deformity of the limb in our patient is certainly the result of a spasmodic contracture; and now it remains yet for us to show, as stated at the beginning, that the contracture in question is of an hysterical nature.

It may be mentioned that there exists among hysterical patients quite a number of spasmodic contractures—and the patient with whom we are occupied offers an example of this kind—which, at least from the point of view of physiological mechanism, do not differ fundamentally from those which are developed as a consequence of organic lesion of the nerve-centres; lesions, as you know, differing both in their nature and in their situation, but presenting this feature in common, that they are accompanied by secondary degeneration in the pyramidal bands. In both cases, no doubt, the spasmodic rigidity occurs at the same time in antagonistic muscular groups, extensors and flexors for example; it is accompanied by an exaggeration of the tendon-reflexes; by an epileptoid trepidation, produced especially when the lower limb is involved; and finally, under the influence of chloroform pushed sufficiently far, the resolution of the contracture becomes complete. Such are the close resemblances which connect these two groups of cases. Nevertheless, in spite of this, hysterical contractures may often be distinguished from contractures due to a material cerebral or spinal lesion, even apart from the symptoms found in other parts of the body, by the aid of certain clinical characteristics which they bear. Thus for example, in the former, the rigidity of the limb is generally very marked; and sometimes moreover it persists in the same condition during sleep, even the most profound sleep; whereas in the latter, the contracture, generally less accentuated, reveals as a rule a manifest relaxation when the patient sleeps, and this relaxation lasts for several hours after waking. And again, anæsthesia, which is generally but little pronounced or altogether absent in the contracted limb due to an organic lesion, may on the other hand be found to occupy in a very marked degree not only the skin, but also the deeper parts, and accompanied by a more or less complete loss of the muscular sense, when we have to do with hysteria. Now these local distinctive features of hysterical contracture we shall find very markedly, as you will be able to see for yourselves, in the patient Dum—, and will lead us naturally to the supposition that hysteria is the origin of the deformity of the limb.

We must not allow ourselves to be drawn away from this conclusion by the existence, as I have pointed out to you, of a certain degree of muscular atrophy and of coldness of the integuments. These may be explained by the prolonged rest; and in this respect I may be allowed to recall to you the results of recent investigations by my chef de clinique, Dr. Babinski, which were set forth first in the 'Progrès Médicale,'[1] and afterwards in the memoir that appeared in the 'Archives de Neurologie.' These investigations have induced me to recognise—contrary to the prevalent notion, to which I had hitherto subscribed without reserve—that hysterical motor paralyses appear to be ordinarily marked by a certain degree of muscular atrophy; and that this condition, always without accompanying reaction of degeneration, may perhaps be very extreme and become developed with remarkable rapidity.

However, the diagnosis towards which we are tending becomes more and more legitimate, especially in the absence of all the symptoms belonging to a focal organic lesion of the nervous centres, by the results we derive from a search for hysterical stigmata. There exists on the left side—that is to say, on the same side as the contracture—complete analgesia; and on the same side a fairly marked deficiency of the hearing, smell, and taste, and also a very manifest retraction of the visual field. Finally, the attacks themselves are represented by the following symptoms: from time to time there occurs in the contracted limb the sensation of an aura which mounts

[1] Babinski, "De l'atrophie musculaire dans les paralysies hystériques" ('Progrès Médical,' 1886, Arch. de Neurol.,' T. XII, Nos. 34 et 35); and also Appendix IV.

towards the pharynx and produces there a feeling of suffocation. Several times this semblance of an attack has been followed by an aphonia lasting for several days.

I think that sufficient has been said to show you not only that our patient is under the ban of the hysterical diathesis, but also that the contracture of the left superior extremity is no other than one of the numerous manifestations of hysteria.

During the preceding exposition it is more than likely that many of you have had in your minds the following question: Why has the flaccid monoplegia produced in this man by an injury, and comparable in every respect, both in its clinical characters and in its mechanism, to the hystero-traumatic monoplegiæ which we have studied in the preceding lectures;[1] why, I say, has this paralysis, flaccid at the outset, become subsequently transformed into monoplegia with contracture?

Well, gentlemen, in my opinion the application of the bandage to the fractured limb is the circumstance which has caused this change. It is, in other words, the pressure exercised for a certain length of time by this bandage that has caused the appearance of spasmodic rigidity in the muscles; a moderate pressure, undoubtedly, for we have here a muscular spasm, and not, as I have attempted to show you, that kind of fibrous alteration described by M. Volkmann as supervening on the application of an over-tightened bandage (p. 349).

I hope to be in a position to furnish you immediately with proof of the proposition that I have just formulated. Here is another patient whom you already know. The man named Mouil—, a well-built labouring man twenty-five years of age, employed as a workman at the railway station. I have presented him to you before as offering a fresh illustration, very typical moreover, of hystero-traumatic monoplegia.[2] The paralysis came on after a slight blow ["tamponnement"] on the right shoulder. You see that the monoplegia thus produced, and which has existed for six months, is still pronounced; and that there is not only cutaneous and deep-seated anæsthesia, but also, and this is the point I want you specially to notice now, the paralysis is attended with perfect flaccidity

[1] See especially Lectures XX, XXI, and XXII.

[2] See Appendix I, Case 2.

of the limb. Well, gentlemen, I think that if a fracture of the bone of the paralysed limb had been produced by the slight injury which happened to Mouil—, and if the application of a bandage had been rendered necessary thereby, we should have had before us to-day not a flaccid monoplegia, but a monoplegia with contracture comparable with that we have observed in Dum—. This proposition may, as you will see, be justified to some extent experimentally. Thus, I will now apply a few turns of Esmarch's ligature to the paralysed and flaccid forearm of Mouil—, and almost immediately you see a spasmodic contracture occurs in the wrist and fingers of the hand. This contracture in truth disappears very soon after the bandage is removed. But, with a full knowledge of the facts to which I shall call your attention in a moment, it appears to me legitimate to admit that the contracture in question may become durable like those of Dum—, if the application of the bandage is repeated several times or maintained in position for a long enough time.

To return now to Dum—, we may presume that there exists in him a tendency to contracture in the paralysed limb, analogous to that which has just been produced in Mouil— by the application of a ligature; and that this tendency has become developed under the influence of the pressure exercised by the bandage applied to the fracture. In favour of this presumption it may be mentioned that the tendency to the contracture exists in Dum— at this very time in his left lower extremity, that is to say on the same side on which the upper extremity is contracted. You observe in fact that the application of several turns of an Esmarch's ligature to his lower extremity below the knee produces rigidity of the leg; and that the same applied a few centimetres above the foot determines the formation of a veritable equino-varus. Consequently there is nothing astonishing in the fact that the prolonged application of a bandage to the fractured limb has been able to determine a permanent muscular contracture in the patient Dum— such as that you have before you now.

This development of a spasmodic contracture under the influence of a circular compression of the limb, of which I have just shown you two examples, is assuredly a very curious circumstance, and merits, both from the point of view of its novelty and of its practical importance, your careful attention. On many occasions and under many different circumstances have we insisted on the frequent existence in hysterical subjects of contractures supervening under the influence of various traumatic causes; or artificially produced at will by the observer, even in the waking state, by the operation of certain manipulations.[1]

As for the last-named condition, that is to say contractures artificially produced in the waking state, the recent investigations which we have made into this matter in connection with the case that we have just been considering have convinced us that the subject is one which has not yet been sufficiently brought out, and which merits further study. Up to the present time we have been able to affirm, after having investigated a great number of patients, that the artificial production of contractures is an occurrence frequent enough in hysterical subjects of both sexes; that the occurrence is not usual in healthy subjects; and that consequently we have here a stigma which, in the same way as the retraction of the field of vision, the sensitive and sensorial hemianæsthesia, &c., enables us to discover in certain difficult cases the existence of the hysterical diathesis. The proceedings which may be employed to determine these contractures are very different, but we will confine ourselves to mentioning the following: repeated percussion of the tendons, traction exercised on the fingers, application of a vibrating tuning-fork, whether to the tendons or to the fleshy parts of the limbs, faradization, &c. But of all these means, the most efficacious beyond doubt is the application of two or three turns of an Esmarch's ligature or some other band.

With the assistance of my house physician, M. Berbès, the application of the ligature has been made in the course of the last month on a total of seventy hysterical subjects (43 women,

[1] See on this subject Charcot, "De l'influence des lésions traumatiques sur le développement des phénomènes d'hystérie locale," 'Maladies du système nerveux,' T. I, p. 449, Appendice.—Ib., T. III, 3e, 7e, et 8e leçons; Ch. Richet et Brissaud, 'Progrès Médical,' 8 Mai, 1880; Paul Richer, 'Mémoire inédit présenté à l'Académie de Médecine,' 1883 (Prix Civrieux); P. Descubes, 'Étude sur les contractures provoquées chez les hystériques à l'état de veille,' Thèse de Bordeaux, 1885.

27 men), some now under treatment in the clinical wards, some frequenting the out-patient department. Here is a summary of the most important results that we have obtained in this series of investigations.[1] The existence of motor paralysis in the limb tested is not necessary in order to obtain the contracture; in hemianæsthetic subjects the contracture is most frequently obtained exclusively in the limbs on the anæsthetic side; it may nevertheless sometimes be obtained in subjects equally well on the side which retains its sensation, but in such cases the contracture is always more pronounced and more easily produced on the anæsthetic side. We have observed in a large number of the patients that *the contracture produced in the limb was much more accentuated, and much more durable after the cessation of the constriction, when the experiment had been often repeated and had been continued for a longer time.* The rigidity was sometimes confined to the limb to which the compression was applied, and was limited to the parts situated below the ligature, but most often it extended to the entire limb, and in a certain number of cases it extended to all the limbs and even to the face. These last-named circumstances demonstrate, I think, that the contracture in question is not the consequence of an ischæmia produced in the limb by the application of the ligature. On the contrary, one sees in it the result, without any doubt, of a peripheral irritation involving a participation of the nervous centres after the mechanism of reflex acts. Viewed in this light, in combination with the whole of the clinical characters, the contractures produced in hysterical subjects in a waking state do not probably differ from the contractures produced in the lethargic period of great hypnotism, except in the intensity of the phenomena, which are much greater in the latter case. Moreover, the contractures produced in hysterical patients, like those of lethargic hypnotism, generally disappear very easily under the influence of a moderate pressure on the muscles antagonistic to those in action; or again under the influence of a slight friction of the skin of the rigid limb.

[1] For further details on this subject see P. Berbès, 'Sur la diathèse de contracture et en particulier sur la contracture produite sur les sujets hystériques (hommes et femmes) par l'application d'une ligature' ('Progrès Médical,' No. 41, 9 Oct., 1886).

However, one must not be too reckless in these experiments and, to speak only of the contracture of hysterical patients in the waking state, it is important not to forget that resolution is more difficult to obtain when the ligature which produced it has been maintained longer in position. In fact, gentlemen, these experiments should never be undertaken except with great discretion.

But I must not dwell longer on this subject, although it offers many points of interest, and merits special and thorough investigation.

Three or four days after the lecture that has just been concluded, Dum—, influenced by one of those strange caprices so common in hysterical subjects, even in male ones, determined to quit the hospital. The very day of his going out the contracted limb was submitted to methodical massage; light frictions [frôlements] were practised on the different segments of the limb, by the aid of the hand moistened with glycerine, at the same time as attempts were made by means of traction to straighten the fingers and to move the wrist, the elbow, and the shoulder. This operation, which lasted about ten minutes, provoked at first rather severe pains along the palmar surface of the fingers where the anæsthesia was not complete; but it was followed by a very satisfactory result, for the contracture became very manifestly lessened, the fingers became straighter, and the patient was finally able to produce fairly extensive movements of his wrist, his elbow, and his shoulder.

He left the hospital that same day, and we lost sight of him for several months. He returned to us a few days ago, and then informed us that, the contracture having to some extent returned a few days after going out, he consulted a doctor in the town, who treated him by Dr. Burcq's method. To-day (October 16th, 1886) he has returned to us with his hands and fingers covered with plates and rings of copper, which he has had on nearly ever since he left us.

This is the condition of the patient at the present time. In the left upper extremity the sensibility has reappeared; it even seems to be exaggerated, especially on the palmar surface of the hand, where the application of a cold substance produces a sensation of heat. The deep sensibility and the muscular sense are normal. The general sensibility elsewhere presents no anomaly, and as for the special senses, we have discovered that the taste, hearing, and smell are as active now on the left as on the right, and that the left visual field has no trace of concentric retraction. On every point amelioration is manifest, and I may add that the phantom attacks do not now occur.

But as much cannot quite be said with respect to the movements of the left upper extremity. The movements of the shoulder, the elbow, and the wrist have returned almost to their normal condition, and are nearly as extensive as the corresponding movements in the limb of the opposite side, which without doubt is an important result. But the movements of the fingers, fairly energetic during flexion (dynamometer, left 25, right 85), are very limited during extension; and consequently the hand remains deformed, the fingers being bent so as to form an angle of about 90 degrees with the palm of the hand

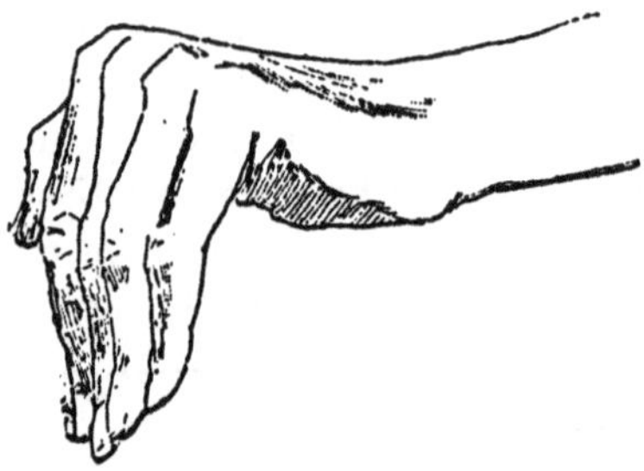

FIG. 82.

(Fig. 82). It is impossible to produce much modification in this angle by extension, and all attempts to straighten the hand give rise to severe pain. In this respect, therefore, the cure is far from being complete, and it is to be feared that the cause which prevents extension of the fingers is now not only the spasmodic contracture of the muscles, but also, as we have observed in other cases under analogous conditions,[1] the presence of fibroid tissue undergoing retraction

[1] Lecture X.

in the palm of the hand. That, however, is a point which cannot be completely elucidated except by the employment of chloroform.[1]

[1] On the 18th Oct. last the patient was submitted to chloroform. The sleep was made as profound as possible, and at no time was it possible to obtain a resolution of the deformity of the fingers just described. Evidently it is no longer a simple spasmodic muscular contraction.—J. M. C.

LECTURE XXVI.

A CASE OF HYSTERICAL MUTISM IN A MAN.

SUMMARY.—*Description of hysterical mutism.—It consists of a very characteristic group of symptoms [Syndrôme]; aphonia, impossibility of whispering, motor aphasia.—Preservation of the general movements of the lips, tongue, etc.—The intelligence is not affected; patients preserve the faculty of writing fluently, and conversing by signs.—Diagnosis of hysterical mutism.—Its importance in certain cases.—Malingerers.—It is generally very easy to detect them.—Experimental production of* hysterical mutism *in hypnotisable hysterics.*

GENTLEMEN,—It is in order to compare one with the other that I present to you two patients whose diseases imply a prognosis so essentially opposed. In the first, the recovery will be complete, that is absolutely certain, and I may add that in all probability it will happen quite suddenly in a few days, perhaps to-morrow. In the second, on the other hand, the verdict is *prognosis pessima, exitus lethalis,* and I might also add *properatus,* for the execution of the sentence will certainly not be postponed more than three or four months; this patient is suffering from a permanent organic bulbar lesion, running a fatal course; whereas, in the other the lesion is probably of cortical origin, and in any case is of a purely dynamic order, and as experience shows every day, of an essentially transitory nature.

However, gentlemen, the affections from which they are suffering present certain traits in common, and on certain points they have such marked resemblance that even an experienced physician may be excused for confounding them.

[1] Lecture edited by M. Gilles de la Tourette. The same lecture has been published in the Gazetta degli Ospedali of Milan, VII, Nos. 75 and 76, by Dr. Melotti.

It is precisely for this reason that I have brought them before you at the same time on the present occasion. This juxtaposition, moreover, will certainly have the advantage of enabling us to accentuate the contrasts and to bring out clearly the distinctive clinical characters of the two affections.

Briefly the features possessed by both are as follows. In one of the patients it is absolutely impossible, and in the other almost impossible, for him to express his thoughts in articular language, and both of them are aphonic. The aphonia of the first is absolute; he is scarcely able to emit the smallest hoarse cry, and that only with much effort. The second is still able to give vent to a few grunting sounds. I may add that both of them have preserved the power of conversing by gesture to perfection. We are able to converse with both of them by signs; but it is easier to communicate with them by means of writing. In fact, both our patients are not only in full possession of their intelligence and understand admirably all that is said to them, but they are quite able to render their thoughts in writing exactly as they could before the development of the disease; that is to say in a style and with an orthography quite in keeping with the education that they have received.

Such are roughly the features of resemblance; as for the distinctive characters we shall reserve them for future consideration.

The first patient is the principal object of our lecture today; the second only having been placed beside him by way of comparison. Gentlemen, I may at the onset state that in my opinion this man, thirty-three years old, a gas-fitter by occupation, is a very good example of what is generally termed *hysterical mutism.* But before entering into the account of his history and attempting to justify that diagnosis, I think it may be useful, in order to render the demonstration clearer and more profitable, to indicate to you in few words the most important facts that are known about this singular affection. You will remember that it is a subject that we have already dealt with in December last, and Dr. Cartaz, who gave us his aid in making the laryngoscopic examinations, has made known the substance of my lectures on this subject, adding thereto a few of his own observations in an interesting memoir based on twenty cases, of which six were in my wards.[1]

Hysterical mutism is not an extremely rare affection; it has often been described, and you will find it mentioned in all writings devoted to hysteria. However, I think that the characteristics of the disease were not sufficiently isolated until the delivery of the lectures to which I have just made allusion. And the details into which we shall now enter may possibly present to some of you the appearance of novelty.

The chief characteristics which in my opinion distinguish hysterical mutism and establish it as a true clinical entity, recognisable by all, are as follows. The facts as I am about to present them to you are founded, partly on cases that I have observed myself, and partly on those published by others.

In the great majority of cases hysterical mutism *comes on quite suddenly*. It often follows a fright or a violent emotion of some sort; sometimes it comes on immediately after an hysterical attack; or again without any apparent exciting cause it may supervene in the course of hysterical aphonia. Lastly, it may become developed in the course of ordinary laryngitis.

Its *duration* is extremely variable, sometimes it lasts for several hours or for several days—in our patient it has existed for three weeks. It has been known to extend over months or even years.

Recovery generally occurs, and the disappearance of the mutism is almost as sudden as was its appearance. It happens suddenly and like the onset very frequently follows some violent emotion. Relapses are frequent.

These are the characters as a general rule. But there are not a few exceptions. Thus, in certain cases the patient is unable to completely recover, in its entirety, the faculty that he has lost. He may be able perhaps to whisper, or to speak in a low voice, although he remains aphonic; he may be unable to speak aloud for a long time. Sometimes—and this is perhaps most frequently the case—before recovering complete

[1] See Appendix V.

possession of his speech the patient passes through a period distinguished by a peculiar stammering, consisting of the frequent repetition of the same syllables. This defect appears especially when the words he uses are of a certain length.

Now I come to the exposition of the constituent elements of the syndroma [group of symptoms]. Although the patient has preserved the integrity of the ordinary movements of the tongue and lips so that he can move these organs with agility in all directions, and so that he can blow or whistle as in the normal state, *yet it is impossible for him to articulate a word even in a low voice, or otherwise expressed, to whisper.* Nor is it possible for him, even by paying the greatest attention, *to imitate the movements of articulation which he sees before him.* The patient therefore is *mute* in the most rigorous acceptation of the term, for he cannot pronounce a single word. It may be said even that he is *more than mute,* for whereas it is possible for a deaf-mute to give utterance to very loud inarticulate sounds, the hysterical mute, note well this singular character, the hysterical mute is *aphonic,* in general absolutely so; or at most, like our patient, he can only emit, with the greatest difficulty, a little hoarse sound such as that which you will hear in a minute.

Is not this, gentlemen, a very remarkable association of symptoms? Some people will perhaps think directly that in such a case the mutism is a natural consequence of the aphonia pushed to a very high degree. The patient is mute because he has no voice, because the larynx and the vocal cords do not vibrate properly. Nevertheless with a little reflection you will at once recognise, with me, that this hypothesis involves a serious error. Hysterical patients who are simply aphonic—a frequent enough condition—are, it is true, unable to emit loud sounds, but they can make themselves perfectly understood by whispering, and by speaking in a low voice.

Whispering is nothing else than spoken and articulate language. The phenomenon is, note it well, absolutely independent of the laryngeal voice. The truth of this fact was demonstrated experimentally in the laboratory of M. Marey, in 1876, and again in 1879 by M. Boudet, of Paris. These authors have clearly shown by means of the graphic method that the larynx takes no part in whispering; the vocal cords do not vibrate, the air traverses the larynx as it traverses the trachea, it passes along a motionless tube, nothing more.

This it is which reveals, perhaps more than anything else, the truly special character of hysterical mutism. If the individual suffering from the affection is unable to whisper, it is not because he is aphonic, or rather because his larynx does not vibrate; it is not because he has lost the common movements of tongue and lips—you have seen that this patient was perfectly able to blow and to whistle; it is because he lacks the ability to execute the proper specialised movements necessary for the articulation of words. In other terms he is deprived of the motor representations necessary for the calling into play of articulate speech.

We have, therefore, to do with a *motor aphasia* and I may add a purely *motor* one. It is a rare kind, very rare in the domain of ordinary organic aphasia. With it other affections of interior language are mostly associated, in different proportions, such as word-blindness or word-deafness, or agraphia, or finally a diminution of intellectual power more or less pronounced.

We shall see that our hysterical mute does not come within this latter category. I should like you moreover to remember —this is a practical feature of the highest importance—that, even in the most complete organic motor aphasia the patient is able to call out, to enunciate a few syllables in a loud voice, even to pronounce a few words, albeit not appropriate ones, but perfectly distinct. On the other hand, in labio-glosso-laryngeal palsy (of which our second patient offers a complete example), although there exists paralysis of the general movements of the lips, tongue, and larynx, the voice and the articulation of words, although feeble and in the last stage most indistinct, are generally present in some degree even up to the end of life. I insist again on these characters, because in hysterical mutism as I say the patient is dumb, perfectly dumb, at the same time as he is without vocal power.

There are some other equally characteristic signs. The hysterical mute has not only preserved all the faculties of his intellect, not only does he readily comprehend all that is communicated to him by means of his ear or his eye, but he is perfectly able, as I said at the commencement of this lecture, to make himself understood by pantomimic signs, and of communicating his thoughts by writing. All these phenomena may be met with, no doubt, in a case of labio-glosso-laryngeal paralysis of bulbar origin—and in this respect we cannot establish very much distinction between the two affections—but in organic aphasia the symptomatology does not assume, as you know, the same characters.

You are aware how rare are cases of pure motor aphasia without complication among organic lesions of the brain. Together with the loss of motor representations of articular language, there are nearly always superadded, as I have just said, in a general fashion or in variable proportions, other perversions of interior language. The aphasic is quite unable to read, or reads only with difficulty; he does not generally understand, or understands only imperfectly, what is communicated to him through his ear, although he is not deaf, and he may have preserved his intelligence completely. But, even when none of these complications exist, it will generally be found that he has lost, at least in great part, the faculty of making himself understood by gesture. You will recall how difficult it is to converse in this way with this kind of aphasic patient. Moreover, in all probability he is unable to write, for you know how exceedingly rare it is to find people aphasic from an organic lesion who can write, and in these individuals the act of writing, if it persists to a certain extent, is slow, difficult, and very imperfect.

It is quite otherwise in the hysterical mute. He has lost nothing, absolutely nothing, of his former education, nor of his intelligence, nor of his faculty of writing. When questions are put to him he grasps a pen or pencil with singular readiness, and renders his thoughts in writing with perfect clearness. The gestures of the patient in such cases are strikingly graphic, and this feature, jointly with symptoms of loss of voice and articulate language, enables one to recognise hysterical mutism almost immediately and without further examination.

I have before narrated, in connection with this subject, the history of a young Spaniard whose case you will find *in extenso* in the memoir of Dr. Cartaz. He was presented to me as having been attacked for more than a year with syphilitic epilepsy, in accordance with which view he had been treated. I was further informed that very often he would remain aphasic for several days after the fits. When I saw him he was suffering from one of these attacks of supposed aphasia. When I approached the patient he made a sign to me by carrying his hand to his throat—a very ordinary gesture of hysterical mutes under these circumstances—that it was impossible for him to articulate a single word. "Speak in a low voice," I said to him. With great difficulty he was able to form with his lips a few silent movements of articulation. "Cry out," I said to him. He was unable to emit a single sound. Then I ascertained that the patient was able to put out his tongue, to blow, and to whistle as in normal conditions. After this the young Spaniard, nettled and impatient at my questions, seized a pen and gave me, with remarkable promptitude by means of writing, some of the details of his history as clearly as it was possible for me to desire, although he wrote in French and not in his mother tongue.

My diagnosis made, I declared him to be a hysteric, which my colleague thought to be a very imprudent proposition, probably because he deemed it too precipitate; but further examination only confirmed it. There existed in this young man a hemianæsthesia, with choreïform trembling on the left side; a retraction of the visual field and a deficiency of hearing on the same side, and pharyngeal anæsthesia; in a word, all the series of stigmata which left no doubt whatever as to the existence of an hysterical basis. I may add that the description of the attack which was then given to us was very characteristic. It was true hystero-epilepsy, and neither epilepsy proper nor symptomatic epilepsy; and by a more thorough investigation of the antecedents we discovered that syphilis had never existed, except in the imagination of the patient, and in that of the physician. The sequel of this case proved in the most peremptory way that it was with hysterical phenomena we had to deal, and nothing else.

Founded on the preceding considerations, and on all that I have since learned of this subject in an experience by no means short, I think that I am justified in affirming that the condition, *hysterical mutsim*, is sufficiently well charactorised, sufficiently original, to be recognised by itself, even in the absence of all information furnished by concomitant symptoms.

And you also, gentlemen, when you have become thoroughly acquainted with the characteristics, you in your turn will achieve diagnoses of such rapidity as to be considered by the unitiated as a sort of magic. Nevertheless it is evident that the case would remain incomplete if the examination of the patient was not conducted further. Now, it is very rarely that the permanent phenomena of hysteria, which for the sake of brevity we call stigmata, are completely wanting; even the attacks also frequently exist, the retraction of the visual field, the single or double hemianæsthesia, the divers sensorial troubles, pharyngeal anæsthesia,—these are the phenomena which you ought to carefully search for. Their presence will greatly contribute to confirm your diagnosis. I may also mention that the contracture of a limb produced experimentally by a circular ligature is an additional stigma which our recent researches have enabled us to add; the frequency of which, both in men and in women, is much greater than is generally supposed.[1]

However, one must not forget to mention that, although the hysterical affection in one subject may take on a polymorphous form, it may be found in another reduced to a single symptomatic element. Thus it is with hysterical mutism; it may be sometimes met with completely isolated, the only evidence of the malady, and this is exactly the case with the patient that you now have before you.

It is just for this very reason, gentlemen, that it is necessary to attach a great importance to an exact knowledge of each of these hysterical syndromata taken by themselves, for it is this knowledge alone which renders it possible to diagnose the affection when it is met with as an isolated condition. It is fortunate that the natural history of the symptoms in the condition we are now considering offers, as a general rule, features which by themselves are sufficiently characteristic to enable one to decide, even under relatively unfavorable conditions, without great chance of error.

[1] See Lecture XXV.

If I insist so much upon this clinical fact, it is because hysterical mutes, more perhaps than individuals attacked with other manifestations of the neurosis, are in a large number of instances, I know not why, considered as malingerers, although in my opinion—I am obliged to say it again and again—the idea of simulation is only too often based under these circumstances on the ignorance of the doctor. Possibly the error is not of such great importance when it is a question of diagnosis in private practice or in hospital; under such circumstances the mistake may be made without very grave inconvenience to the patient.

But if the case occur in the army, or when it comes in some way within the jurisdiction of the law, the results are very different. Under these circumstances, the ill-founded idea of simulation may lead to far more serious consequences, to grave injustice, and possibly to the employment of barbarous means of treatment. For example, very powerful faradization of the larynx is, as you know, not by any means without danger. Moreover, it is my duty to point out to you that in these particular cases simulation is perhaps more easy to dispel than is generally believed. There are very few simulators, be it known, who have sufficient intelligence to combine and display, with the object of deceit, all the symptoms that belong to the natural history of hysterical mutism, without taking from or adding in any way to this group of symptoms, at once so special and so complex.

Generally speaking the malingerer may be considered to be a fantastic person. He gives the reins to his imagination, and he adds all sorts of embellishments. Recall to your minds the conversation between Sganarelle and Lucinde, who may perhaps be considered as a perfect simulator.[1]

"Sganarelle.—'What is the matter? What pain is it that you feel?'

"Lucinde (*replying by signs, carrying her hand to her mouth, to her head, and to her chin*).—'Han, hi, hon, han.'

"Sganarelle.—'Eh! what do you say?'

"Lucinde (*continuing the same gestures*).—'Han, hi, hon, han, han, hi, hon.'

"Sganarelle.—'What?'

[1] "Le Médecin malgré lui," Scène VI.

"Lucinde.—'Han, hi, hon.'"

Well, gentlemen, these han, hi, hon, han, are evidently superfluous, and reveal simulation. The legitimate mute remains silent, as I have told you, and if he carries his hand often towards his throat, it is to show you where in his idea the obstacle is; he would not point to his head and to his mouth. This is the way, as it seems to me, by considerations of this sort, that simulation often unmasks itself.

Under certain circumstances, gentlemen, simulation may appear very probable, at first sight, though a more attentive examination shows that in reality the symptoms are perfectly legitimate. As an illustration of this I may mention the following case which I had tho opportunity of observing in the prison of St. Lazare, thanks to the kindness of my colleague, Prof. Brouardel. Hélène G—, a young prisoner of about twenty-four years of age, had directed to a priest, who she believed had wronged her, the dead body of a newly born child well wrapped up and placed in a basket. The parcel, labelled *cheese*, arrived by post just at the moment when the priest was receiving friends. Enclosed with the body was a small note, thus worded:—"*Pray for what you have lost.*" Was not that the act of an hysterical lunatic?

Arrested soon afterwards, Hélène G— suddenly lost her speech after the very first interrogation. This time you will say the mutism was evidently simulated. Well no, gentlemen, it was not so in my opinion, and this was also the opinion of my esteemed colleague, M. Brouardel.

This was my argument; the natural history of hysterical mutism, though very little known by the laity, was well depicted here. Hélène G— was mute and aphonic; she did not emit the least sound even when startled or excited to laughter by surprise. Not the least sound, no hin, hi, hon, han; not the least unnecessary gesture. The onset was quite sudden. The hysterical stigmata were, moreover, very pronounced, and of such a nature as did not admit of simulation; complete general anæsthesia; anæsthesia of the pharynx; retraction of visual field, &c. And lastly, there was a feature that is absolutely peremptory; as in the case of other hysterical mutes. *The patient wrote fluently and correctly, and it was in this way that she was able to communicate with the magistrate, and, at least in great part, confess her crime.* A malingerer, without any doubt, would have pushed matters to the bitter end, she would have ceased to be able to write, whereas this girl wrote without any flaw. The autopsy of the body of the child having demonstrated that it had lived, Hélène G— was convicted of infanticide, and condemned to three years' imprisonment.

But it is time, I think, after this digression, to return to the demonstration of our case. After the foregoing we shall be able to complete this rapidly.

The patient is thirty-three years of age. After having followed many kinds of occupation, he is now in the service of the Gas Company. There does not seem to exist any nervous heredity in his family history, nor has he suffered from any illnesses worthy of note, although during a period of *six years*, from twenty-four to thirty years of age, he had attacks of which he gives us a very graphic description by the aid of pantomimic gestures. The attacks began with an aura, and included, amongst other features, the "arcs of a circle," and great movements; he assures us that he did not lose consciousness. However, several years previously, when he was twenty years old, he momentarily lost the use of his senses after hearing a very loud noise which gave him a great fright. He was married three years ago, and since then the attacks have ceased. Shortly afterwards, without known cause, other than a laryngitis accompanied by aphonia, he became suddenly mute. He went under the care of M. Rigal, who cured him at the end of a few weeks quite suddenly by the application of a laryngoscopic mirror. It was three weeks ago, and following the same cause, namely, a laryngitis of only a few hours' duration, that the mutism again occurred.

You see that our patient presents all the classical characters of hysterical mutism, such as I have been describing. When told to call out, to speak, or to whisper, he is absolutely unable to comply. When I persist, he makes the characteristic gestures, and points with his hand to his throat as though he would tell us that the difficulty lies there.

However, he moves his tongue and his lips perfectly in every direction. He is able to write and render his ideas very well, and in a style that corresponds with his incomplete education. In this case, beyond the special characteristics of the mutism, the fits from which he formerly suffered are the only symptoms in favour of hysteria, for the patient is quite free from all hysterical stigmata. Here then the mutism occurs as a solitary hysterical symptom, *mono-symptomatic*, and yet we do not hesitate in the diagnosis for a moment, for the reasons that I have pointed out and, I hope, sufficiently made clear to you.

Now let us turn to the second patient. I need not make a great point of his age—seventy-one years—because a bulbar affection may become developed at twenty or younger, and we know of hysterical men of forty years and more. But what I would emphasize is the slow and progressive onset of his difficulty of speech. And again, although he cannot speak, this patient can at any rate cry out. There is paralysis and atrophy of the tongue; his mouth is widened, his lips are pendent, and he has the aspect of one who is weeping. In spite of all this the articulation of words is not completely lost; he can still—though in truth with great difficulty—pronounce some indistinct words. In his case there is not loss of memory of the movements of articulation, nor is there motor aphasia, but we have to do with *anarthria*, consequent upon the paralysis of the general movements of the tongue and of the lips.

I may add that the saliva dribbles involuntarily away, the deglutition is very difficult, and when he drinks liquid it returns by the nose; and finally, at night he has attacks of suffocation.

You see, gentlemen, from this comparison, that between these two patients there only exists a rough resemblance. And although in both of them there is a marked contrast between the faculty of writing easily, which remains, and the impossibility of making their articulation heard, it may be pointed out that this last phenomenon is not of the same order in the two cases, but is due to absolutely different mechanisms.

I will terminate this lecture by an experimental demonstration, and present to you two cases of artificially produced mutism in two hypnotisable, hysterical subjects. Prior to the experiment to which they have been submitted, these two women have never been in communication with hysterical mutes, although, on the other hand, they are daily in contact with patients who are affected with anarthria due to labio-glosso-laryngeal paralysis. Nevertheless, you will recognise without difficulty in both of them characters identical with those which have been described just now in spontaneous hysterical mutism. These women are unable to cry out, to articulate a single word, or even to whisper; and yet the general movements of the tongue and lips are quite free from any affection; they continue to be able to express themselves by writing and by gesture, and their intelligence is quite unaffected.

I bring them before you now, awake, but still mute; I ought to tell you how the phenomenon of mutism may be artificially produced. The patient being plunged into the somnambulic stage of hypnotism, you commence by conversing with her for a few minutes, then gradually you approach closer and closer to her, and finally pretend neither to hear nor to understand her. She makes further efforts to speak louder, but you continue to practise the same ruse, and appear not to understand any better than before. Then it happens that the voice of the subject becomes progressively lower, and in the last stage aphonia becomes complete and there is an impossibility of articulation. Artificial mutism, obtained during the somnambulic period, persists as you see, in the waking state. I dare not allow this experiment to be prolonged too much, for I have remarked on many occasions that hysterical symptoms artificially produced during hypnotism are more difficult to be made to disappear in a waking state in proportion as they are allowed to persist for a longer time.[1]

[1] The hysterical patient who formed the main subject of this lecture, and who was present part of the time, seemed to be vividly impressed by all he had heard. The following morning, shortly after waking, he suddenly regained his speech.

Gentlemen, the possibility of giving rise to the syndroma *hysterical mutism* artificially by means of suggestion, appears to us to indicate sufficiently clearly the point of departure of all the phenomena; and one is thus able to suppose the mechanism of its development. It is in the grey cortex of the cerebral hemispheres that we must seek for the dynamic lesion whence emanate the symptoms in question; and the mechanism that is to be invoked in such conditions is none other than that which acts in the production of psychical, or, if you like it better, mental paralysis.

This theory, which is now founded on a considerable number of facts and on experience, is applicable, as you know, to a large number of hysterical affections, particularly those which arise under the influence of an occasional cause, such as a violent emotion, a traumatism, &c. It is a subject that has occupied us many times in several of the preceding lectures, to which I would refer those amongst you who wish to acquire further information in the matter.[1]

[1] See particularly Lectures XXI and XXII.

APPENDIX

I.

TWO ADDITIONAL CASES OF HYSTERO-TRAUMATIC PARALYSIS IN MEN.

Part of a Lecture by M. Charcot (1886), *edited by Messrs. Babinski and Berbèz.*

(Appendix to Lectures XX, XXI, XXII.)

I. *A case of hystero-traumatic paraplegia supervening on a street accident.*[1]

THE man named Le Log— was born in a little village of Brittany, and he is now twenty-nine years of age. One of his first cousins was subject to epilepsy (a falling down, calling out, biting of tongue, &c.). One of his sisters, who finally died of typhoid fever, had had "nervous attacks."

The patient has also suffered from typhoid fever, and after this he remained *aphonic* for several months.

He came to Paris when twelve years old, knowing but little French; at the present time he is able to read, but he can only write with difficulty. People who know him have given him a very good character. He has always been amiable, and obliging. He is a steady lad. He is not gloomy, nor is he alcoholic. By occupation he was formerly a cook's assistant, but lately, for want of better work, he went into the service of a florist in the market. His work consisted in selling in the market during the morning, and in the afternoon, every second or third day, he went to a horticulturist at St. Cloud to fetch plants. These he brought back on a

[1] The notes of the case are by M. Berbèz, Interne du Service.

little hand-barrow, which he drew, while his master's son, young Conr—, helped by pushing behind.

It was on returning from St. Cloud in this fashion on October 21st, 1885, about 6 o'clock in the evening, that the accident happened which was the cause of all his troubles. On this evening, when it was very nearly dark, Le Log— was dragging his barrow along the road beside the Seine. He had arrived at the top of the Pont des Invalides, when all of a sudden, a heavily laden laundryman's van, driven by some drunken men at railway speed, charged into him. The wheel of the hand-barrow was struck, and Le Log— was violently thrown on to the footpath, from which he was picked up absolutely unconscious. The horse of the laundryman's van did not touch Le Log—, and its wheels *did not pass over him.* There was no apparent wound, nor was any blood discovered about his person. Le Log— was placed upon his own barrow and was taken in the first place to a chemist's shop, where he remained for about twenty minutes, and was then carried, still unconscious, to the Beaujon Hospital.

The preceding details were given by young Conr—, and confirmed, moreover, by a man named L—, a post-office official at the Palais de l'Industrie, who was present during the collision. The account which Le Log— himself gives of the affair when he is questioned is a very different one. *He has made out a long history of the accident* in which he firmly believes, and of which the circumstances appear to him from time to time *in his dreams.* The laundryman's van came charging along with much noise; the horse fell right upon him, and struck him in the breast with its head. He fell down, struck his head violently on the ground, and finally the heavy van *passed completely over his body, across the upper part of the thighs.* Generally, when his dream arrives at this point, the patient wakes up suddenly screaming. At the Hôtel Dieu, and here also at the Salpêtrière, he has often been heard to cry out "Stop! don't drive on, the horse is going to crush me."

As a matter of fact, the patient has completely lost all recollection of what passed at the moment of the accident. It is very probable that he was affected at the time by an *intense cerebral commotion,* followed by a form of amnesia which MM. Ribot and Azam have described under the name of *traumatic retrograde amnesia.*

He was transported to the Beaujon Hospital, where he remained during five or six days without consciousness. Leeches and sinapisms were applied, and an ice-bag was put on his head. When his consciousness returned he was very surprised to find himself in the hospital; he remembered absolutely nothing of what had taken place. It was only after he had heard the history from those around, as he himself confesses, that the circumstances of the accident as he narrates them occurred to his mind.

Several facts relative to his state in the Beaujon Hospital are worthy of being mentioned. (1) *His lower extremities seemed to him as though they were dead.* At first he was unable to lift them from the bed, except with the aid of his hands, but at the end of a few days he was able to leave his bed, go out of the hospital, and walk part of the way home on foot. (2) He had several large bruises on the hip, the right groin, and over the lower abdomen. (3) He suffered with his head in the same way he does now.

After leaving the Beaujon he remained for a week laid up at home. At that time he had some profuse epistaxes, which were only arrested by plugging, and which have since recurred several times.

He left his house one day to go and see some friends, and while there was seized with a severe attack, preceded by a sensation of a ball rising in his throat, and during which he lost consciousness. He was then placed on a stretcher, and taken to the Hôtel Dieu.

There he came under the care of Dr. Capitan, Chef de clinique de la faculté, who has given us the following information concerning Le Log—'s condition during his stay of two months at the Hôtel Dieu: "During the first week the patient was in a state of continual coma. After waking from this he presented for two days all the symptoms of hysterical mutism. Frequent epistaxes occurred, and were only stopped by plugging. The *motor weakness* of the lower extremities, imperfect at first, gradually became complete."

On the 25th March Dr. Capitan had the kindness to send the patient to us. The following are the prominent sym ptoms that we have observed in him, in addition to the *crises* which will be described by-and-by.

On admission, the patient was lying in a prostrate condition of dorsal decubitus, silent, as though he were preoccupied, replying but slowly and unwillingly to the questions that were put to him. From one day to another he has varied in his account; evidently his memory and intelligence are considerably affected. The physiognomy, moreover, is expressive of sadness, hebetude, and from time to time even stupor, and the speech is embarrassed.

He complains of a dull aching pain in the head, and when the head is lightly touched or the scalp stroked, he seems to suffer acutely. He states that at night-time he has flames before his eyes, and terrifying dreams, and all the while beatings in the temples and dizziness in the ears.

On examining the face it is remarked that the left labial commissure is raised, and on this side the mouth is partly open. This was at first thought to be due to paralysis of the right inferior facial. But on further examination it is recognised to be due to a spasm of the muscles on the left side of the face, as is evident by the tremors, sometimes slow, sometimes fast, in the labial commissure of this side. When the tongue is protruded there is no deviation.

The patient is thin; his pulse is feeble. The skin of the extremities is warm and always covered with sweat; the perspiration over these parts is from time to time extremely abundant. The tongue is natural and the temperature normal. The patient has been able to eat, though he eats but little.

The upper extremities do not present any trace of paralysis nor of insensibility, although the dynamometric force of the hands is rather weak (right 40, left 35). It may be noticed also that the hands present slight trembling, which is much accentuated when the patient carries a glass to his mouth.

But it is the state of the lower limbs that especially claims our attention. Their voluntary movements are so feeble that Le Log— is scarcely able to raise them from the bed. He is able to offer very little resistance to passive movements of the different joints, though certainly the limbs are not in a state of flaccidity, for they do not fall like inert masses after having been raised. Standing upright is possible when he is supported on each side, but he oscillates and would probably fall when told to shut his eyes. It is impossible for him to make a single step forward; in spite of his best efforts the feet remain literally fixed to the ground. Although the limbs are not flaccid they do not present any of the characters of spasmodic paralysis; no exaggeration of the patellar reflexes, no trepidation on bending upwards the point of the foot.

The *perversions of sensibility* observed in the lower limbs are quite peculiar. They involve both the skin and the deeper parts. As for the latter, torsion and traction, however vigorously exercised on the different joints (hip, knee, ankle, &c.), do not produce the least pain, not the least sensation. When the eyes are closed the patient is absolutely ignorant of the position given to the different segments of the lower extremities. For example, when one of the limbs is raised or flexed at the foot, or one knee is placed over the other, the patient is quite unconscious of it. Pricking, pinching, the application of cold and heat to the skin, are not perceived. By reason of their wide extent and their accentuated character, the perversions of sensibility offer a marked contrast with the motor troubles. There is no atrophy of the muscles, and the electrical reactions are normal. No traces of paralysis of the bladder or rectum.

The search for hysterical stigmata gives the following results. Absolute anæsthesia of the pharynx; one is able to push the finger as far as the epiglottis, and to keep it there for a long time without provoking the least reaction. Taste is absolutely lost; a morsel of sulphate of quinine applied to the tongue is not detected by the patient. There is also anosmia; diminution of hearing on both sides; concentric retraction of the visual field very pronounced on both sides (Fig. 83).

We have already pointed out the permanent hyperæsthesia of the scalp which is elicited by the slightest touch or friction. Friction produces an attack of beating in the temples and noises in the ears.

The attacks are represented by the following symptoms:—Pain in the pharynx, sensation of a ball rising in the throat, a stifling sensation, beatings in the temples. Very often epistaxis terminates the scene; but these symptoms do not go any further.

Now it is necessary to point out more particularly the

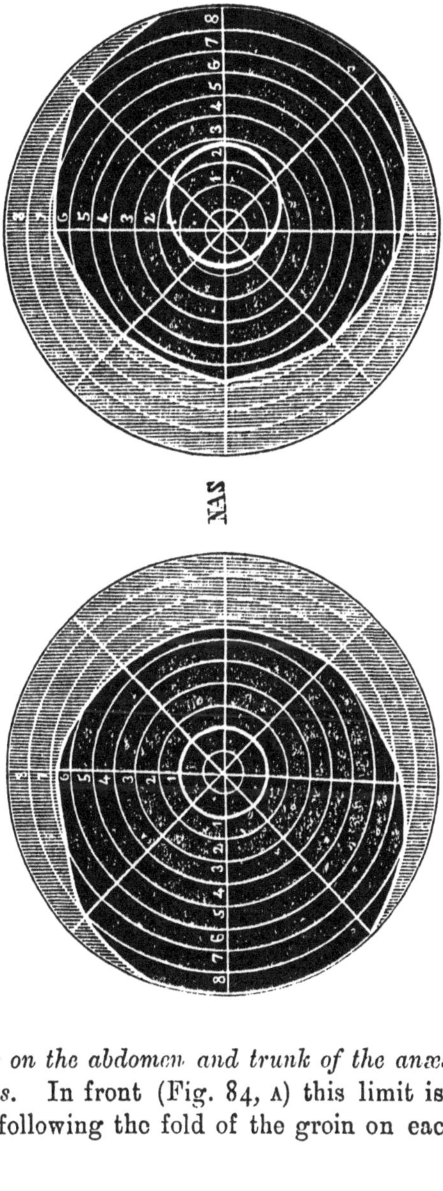

FIG. 83.—Le Log—'s visual fields.

boundaries on the abdomen and trunk of the anæsthesia of the lower limbs. In front (Fig. 84, A) this limit is represented by a line following the fold of the groin on each side as far as the anterior iliac spine, excluding the genital organs. Behind (Fig. 84, B) it is represented by a line following the

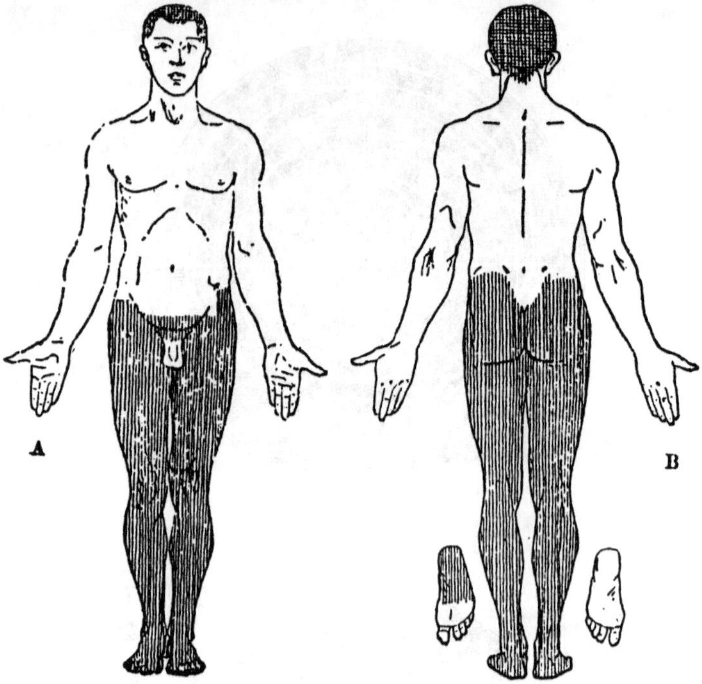

A B

FIG. 84.—Distribution of the anæsthesia in the case of Le Loз—. On the head is a large patch of hypæsthesia.

origin of the gluteal muscles, excluding a V-shaped space in the middle, which corresponds to the sacrum.

* * * * *

The presence of the classical stigmata and the attacks, albeit rudimentary, though sufficiently characteristic, enable one to establish in a peremptory way the existence in the patient of an hysterical basis. But one can go further, and show that the paraplegia itself reveals all the characteristics of psychical or mental paralyses as they may be called. In support of this hypothesis, in the first place there is the delimitation towards the abdomen of the anæsthesia of the lower extremities. In front the upper limit follows, as has been said, the line which passes along the fold of the groin, excluding the genital organs, and reaching to the iliac spine; and behind the boundary line follows the origin of the gluteal muscles, excluding a V-shaped space in the centre which corresponds to the posterior surface of the sacrum (Fig. 84, A and B).

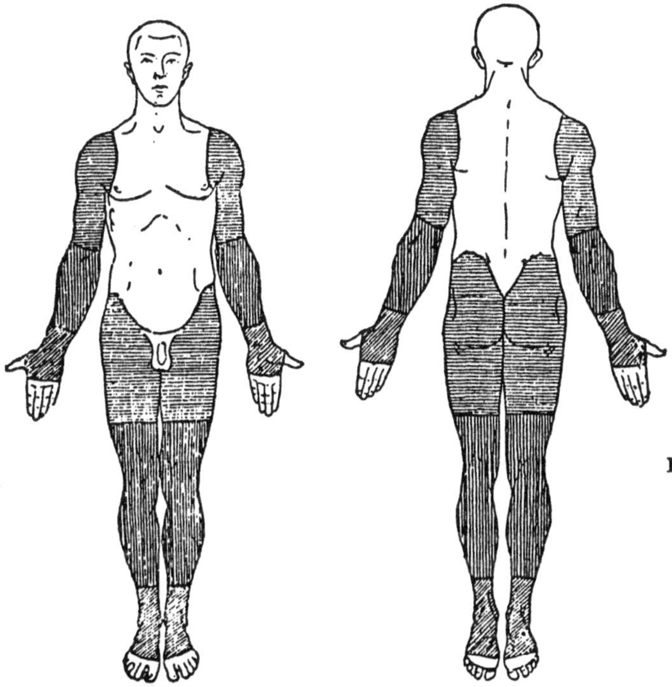

A B

FIG. 85.—Distribution of the anæsthetic zones in a case of partial paralysis of the different segments of the limbs, artificially produced by suggestion in hypnotisable hysterical subjects (somnambulic period).

This disposition is obviously different from that which is found when the anæsthesia of the lower limbs is consequent on an organic lesion situated, for example, about the middle dorsal region, and involving more or less profoundly the grey central matter. Then the anæsthesia of the lower limbs extends over the lower part of the abdomen, and is limited by a line perpendicular to the axis of the trunk passing through the neighbourhood of the umbilicus. On the other hand, the limitation of the anæsthesia in this patient exactly reproduces the disposition which—as the result of numerous investigations by M. Charcot on this subject—is to be found when, *by means of suggestion in the somnambulic period, complete motor and sensory paralysis of the lower extremity of the non-anæsthetic side is produced in hypnotisable hemianæsthesic hysterical subjects* (Fig. 85).[1]

It should be added that in Le Log—, as in hysterical subjects in question, the anæsthesia extends to the deeper parts, and all notions relative to the muscular sense are completely abolished, and that the loss of motor power is very pronounced.

Hence, as far as concerns the paralysis, the case of Le Log— does not differ clinically in any essential particular from the case of hypnotisable hemianæsthesic hysterical subjects whose lower limbs have been paralysed by means of suggestion. This renders it very probable that in the two orders of facts the mechanism of production both with reference to the paralysis of motion and of sensation is the same. Now, when in a somnambulic subject one suggests by speech the idea of the motor weakness of a limb, and one sees this idea effectively realised under the special form of paralysis which has just been described, one can hardly in the present state of science refuse to admit that it depends upon a dynamic lesion affecting the motor and sensory zones of the grey cortex of the brain which in a normal state preside over the functions of that limb. Consequently we are in this way led to propose as a very plausible hypothesis that in Le Log— the production of the paralysis is due to an analogous process.

Without doubt, the objections may be raised to this ex-

[1] Just as has been seen in the case of the upper extremity (Lectures XXI and XXII), one is able in hypnotisable anæsthetic subjects during the somnambulic period to determine by a blow a total or partial paralysis of the lower limb. When partial paralysis of the movements of the joint (hip, knee, ankle, &c.) occur the loss of motor power of that joint carries with it almost necessarily—just as in the case of the upper extremity—cutaneous and deep anæsthesia of the corresponding segment of the limb. The limits which separate the different zones of anæsthesia thus produced are represented here also by circular lines following an imaginary plane at right angles to the long axis of the limb (Fig. 85, A and B).

planation that in the first place the patient had not been hypnotised, and in the second the conditions of a suggestion cannot be found in this case,—at first sight at any rate. But in reference to these two points the following circumstances may be mentioned.

It is certain that the mental state which is to be found in the somnambulic period of hypnotism does not constitute the only condition where, in consequence of the obnubilation of consciousness, of the facile dissociation of the *ego*, it may be possible to awake in the mind an idea or a group of associated ideas which, freed from all control, all opposition, may become developed into an autonomous condition which acquires by that very fact an enormous force, and a power of realisation which is almost without limits.

Among the unconscious or subconscious mental conditions in which, apart from hypnotic somnambulism, suggestions are thus easily able to become realised, may be mentioned certain intoxications, as of haschich for example (Ch. Richet) or of alcohol (Magnan). And one may mention also, according to M. Page, emotions, physical commotions, traumatic shock, with or without direct injury of the cranium, that is to say with or without cerebral commotion, using this last term in its surgical acceptation. In fact, experience has shown for a long time, that under the conditions just named it is by no means rare to find paralysis clinically comparable with those we are now discussing.

That being so it will be easily recognised that in Le Log—'s history are to be found all the circumstances requisite for the production of the particular mental state favorable to the objective realisation of suggestion. It will be remembered that, thrown violently on to the pavement, Le Log— lost consciousness immediately; that he remained comatose for several hours, and that afterwards he was plunged, for the two or three days which followed the accident, into a state of veritable intellectual torpor; in a word, he presented at that time the condition of psychical obnubilation suitable for the efficacy of suggestions.

But now it may be asked what it was, in the patient thus prepared, which formed the point of departure of suggestion, if suggestion there was. This is a good opportunity for remarking that all suggestions are not brought into play by means of speech. There are those which become developed in consequence of the perception of an odour, a taste, or sight of a particular object; or in a word after any sensation whatever. And although it most frequently happens that they are produced by external objects, nevertheless they often occur in consequence of a sensitive or sensorial modification developed either spontaneously or accidentally in the patient himself in a way that is known as *auto-suggestion*.

In reference to this matter M. Charcot draws attention to the arguments which have been mentioned in the preceding lectures[1] relative to the mechanism of the development of hystero-traumatic paralyses; a mechanism in which auto-suggestion plays the principal part. It may be well here to advert in the first place to the phenomena of *local shock*[2] described by some authors. This consists of a contusion of a limb, for example, which whether of small or great intensity, produces divers transitory affections of sensibility and movement; such as a sensation of weight, sometimes true anæsthesia or motor paralysis more or less accentuated either in the single part of the limb which was the seat of the blow or of the entire limb. For a shock of a given intensity, the results vary considerably in different subjects. Thus in a vigorous man of stable mental equilibrium a blow with the fist of moderate force upon the shoulder—and what is said of the shoulder will equally apply to the buttock or the thigh—will barely produce a transient numbness or heaviness limited to the contused spot; whereas in all probability in an hysterical woman the numbness will be replaced by much more accentuated, more extensive, and more durable perversions of sensibility. There will be, for example, in this last, simultaneously with the feeling *of absence of the whole limb*, a generalised anæsthesia of the limb, and a paresis perfectly appreciable to dynamometric exploration. It may be added also that if the same hysterical subject had been plunged into a somnambulic state the same shock would have determined, almost to a certainty, a complete monoplegia involving both sensibility and movement, presenting in a word all the char-

[1] See Lectures XXI, XXII, and XXIII.

[2] Groeningen, Fischer, Billroth, &c., see Lecture XXVI.

racters which distinguish hystero-traumatic paralyses in their most perfect type of development.

It is evident that the different instances that have been mentioned represent stages of the same series, and that the explanation which is invoked for one of them applies equally to them all. It will suffice to consider, for example, the case of the hypnotised subject where the symptoms are carried to the highest degree, and occur, moreover, under conditions which are more accessible to analysis. Now, in this condition, M. Charcot submits that in the very fact of local shock, and particularly in the sensory and motor phenomena attached thereto, must be sought the point of departure of the suggestion. The sensation of heaviness or even absence of the limb struck, and, again, the paralysis which is never wanting, in some degree at any rate, will give rise quite naturally, as it were, to the idea of motor weakness of the limb. And this idea, by reason of the somnambulic mental condition so completely favorable to the efficacy of suggestion, comes to acquire, after a period of incubation, a considerable development, and is finally able to become realised objectively in the form of a complete paralysis.

It is quite conceivable that this theory is capable of application, in a most perfect manner, to the interpretation of the mode of development of hystero-traumatic paralyses which occur in the waking state, quite apart from any hypnotism. Here the necessary mental modification is determined by the general nervous commotion (*nervous shock*) which is sure to attend the accident. And as for the suggestion itself, it is the direct consequence, the amplified prolongation, as it were, of the phenomena of the local shock. In this way it is easily understood why psychical paralyses consequent on a contusion so frequently occupy the limb which received the blow.

A large number of the cases of paraplegia determined by an emotion, by fear in particular (Schrecklaehmungen of German authors),[1] are capable of explanation without any doubt on the hypothesis just mentioned.

[1] *On emotional paralyses* see especially R. B. Todd, 'Clin. Lect.,' ed. by Beale, London, 1861, p. 779; O. Berger, "Emotions neurose;" 'Deutsch. Zeit. f. prakt. Med.,' 1877, Nos. 38, 39, Leyden; 'Ruckenm. Kr.,' I Bd., pp.

It is well known that in man a sudden and violent emotion, fright, for example, is followed almost necessarily by a feeling of powerlessness in the lower limbs which may attain a very high degree, and all without departing, so to speak, from physiological conditions, yet amounting to a veritable paraplegia, accompanied, may be, by tremor.[1] The cerebral nervous shock inseparable from such emotion produces, in a subject predisposed, a mental modification which renders possible the transformation from an emotional, transitory, "physiological" paresis into a veritable paraplegia complete and lasting. In this way probably it would be possible to explain a large number of the cases of paraplegia from thunder.

Coming back again to the case of Le Log—, it only remains for us now to inquire how it is that this hystero-traumatic paralysis became developed in his lower extremities. It may be remembered that in the early days after the accident large ecchymoses were noticed upon the anterior surface of the right thigh and on the lower part of the patient's abdomen. It will be remembered also that at this time he complained of a feeling of heaviness, of weight, almost a sensation of *absence of his legs,* and, moreover, the lower extremities were notably paretic. It was very probable that these phenomena, together with the presence of the ecchymoses, gave rise to the conviction in Le Log—'s mind that the wheels of the van which knocked him over "passed over the body," as he puts it. Nevertheless, this conviction, which has even appeared to him in his dreams,[2] is absolutely erroneous. We know it to be so from the most accurate information furnished to us by eye witnesses of the scene. But although the thighs and the pelvis were not crushed by the weight of the wheels it is scarcely to be doubted, on the other hand, that these parts, at the time when the unhappy man was thrown upon the pavement, were very severely contused in the fall. And it is precisely the consequences of this local shock which

172, 173, and 174; R. Lippe, 'Zur Casuist der Schrecklaehmung,' Inaug. Diss., Breslau, 1877.

[1] Ch. Darwin, 'L'expression des émotions,' p. 30, *et seq.*, Paris, 1877.

[2] See a case of paraplegia consequent on a dream, communicated to the Société de Biologie par M. Feré (Séance, 20th Nov., 1886).

have determined the auto-suggestion whence results the paraplegia. It is worthy of remark that in the case of Le Log—, as in others of the same kind, the paralysis was not produced at the very moment of the accident, but it was only after an interval of several days, after a sort of incubation stage of unconscious mental elaboration.[1]

Besides the phenomena of an hysterical kind that have just been described in Le Log—, there are others which do not belong to the same category. We have seen that the patient suffers from a permanent headache of a constrictive character, producing the sensation of a heavy helmet pressing all parts of the head. All kinds of sound are painful to his ear, and he does his best to avoid them. It is impossible for him to fix his attention to any matter, or to devote himself to anything without speedily experiencing very great fatigue. Moreover, he is silent, and only replies slowly to questions addressed to him, and as though he resented them. Generally speaking, he is sad, melancholic, almost stupid, frequently anxious. He is irascible, resents the smallest observations made to him, and is incessantly asking to have his place changed in the ward where he sleeps, complaining of his neighbours, who, he says, annoy him. He has insomnia, and is frequently tormented by horrible dreams, relative to the imaginary details of his accident. Further, his memory appears to be considerably weakened; he does not even remember the accident itself, whatever he may say, and there is every reason to believe that everything he states, and his dreams, are inventions founded more or less on what he has heard stated with reference thereto. The same may be said

[1] We have here a phenomenon of unconscious or sub-conscious cerebration, mentation or ideation. The patient, in a case of this sort, is aware of the result, but he does not preserve any recollection, or he only preserves it in a vague manner, of the different phases of the phenomenon. Questions addressed to him upon this point are attended with no result. He knows nothing or almost nothing. Briefly one can compare the process in question to a sort of reflex action, in which the centre of the diastaltic arc is represented by regions of the grey cortex, where the psychical phenomena relative to voluntary movements of the limbs are situated. By reason of the easy dissociation of the mental unity of the *ego* in cases of this kind, these centres can be set in operation without any other region of the psychic organ being interfered with or forming part of the process.

of occurrences before the accident, and there are in the tablet of his memory large vacant spaces. He cannot, for example, name any of the masters for whom he has worked, nor can he say where they lived.

These different phenomena correspond on all points with the psychical troubles which, with or without the accompaniment of hysterical manifestations, so frequently appear in consequence of a nervous shock, more particularly when the shock has been preceded or followed by a physical cerebral commotion. These symptoms have been perfectly described by MM. Skae, Page, Westphal, Moeli, Krafft-Ebing, and quite recently by M. Guder.[1] It is evident that these conditions greatly aggravate the situation, already sufficiently complicated, in the case of the unfortunate Le Log—. Hysterical conditions in men are of themselves often very serious, especially when they are of traumatic origin, by reason of their tenacity, their duration, and their resistance to rational treatment. The existence of traumatic psychosis [psychose traumatique] adds still more to the gravity of the prognosis, for it would not be difficult to cite examples where this state became incurable, and terminated in dementia.

The preceding details of Le Log—'s case extend to April 19th, 1886. The following is the progress of the case since that time. There was no appreciable change during the months of May and June; the attacks and the nose-bleedings were both frequent and severe; his bad tempers continued, and sometimes stupor. He also had some anuria from time to time. The patient's nutrition was bad. He vomited frequently, and had profuse sweats. About the middle of July the attacks took on a more accentuated spasmodic character. He struggled more, assumed arcs of circles, tore his clothes; and he was obliged to be tied down, yet notwithstanding his violence, the lower limbs remained quite immovable. The epistaxis became rarer and less profuse in proportion as the convulsions became more severe. On the morning of the

[1] Westphal, 'Charité Annalen Jahr. 1878,' S. 379; Kiegler, 'Die im Eisenbahndienste Vork. Berufskrankh.,' Berlin, 1888; Moeli, "Ueber physische Stoerungen nach Eisenbahnumfallen," 'Berl. klin. Woch.,' 1881, No. 6; Krafft-Ebing, 'Lehrb. der Psychiat,' 1883, p. 188; P. Guder, 'Die Geistesstörungen nach Kopfverletzung,' Jena, 1886.

15th August, 1886, the patient had a convulsive seizure of great severity. There had been no epistaxis. During the attack, all in a moment, it was noticed *that the lower extremities were being thrown about, and the feet struck the bar at the end of the bed with so much force that it became displaced. The attack terminated; the patient got up from his bed and commenced to walk,* at first with a certain amount of hesitation, supporting himself along the wall and by means of surrounding objects, but at the end of a few hours his powers of walking became absolutely normal.

Nevertheless, the cutaneous and deep anæsthesia persisted still in a very pronounced degree in the lower extremities. The other stigmata, namely, the retraction of the visual field, pharyngeal anæsthesia, &c., had not undergone any appreciable modification.

Since this epoch the attacks have become less frequent and less intense. The amelioration in the movements of the lower extremities has continued, and the patient walks better and better each day. He has gone out of the infirmary several times to see his friends, and can accomplish fairly long distances without too much fatigue. Nevertheless the cerebral torpor still remains to a certain extent, and the stigmata and anæsthesia of the lower limbs are not materially modified (November 1st, 1886).

The *sudden disappearance* of the paraplegia after an attack which presented all the characters of an hysterical seizure confirms in a very decisive manner the opinion expressed concerning the nature of the complaint. Nevertheless, the patient although it is a year since the accident, cannot be considered as cured, in that the hysterical stigmata persist in almost the same condition as they were before.

II. *Case of hystero-traumatic brachial monoplegia consequent on a blow on the shoulder.*[1]

The man named Mouil—[2] is robust, vigorous, and well developed. He is 25 years of age, an agricultural labourer.

[1] Edited by M. Babinski, Chef de Clinique de la faculté.

[2] See Lecture XXV, p. 353, *et seq.*

He was born in the department of Doubs, not far from Besançon. A little less than a year ago he was a farm labourer. Since the month of May, 1885, he has been in Paris and employed at the railway station in various ways. He had never been ill before this. He had never been nervous, and he does not know what it is to have nervous attacks. He is rather slow, apathetic, somewhat silly, and as far as one can judge during the eight months he has been in the wards, his imagination does not seem to be of a very active kind. There is no nervous malady known to exist in his family.

Mouil— was in his usual state of health, when on December 1st, 1885, at six o'clock in the evening, while he was working on the line, his right shoulder was squeezed between the buffers of a waggon and an engine. The contusion was certainly very slight, for it was not followed by any serious surgical injury. Nevertheless, under the influence of the shock the patient immediately lost consciousness and fainted. He was carried to the station-master's office, and he did not regain his senses till about twenty minutes afterwards.

It is interesting to note the phenomena which, according to him, existed immediately after his waking.

1. Respiration was very difficult, and it seemed to him as though his right upper extremity, the one injured, *was absent, replaced by a heavy body which hung lifeless by his side.*

2. There was no immediate tumefaction of the parts.

3. Movements in the shoulder and the elbow were impossible though he was able to move the fingers both at the time and for three or four days subsequently; hence it may be said that the motor paralysis was not immediately complete.

4. He suffered from general weakness, so that he found it impossible to stand upright or even to raise himself. He was only able to get up and go out at the end of thirteen days.

The patient was carried to the Lariboisière Hospital, the one nearest to the Northern Railway Station, on the very day of the accident, about 8 o'clock in the evening, and was placed in the wards of Dr. Brun. The next morning they discovered a slight swelling of the shoulder, and an extensive ecchymosis over that joint, the subclavicular region, and part of the face. The right upper extremity was completely deprived of all movement excepting the fingers, and the limb was also anæsthetic, insensibility to pricking was absolute everywhere; but at this time the deep-seated sensibility was probably not yet affected, for the movements imparted to the limb in order to ascertain whether there was a dislocation or fracture were rather painful. The result of these explorations was completely negative.

It was only on the thirteenth day that the patient was able to leave his bed. He left the hospital, and shortly afterwards went into the Hôtel Dieu into the wards of M. Merklen, on the 13th January, 1886, that is to say six weeks after the accident. There they recognised all the characters of the monoplegic affection about to be described, and the diagnosis of M. Merklen, like that of Dr. Brun, was that the case was one of hystero-traumatic monoplegia. A fact which is well worthy of your attention is that at the time of his admission into the Hôtel Dieu, a month after the accident, there existed in the paralysed limb, both of the arm and forearm of the right side, a very notable diminution of the volume. During his stay of more than a month in the Hôtel Dieu, faradic treatment was continued without interruption, and without any result.

The examination of the patient at the time of his admission into the Salpêtrière, March 2nd, 1886, gave the following results. Monoplegia of the right upper extremity, without any trace of participation in the face or the lower limb (it seems certain that the face has never been involved). The *motor monoplegia* was complete, the trapezius alone was able to raise the shoulder. The paralysis was of a flaccid kind, the tendon-reflexes were not increased, indeed they were rather diminished.

Affections of sensibility.—1. Cutaneous sensibility of all kinds was absolutely lost, cold, pinching, &c. The cutaneous anæsthesia occupied the entire prominence of the shoulder; limited on the thorax by an unbroken line following a circular plane perpendicular to the long axis of the limb when it was extended (Fig. 86, A and B).

2. The anæsthesia extended to the deeper parts; torsions,

twistings practised on the different segments of the limb were quite unperceived.

3. Notions of muscular sense were completely lost; the patient was unable to say where his limb was, and he could not tell which finger was moved, &c.

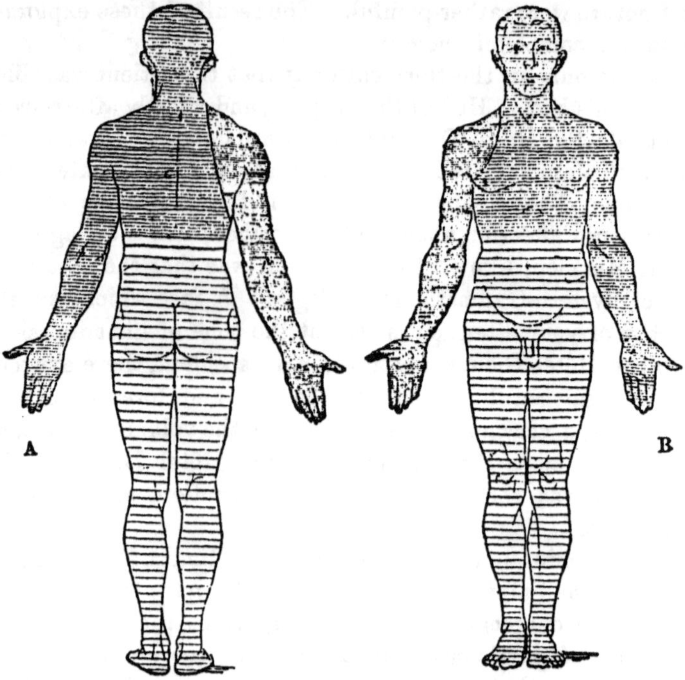

A B

FIG. 86.—Distribution of the anæsthesia in Monil—.

Trophic changes.—The wasting of the limb has already been mentioned. It should be added that the fingers are purple and cold, like those observed in certain organic paralyses. However, the muscles present absolutely normal electrical reactions, and the same with the nerves. Faradization, which produces an energetic contracture of the muscles, produces absolutely no sensation.

The patient has at no time ever had anything resembling hysterical seizures, but the permanent sensitive and sensorial troubles (*hysterical stigmata*) are very pronounced. There exists an analgesia over the whole of the right side of the body and face, and everywhere the patient is unable to perceive cold (Fig. 86).

The *sensorial troubles* are very noteworthy.

1. Very pronounced retraction of the visual field on both sides.

2. Monocular diplopia.

3. Diminution of hearing on both sides.

4. Diminution of smell on both sides. Taste is absolutely lost, and one can push the finger far into the pharynx and maintain it there without determining the least reaction. The patient is not hypnotisable.

On November 1st, 1886, eleven months after onset, in spite of different methods of treatment, the monoplegia is not modified in any way. The stigmata persisted in exactly the same condition. The general condition is excellent. It has been discovered that the application of a circular ligature produces very pronounced and durable contractures in the lower limbs of Mouil— [contracture diathesis].

It is not necessary to dwell at any great length on this case of hystero-traumatic monoplegia, for it is, so to speak, a reproduction, even in the most minute details, of the classical types already described by M. Charcot.[1]

It is only necessary, therefore, to again remark that the sensations produced by the local shock were evidently here the starting-point of the suggestion which has resulted in the production of a complete sensory and motor monoplegia, which has persisted as it is now for eighteen months. As for the state of suggestability, it has doubtless become developed by the cerebral commotion produced by the nervous shock. It is a fact worthy of being noticed that the motor paralysis was not complete at first, and that consequently in this case, as in others of the same kind, the motor weakness was only completed after a sort of unconscious mental elaboration.

The amyotrophy, without modifications in the electrical reactions, occurred somewhat rapidly in this patient. This rapidly developed hysterical amyotrophy has been recently

[1] See Lectures XX, XXI, and XXII.

pointed out several times by M. Charcot, and it has formed the subject of an extensive work published by M. Babinski in the 'Archives of Neurology.'[1] A brief summary of Mouil's case appears in the former part of this volume (p. 353).

[1] See J. Babinski, "De l'atrophie musculaire dans les paralysies hystériques" ('Arch. de Neurologie,' Nos. 34 and 35); see also 'Progrès Médical,' 1886, No. 6, et l' Appendice, IV.

APPENDIX

II.

NOTIONS OF MUSCULAR SENSE AND VOLUNTARY MOVEMENT.

(Appendix to Lecture XXII, p. 303.)

I AM constrained to admit with many authors that the *motor representations*, which of necessity precede the accomplishment of a voluntary movement, take place in the cortical motor centres, their more exact organic substratum being in the motor cellules of those centres. These motor representations are chiefly constituted by the "sentiment of innervation," of "nervous discharge," as it is still sometimes called, which has its seat in the central organism.

On the other hand, the notions furnished by what is properly called "*muscular sense*" (kinæsthetic sense of Bastian) consist of impressions coming from the periphery, namely, from the skin, muscles, aponeuroses, tendons, and articular capsules. These impressions become registered [s'emmagasineraient] in the cortical sensitive centres, where their ideal recall can take place.

The first alone of these representations is indispensable to call voluntary movement into operation. The other kind, in general, intervenes only in a secondary, though very effectual fashion, in order to complete, direct, and, so to speak to perfect the movement which is already in process of execution. We know besides by numerous proofs that the visual image of voluntary movement contributes powerfully towards the same result.

It follows, therefore, that if the motor representations happen to become defective in consequence of a lesion occurring in the nerve-cellules of the cortical motor centre of a limb, or in the prolongations which connect them with the centres of ideation, although the kinæsthetic and visual representations may persist, then a complete paralysis of the voluntary movements of the limb results. In a forgotten book which my eminent colleague Professor Janet has courteously brought under my notice, I find that Rey Regis, of Montpellier, recognised in 1789 the existence of *motor paralysis* depending on a loss of the *memory of motor force*, due to lesion of certain parts of the brain ('Natural History of the Soul,' London, 1789, pp. 26—28).

From the preceding statements it will be understood that the suggestion of loss of power should be capable of determining in certain subjects a complete motor paralysis, without the accompaniment of any affection whatever of sensibility either cutaneous or deep (as I have already mentioned, p. 303), and more particularly without any loss of the notions furnished by muscular sense. But we have observed that more frequently a suggestion of this kind, at least when addressed to "hysterics" anteriorly hemianæsthesic, and not accompanied by any injunction relative to sensibility one way or the other,—this suggestion, I say, is followed, according to our experience, not only by paralysis of movement, but by loss of sensibility in all its modes, including muscular sense. It may be said therefore, that under these circumstances, paralysis of the fundamental apparatus of voluntary movement carries with it in some way paralysis of the "perfectioning" apparatus. It is further probable that in these cases of paralysis by hypnotic suggestion—as in a large number of hysterical paralyses with flaccidity, which are in like manner of psychical origin—the subcortical and bulbar grey nuclei, as also the spinal nerve-cells (which in the normal state are all in direct or indirect relation with the cortical motor centres) may become more or less profoundly affected in consequence of a diffusion of the lesion from the higher cerebral centres. The loss of automatic movement, whatever its origin, and the abolition or diminution of acts of a purely reflex order, which under these conditions accompany the paralysis of voluntary movement, would seem to testify to this.

The following passages appear to me sufficient to indicate the ideas of the authors whence they are taken, as to the nature and seat of the psycho-physiological process which originates deliberate movements. "If the idea tends to produce the fact," says Bain ('The Senses and the Intellect,' translation of Cazelles, 1874, p. 298), "it is because the idea is already the fact in a more feeble form. To think is to restrain oneself from speaking or acting."

"Mental actions take place in the same centres as physical actions. Ordinarily, simple volition suffices to carry them to a point at which the muscles are set in action" (loc. cit., p. 305). "As the nerves which the muscles receive are principally motor, which convey to them the stimulus emanating from the brain . . . . we cannot do better than suppose that the concomitant sensation of muscular movement coincides with the centrifugal current of nerve force, and not that it is the result, as in a sensation, properly speaking, of an influence transmitted by the centripetal nerves" (loc. cit., p. 59). "In a voluntary act, considered in its simplest form," says Herbert Spencer ('Principles of Psychology, vol. i, translated by Ribot and Espinas, p. 539), "we are unable to find anything save the mental representation of the act followed by its accomplishment—a transformation of that nascent psychical change, which constitutes at once the tendency to the act, and the idea of the act, into a positive psychical change which constitutes the accomplishment of the act in so far as it is mental. The difference between a voluntary and involuntary movement of the leg, is that, whereas the involuntary movement is caused without any antecedent consciousness of the movement to be made, the voluntary movement is produced only after it has been represented in consciousness. And since that representation is no other than a feeble form of the psychical state which accompanies the real movement, it is nothing else than the nascent excitation of all the nerves participating in this function; which precedes their actual excitation."

Further ('Premiers Principes,' p. 216). "Volition is an initial discharge along a line which has become, as the result of antecedent experiences, the line of most feeble resistance. The transition of volition to action is but the complement of the discharge." According to Wundt ('Physiology,' Fr. transl., p. 447), "The seat of the sensation of movement does not appear to be in the muscles, but in the motor cellules. . . . . We have not only the sensation of a movement executed, but that of a movement to be executed. The sensation of movement is therefore limited to a motor innervation, and hence we call it the sentiment of innervation ('Innervationsgefühl.') Herr Meynert expresses himself thus: ('Psychiatrie,' p. 312). "Ich glaube der erste gewesen zu sein welcher sich dahin aüsserte, dass die Innervationsvorgänge von den Hemisphaeren aus, welche man Willensacte nennt, nichts weiter seien als die Wahrnehmungs und

Erinnerungsbilder der *Innervationsgefühle*, indem solche, jede Form der Reflexbewegungen begleitend, in die Hirnrinde übertragen werden, als die primare Grundlage secundär von dem Vorderhirn ausgelöster aehnlichen Bewegungen. Diese Erinnerungsbilder bekommen dann durch associations Vorgänge die intensität der Kraft zugeführt, durch welche sie für die vom Vorderhirn ausgehenden secundären Bewegungen, als Arbeitsanstoss langs centrifugalen Bahnen wirken." In his 'Clinical and Physiological Researches on the Nervous System,' 1876, pp. 20–37, Hughlings Jackson adheres to the views of Bain, Wundt, and others, that our "consciousness of muscular activity" is in great part initial, central, and realisable in the motor centres. According to Maudsley ('Physiology of Mind,' trans. of Herzen, p. 249), "it appears that it is in the frontal part of the convolutions (cortical motor centres) that the muscular sensations whence we derive our motor intuitions are stored up. The parts of the surface of the brain which act as motor centres are the seat . . . . of the conception of the degree and quality of muscular innervation—that is to say, of what are called *muscular inductions*." Ferrier ('Functions of the Brain,' Chap. XI) expresses himself thus: "In the same manner that the sensory centres form the organic base of the memory of sensory impressions and the seat of their ideal resurrection, so the motor centres of the hemispheres, besides being the seat of differentiated movements, are the organic base of the memory of corresponding movements, and the seat of their re-execution or ideal reproduction. We have thus a sensory memordy an a motor memory, of sensory and motor ideas respectively; the sensory ideas being revived sensations, and the motor being revived or ideal movements. The ideal movements do not form an element less important in our mental processes than the revived sensations of an ideal character." Contrary to these views, Bastian ('The Brain as an Organ of the Mind,' vol. ii., 1882, pp. 209, 165, and Appendix, transl.,) expresses the opinion that the motor centres, wherever they may be situated, are the parts whose activity appears to be absolutely free from subjective concomitant phases. It does not appear that the ideal reproductions ever take place in these centres . . . . It is the changes in the muscle excited and in the contiguous parts—a change occasioned by the movement—that beget a group of centripetal impressions whose *terminus* is the kinæsthetic centre (centre of the sense of movement) . . . . This, then, is really a sensory centre, and *ideal movements* may be revived in it, either isolated or associated with visual impressions pertaining to it . . . . It is only productive of great confusion to attribute the activity of the sensory centres to the motor centres. . . . . The cerebral substratum of mind does not embrace in any manner the processes which take place in the motor centres of the brain, wherever they are situated. In other words, we cannot legitimately regard mental operations as being even in part immediately due to the activity of motor centres."

In support of the theory advanced above, we may recall what is observed in certain subjects, hysterical for the most part, who, deprived of all forms of sensibility in a member, have nevertheless maintained in great part the faculty of moving that member freely when even they are unable to have recourse, the eyes being shut, to the directive and dynamic influence of the visual image of movement. Our patient Pin—[1] offers at the present time a good example of this kind. In him, as we have seen, the cutaneous and deep sensibility are lost over the whole extent of the left superior extremity, and while his eyes are shut he does not recognise any passive movements imparted to the diverse segments of the member nor the position thereby resulting. The eyes being open, general and partial voluntary movements of the member present all the characters of the normal condition both in respect of variety and precision. These movements persist in great part while the eyes are shut, only they are more uncertain and more hesitating, although *never inco-ordinate;* they operate, in a word, as though he were groping. And again, Pin— is able, the eyes being shut, to direct his fingers with a certain precision towards his nose, his mouth, or his ear, or towards an object placed at a distance, and to succeed in his aim, though he very frequently misses. He is not able, generally speaking, when one asks him to do so, to flex one of his fingers singly. Habitually all the fingers are flexed together. Occasionally he is unable to say whether he has flexed his wrist or not, &c. I do not now speak of the dynamometric pressure, which for the affected hand shows 30 K. when the eyes are open, and only 15 K. when they are closed. These modifications occurring in the exercise of movement, in patients of this description, when the co-operation of kinæsthetic and visual representations is wanting, permit us to discern up to a certain point in what the operation of the

[1] Lectures XIX and XX.

fundamental apparatus of voluntary movements normally consists. On the other hand, the study of cases of psychical paralysis where movement alone is involved reveals the truly secondary *rôle*, however important it may be, of visual and kinæsthetic representations in the normal accomplishment of voluntary movements.

Perhaps, moreover, there exists in the normal state varieties in this respect. It is possible, indeed, that at the moment when a premeditated act is about to be accomplished, there is awakened in some people exclusively motor representations properly so called, and in others kinæsthetic and visual representations; in other persons better endowed, sometimes the one and sometimes the other, or both at once. Difference in education, habit, or hereditary predisposition may account for these varieties. We can consequently understand that a lesion of the same nature, of the same extent, and the same localisation, may in different subjects reveal itself by different clinical phenomena, according as individuals belonging to one or other of these categories may be concerned.

APPENDIX

III.

A CASE OF HYSTERICAL HEMIPLEGIA FOLLOWED BY SUDDEN CURE.

(*From Professor Charcot's lectures, by Dr. Marie.*)

(Appendix to Lecture XXII, p. 296.)

Gentlemen,—Among last Tuesday's out-patients a girl presented herself who had been attacked with motor paralysis in a very sudden manner. I have thought it advisable to bring her before you this very day, because it is possible that the patient's symptoms may disappear at any moment.

Henriette A—, 19 years old, has generally enjoyed good health. She is a laundress and follows her calling on a boat on the Seine. Her father, a spectacle-glass maker, who is now fifty years old, had an apoplectic stroke some time back, followed by left hemiplegia, and at the present time he frequently suffers from giddiness. Her mother and sister do not present any nervous abnormalities.

As for the patient herself, at the age of sixteen she had scarlatina, and during convalescence she had "nervous attacks," of which she gives the following description: no aura, loss of consciousness, but no movements of the limbs; on waking, sensation of a ball in the epigastrium and desire to weep; she has never had biting of the tongue nor involuntary evacuations during the attacks. These symptoms only lasted for a year, from sixteen to seventeen years of age; during that time the menstruation was very irregular, but since then it has become quite normal. She has never suffered from rheumatism, nor shown signs of cardiac disease.

Now that you know the antecedents of this young woman, I will narrate to you the circumstances under which the disease developed. During the night of 29th November, while she was asleep, a shelf situated above her bed slipped and fell, with all the articles it supported, on to the head of Henriette A—. She awoke with a start, very frightened by the noise and by the unexpected blow, and for the remainder of the night she was much upset and could not sleep. The fall of the shelf did not produce any injury; Henriette is positive that she had not the slightest bruise. However, the catamenia which she was expecting a few days later, came on in the course of that night.

Next morning, November 30th, she got up as usual, went to the boat and worked as she was accustomed to do without experiencing anything unusual. But, about half-past seven in the evening, when she was going with her bucket in her hand to fetch some water, her right side suddenly gave way and she fell. She was unable to rise, her right leg was useless and the bucket rolled far away from her right hand, which was unable to hold it. There was no loss of consciousness, the very moment she fell she called out for help; no sensation of giddiness or faintness; no convulsions whatever, nor any other cerebral symptom. The paralysis occupied the upper and lower limbs of the right side; but it did not extend to the face—that is a point you should specially observe. The loss of power was so great that she was obliged to be taken home in a carriage.

The following days, 1st, 2nd, 3rd December, the paralysis of the leg improved somewhat; but when Henriette A— came last Tuesday among our patients, she was obliged to be brought in a cab, and it was necessary for her to be vigorously supported when she was brought into the room.

During the four days that have passed since then, the amelioration has become more pronounced, and as you will see directly, mobility has to a great extent returned in the lower extremity.

Let us now turn to the present condition of the patient;

and firstly we will examine the power of movement. The right superior extremity is absolutely paralysed, flaccid, and falls like an inert mass after being raised. Such at least is the general appearance of the limb, but on examining it more closely it may be discovered that, although most of the muscles of the arm and forearm have lost mobility, some have reserved their power. The forearm can be extended (action of triceps), but it cannot be flexed (biceps and brachialis anticus): flexion of the fingers is possible though it is very feeble: pronation and supination of the forearm, are impossible, as also adduction and abduction of the wrist. But there are a few slight movements of flexion and extension of the wrist; the fingers also can be feebly drawn together and placed in the position resulting from contraction of the interossei.

As for the muscles of the shoulder, it will be seen that the deltoid does not contract at all; the pectoralis major has almost preserved its usual power; the trapezius and the other muscles of the trunk are absolutely normal.

The lower extremity has, as we said, almost regained its natural strength. It no longer presents the signs of complete paralysis, but rather of a paresis, more marked in some muscles than others. The patient is able to walk though she limps slightly. The face, you will notice, presents no deviation, no paralysis of the orbicularis oris. Nor is there any paralysis of the muscles of the trunk. In a word, the paralysis in this patient is not properly speaking a hemiplegia, but rather a brachio-crural monoplegia.

The tendon-reflexes, you observe, are not exaggerated; on the contrary, they are less pronounced on the paralysed than the healthy side. We have not, therefore a spasmodic, but a flaccid paralysis.

Next, we must examine the sensibility. There is a fairly marked deficiency of sensation to pricking and heat in the right lower extremity. In the right upper limb there is total anæsthesia extending over the hand, forearm, and arm as high as the acromion. The skin of the chest is sensitive, the limit of separation between sensitive and insensitive areæ being through the middle of the axillary space. There is no modification in the special senses of sight, smell, taste, and hearing. No special point of hyperæsthesia has been found on the body, and no ovarian tenderness.

There remains the muscular sense to examine. For this purpose we instruct the patient, after carefully blindfolding her, to grasp the right (paralysed) hand with the left (healthy) one, and you see, gentlemen, that she is quite incapable of doing so; she seeks it high and low, and on all sides but cannot find it. There is not the same condition in the right lower limb, she has no difficulty in finding with the eyes closed her right foot with her left hand.

The condition of the local temperature is a point of some interest. It is lowered several tenths of a degree on the paralysed side, as revealed by the comparative thermomety of the two sides. There is no abnormality in the general temperature of the body. The general condition in other respects is excellent.

If now, gentlemen, we make a summary of the different phenomena presented by this patient with a view to diagnosis, what do we find? A monoplegia associated with diminution of the tendon-reflexes, without epileptic or apoplectic cerebral phenomena; accompanied by an absolute anæsthesia limited to the arm of the paralysed side and combined with abolition of muscular sense. And all these phenomena appeared in a young girl of nineteen who had previously presented hysterical symptoms.

These are the main features in the case. Are they due to a focal cerebral lesion—a hæmorrhage or softening? One may boldly reply to this question in the negative. These are not the ordinary characters of hæmorrhage or softening; for we have seen that it is not a true hemiplegia in our case but rather a combined monoplegia, without any participation of the face. Moreover, there is anæsthesia which corresponds absolutely both in position and degree with the paralysis of the limbs. Nor is it a hemiplegia of a spinal nature, for under those circumstances the paralysis and anæsthesia ought to be crossed, whereas here, they are not only on the same side, but absolutely superposable so to speak one upon the other.

Briefly therefore, it is unnecessary to hesitate longer or to create imaginary difficulties in the diagnosis. The purely hysterical nature of this paralysis is strikingly evident after a detailed examination of the patient such as we have made; and we may accept it without further discussion as a basis for prognosis and treatment which follow as necessary consequences therefrom.

(Professor Charcot, having remarked that the electrical examination of the muscles had been deferred because it was possible that an attempt of this kind might entail a return of the mobility and sudden cure, and that he wished his audience to witness any such occurrence, proceeded in the lecture room to faradize the muscles of the shoulder and arm of the right side. At the end of a minute the sensibility had entirely returned to this region, without transfer. A minute later the sensibility had returned throughout the entire limb and the paralysis had gone. The patient was then able to use the arm as well as ever, and went round among the audience vigorously shaking them by the hand, desirous of proving how real was the recovery they had just witnessed.)[1]

[1] At that time the weakness of the lower limb, to which no application had been made, still existed. It remained for two days longer and then disappeared spontaneously. From that time the sensibility and mobility have remained absolutely normal.

APPENDIX

IV.

CONCERNING MUSCULAR ATROPHY IN HYSTERICAL PARALYSIS.

(*From Prof. Charcot's lectures, by M. Babinski.*[1])

(Appendix to Lecture XXV.)

Among the diverse characters of hysteria—that neurosis so fertile in all kinds of manifestations—is one of a negative character, which seems to have been regarded hitherto as quite distinctive. It consists in the absence of trophic changes. This negative feature has come to take rank as a law, so that a physician would seem to be justified in rejecting a case from the category of hysteria if it presented any trophic trouble.

Cases recently observed by my master, Prof. Charcot, have tended to show that this is by no means a constant feature, and that it is certainly not a law, if indeed it even be a general rule.

In fact, four patients in M. Charcot's wards, the victims of hysterical paralysis, present in the paralysed limbs an amyotrophy which cannot be attributed to any cause other than hysteria. All these patients have been shown by M. Charcot during his course of clinical lectures. In a future work a complete exposition of the different cases will be given, but in the meantime it will not be without interest, in view of the novelty of the facts, to give a short analysis, briefly depicting the main characters of these atrophies.

[1] See 'Progrès Médical,' 1886, No. 6, and 'Archives de Neurologie, Nos. 34 and 35, 1886.

It should be clearly understood that the characters we are about to indicate are not absolute, for the number of cases observed up to the present time are not sufficient to admit of such a generalisation.

The cases investigated so far are four in number. Two of these were cases of brachial monoplegia; the other two were cases of hemiplegia without involvement of face. In one of these latter, the paralysis and atrophy predominated in the upper extremity; in the other they predominated in the lower extremity.

The following are the characters presented by the muscular atrophy in question:

1. It varies in degree, but it may attain very considerable proportions. In two of the patients there was a difference of 3 centimetres between the greatest circumference of the affected and the healthy arm; and in another patient there was a difference of 5 centimetres between the two thighs.

2. There are no fibrillar tremors.

3. The idio-muscular excitability appears to be normal.

4. The electric contractility is diminished in proportion to the degree of muscular atrophy, but there is no reaction of degeneration.

5. The atrophy may become developed with great rapidity. In one patient it was quite appreciable fifteen days after the onset of the paralysis, and a month and a half afterwards it was very accentuated (3 centimetres difference between the two arms). In the other patients the development of the amyotrophy was also very rapid.

6. The retrocession of the amyotrophy appears to be as rapid as its development. In one case of brachial monoplegia, ten days after the disappearance of the paralysis, which was sudden, the circumference of the arm had already increased one centimetre.

What is the nature of this amyotrophy? It has just been mentioned that there was no reaction of degeneration. It is therefore a *simple atrophy*, that is to say, an atrophy independent of any material lesion of the grey matter of the cord, or of the peripheral nerves. This is a fact of the highest importance, but we must proceed further and seek to ascertain the mechanism of this lesion.

It would seem at first sight quite natural to attribute it to a functional weakness; but on a little reflection such an explanation is seen to be erroneous. It is well known that the wasting of the muscular masses which result simply from functional inactivity of the muscles is slow in its production, that it is never very accentuated, and that it may be completely wanting, even when a paralysis has lasted a long time. Thus it was in the patient named Porcz—, who was affected with hystero-traumatic monoplegia (one of the patients upon whose case M. Charcot founded his description of this variety of paralysis, and which is published at length in the 'Progrès Médical' of 1885),[1] the muscles of the upper extremity, although inactive for a whole year, had not undergone the least atrophy. Now, in the patients in question, the atrophy develops very rapidly, and very soon assumes considerable proportions. These characters clearly indicate that this diminution of volume of the muscles belongs to the catagory of trophic phenomena.

Nevertheless, such an assertion may appear strange; for, is it possible to compare the atrophy we are now discussing with the amyotrophy that results from an organic lesion of the anterior horns of the spinal cord, or of the motor nerves, such as constitutes the type of the trophic lesion? It is necessary without doubt to establish a fundamental distinction between these two varieties. But it is equally necessary to point out that the expression "trophic trouble" does not imperatively imply a material alteration in the nervous system appreciable to our present means of investigation. It simply means that the incontestable influence exercised by this system over the nutrition of the tissues is modified or suppressed. Now, this modification or suppression may be purely dynamic; and it is evidently a phenomenon of this order that we have here.

M. Charcot has, moreover, pointed out that we are already aware of the existence of atrophies quite comparable to these hysterical atrophies. The amyotrophies consequent on articular affections[2] are now-a-days considered by most physicians, in conformity with the opinion which MM. Charcot and

[1] See Lecture XX.

[2] Lectures II and III, *ante*.

Vulpian expressed long ago, as of reflex origin and resulting from a modification in the state of cells in the anterior horns of the spinal cord. It is true that this is as yet only a hypothesis because it does not admit of an absolute ocular demonstration; but it rests on very great probability. In these cases there are purely dynamic alterations of the nervous system; the grey centres of the cord, and the peripheral nerves are normal; and the muscular atrophy is, like that in hysteria, a simple atrophy.

M. Charcot has also compared hysterical atrophy to a variety of atrophy that I have recently described which occurred in a case observed at the Salpêtrière.[1] It was an amyotrophy which occurred on the paralysed side of a hemiplegic patient of cerebral origin followed by descending degeneration, and which was independent of any change in the anterior horns of the cord or the motor nerves. Nor was it in this case possible to doubt the origin of the muscular atrophy, as in cases of articular amyotrophy unattended by autopsy; it certainly depended on the central nervous system. Now, since the anterior horns of the cord constitute the trophic centre of the muscles, and since they are not altered organically, it must surely be admitted that they are altered dynamically. The only difference between this variety of atrophy and hysterical atrophy is that, in the former the dynamic modification of the anterior horns is consecutive to an organic alteration of the brain and the pyramidal bands; whereas, in the latter case *all* the modifications in the different parts of the nervous system are dynamic.

But whatever hypothesis may be invoked in connection with these observations, the important and incontestable fact remains that, contrary to the prevailing opinion, muscular atrophy may be met with in direct connection with hysteria, and that the amyotrophy is a simple one.[2]

[1] Babinski, 'Société de Biologie,' séance du Fev. 20, 1886.

[2] The existence of amyotrophy in a limb affected with hysterical contracture has been very explicitly pointed out by M. F. Kalkoff in his inaugural thesis made under the direction of M. Seeligmuller ('Beiträge zur differential diagnose der hysterischen und der Kapsulären Hemianesthesie,' Halle, 1884).

APPENDIX

V.

ON HYSTERICAL MUTISM.

(*From Prof. Charcot's lectures, by M. Cartez.*[1])

(Appendix to Lecture XXVI.)

Among the many varied manifestations of hysteria is one which, perhaps, up to the present time has not attracted the attention it merits—that is mutism. Prof. Charcot has treated of this subject in his lectures[2] in connection with several patients, whose cases he has been good enough to allow me to report. Side by side with these cases I propose to place several observations collected from French and foreign sources which evidently belong to the same category.

Looking to the number of patients of both sexes attacked with hysteria, it may be stated that mutism is a relatively rare phenomenon. It is scarcely mentioned in older works on this subject, and in a certain number of more recent observations it has been to some extent confounded with aphonia; at least, the interpretations offered by the authors tend to promote this confusion.

If a thorough search were made through all the observations recorded which refer to the hysterical neurosis, in all the historical documents relating thereto, a large number of cases corresponding to this clinical syndroma [syndrome] would undoubtedly be found. The story of the son of Crœsus,

[1] Published in the 'Progrès Médical,' 1886.

[2] Delivered in December, 1885, *vide* 'Gazette des Hôpitaux' of January, 1886.

mentioned by Herodotus, who, though perfect in every other respect, was dumb until one day, when a soldier was about to strike his father, he suddenly recovered his speech—this history is probably an example of hysterical mutism. But we will confine ourselves to more modern observations.

Briquet in his Treatise says that "Aphonia, and more often dysphonia, for the patients are still able to speak in a low voice, is met with from time to time among hysterical subjects." "The aphonia is much more complete than that which results from paralysis of the muscles of the larynx and from paralysis of the diaphragm." However, Briquet cites the following case of mutism recorded by Watson ('Philosophical Transactions,' vol. xiv). A young woman had been for a long time subject to violent convulsions which were frequently followed by temporary paralysis of the muscles that were most severely affected. After one of these attacks she completely lost her sight for five days. On another occasion she lost her speech, which returned, however, at the end of a few days. The convulsions recurred from time to time, and she again lost her speech and remained completely deprived of it for fourteen months, during which time her health became quite re-established. Finally, one day after having danced a great deal, she suddenly regained her speech and was cured.

In the transactions of the 'Académie des Sciences' (1753) is the account of a girl of fourteen who was struck with paralysis and loss of speech after a fright.

Wells ('Medical Communications,' 1790) reports the history of a woman who on recovering from an hysterical attack discovered that she was unable to speak or emit a single sound, although she was in full possession of her intellectual faculties. After a fresh attack she recovered her speech.

In 1855, Sédillot reported a case to the 'Académie des Sciences' of a patient who had suffered from mutism and aphonia ever since the age of fourteen; and who was cured by electricity.

Richter, of Wiesbaden, has published a very curious case of a woman who became aphasic regularly every day; the intelligence remaining quite unaffected. The attack terminated by an abundant evacuation of urine.

Bateman ('Gazette Hebdomadaire,' 1870) relates several cases of hysterical aphasia and mentions that at the Société Médicale des Hôpitaux (1867), when this subject was under discussion, M. Moreau regarded the phenomenon as common. From what I have observed in M. Charcot's wards I do not believe that hysterical aphasia is so common as M. Moreau seems to think. M. Legroux, in his graduation thesis on aphasia, mentions the possible occurrence of this manifestation in hysterical subjects, adding, however, that it must not be confounded with the more or less obstinate mutism of certain patients.

In the interesting case they have published, to which I refer later on, MM. Liouville and Debove appear to connect mutism with a muscular paralysis. "At other times," they say, "it (the paralysis) involves certain muscular apparatus such as that of the larynx, and then, according to its degree, it produces aphonia or mutism."

Professor Revilliod, of Geneva, who had for a long time in his wards the hysterical patient who forms the subject of Case I, seeks for an explanation of the aphonia and mutism presented by the patient in the paralysis of a special nerve. Three other cases which he observed at the same time are published in a most interesting paper which appeared in the 'Revue de la Suisse Romande.'

I have been able to find a certain number of cases of this kind, which, together with those taken from the wards of M. Charcot—the most important observations published up to the present time—amount to twenty. The attentive study that I have been able to devote to these cases enables me to recognise in this mutism a central psychical affection analogous to that which produces the paralysis of a limb, the abolition of all or part of the visual field, &c. It is an aphasia, but as M. Charcot has remarked, an aphasia of a special type, which one is able, as it were, to diagnose at first sight and to distinguish from the different forms of aphasia of organic origin.

I have summarised most of these cases without giving a minute description of the diverse features indicative of hysteria in the patient. However, I have made an exception in the first case, which I have described at length because of the interesting details in the history of the patient and the thorough investigation made by our confrères at Geneva and Lyons.

CASE I (communicated by M. Charcot)—Ch—, 37 years of age, was admitted on November 8th, 1885, into the Bouvier ward, under the care of M. Charcot.

Family history.—Paternal grandfather died of an affection of the œsophagus. The brothers and sisters of the grandfather enjoyed good health; one of them died at seventy-eight. One of his nephews was bad-tempered, somewhat hypochondriac, and finally committed suicide. The paternal grandmother was very nervous, died at seventy-two of a catarrh (?). In her family there was a lunatic who died in an asylum. The maternal grandmother had an inebriate son who was not considered responsible. The father of the patient had epileptic fits and died of laryngeal tuberculosis at the age of fifty-seven. The patient's mother, who was very passionate, died of phthisis. She had eight children of whom Ch— was the eldest. Of his seven brothers and sisters, one brother died of croup at three years of age; two sisters died of phthisis at twenty-four and twenty-six years. One of them was subject to nervous attacks, and attacks of cataleptic sleep; "on waking she was aphonic; she articulated quite clearly, but very low, so low that it required extreme attention to understand her." Four sisters are living; two are delicate but without any definite complaint. One of the latter has a rachitic and choreïc son.

Ch— was always ailing in childhood. When twelve he was confined to bed for five or six months with weakness. The doctor treated him for anæmia. "The least sound," he says, "caused me to faint; they were unable to converse beside my bed." On two occasions when he was at school he had hæmoptysis. He was nicknamed the philosopher on account of his taciturn character. On leaving school he went to a college as assistant tutor; and subsequently went for some time into a large private horticultural establishment.

After some family disagreements and disappointments in love, he quitted Switzerland his native country and joined the Foreign Army Corps. During his sojourn in Algeria he drank absinthe to excess, and contracted intermittent fever. When the war of 1870 broke out his regiment came to France. At Vierzon he remained eight days in a delirious condition, caused, so he says, by an attack of fever. He rejoined his regiment and in the Eastern Campaign he received a bullet-wound in the left elbow (January 17th, 1871) for which his arm was amputated by Dr. Mollière, of Lyons. He then returned to Switzerland and was appointed manager of a post-office. It was at this time (end of 1871) that the first important nervous manifestation made its appearance. While at supper with some friends he was seized, towards the end of the repast, with invincible sleep, and slept with his elbow on the table. His comrades were quite unable to awaken him. Towards the morning a nervous attack came on attended with terrible delirium. The doctor suspected an acute meningitis; and Dr. Mayor, called into consultation, confirmed this diagnosis. The second day afterwards, the patient recovered, but relapsed a few days later. Leeches were applied, but a nervous attack, still more terrible than the first, came on. However, the fever and the delirium disappeared at the end of two days.

Up to the year 1875 nothing abnormal occurred in Ch—'s condition. In this year he departed for Algeria, where he had obtained a post of clerk in the Prefecture of Oran. Shortly before his departure he experienced for the first time sudden and violent attacks of palpitation which would sometimes oblige him to sit down.

Then strange symptoms occurred. "I was unable for whole days to bear any clothes on my body. My skin seemed on fire and I had contractions of all my limbs. When I attempted to put on my clothes it seemed as though I had millions of pins pricking me." During his journey to Lyons on his way to Algeria he was seized with feelings of suffocation, and on going into a chemist's shop he was taken with a nervous fit similar to the preceding, but which only lasted about two hours. In December, 1877, he had a slight attack of smallpox.

"In the spring of 1878, while on circuit with my chief, I was found one morning senseless in my bed. Bleeding and doses of calomel restored me, but my larynx was almost completely paralysed. I continued for seventy-two days to articulate my words with difficulty, though I could make myself understood." The patient allowed himself to indulge in both venereal and alcoholic excesses. To escape the frequent attacks of ague he went to the province of Algiers, and after staying there three years he returned to Geneva.

In 1880 he traversed Europe on foot, staying for some time with his brother-in-law in Prussia. There he was taken a second time with cataleptic sleep, which disappeared under the influence of bleeding. On waking he had paralysis (with insensibility) of the left leg and he had also complete mutism. Not a single word could he speak. "But my intelligence was unaffected, my memory, alone, was a little at fault, for recent events." After this he left Prussia and returned to Geneva.

We take the details of his story in Geneva from the case as published by Dr. Revilliod. On admission into the hospital, February 11th, 1881, the only pathological phenomena he presented were absolute mutism and slight numbness of the left side.

On laryngoscopic examination, which was rendered very easy by reason of the anæsthesia of the pharynx, the following condition was made out (Dr. Wyss). Abduction and adduction of the vocal cords are normally performed when the patient pronounces *e, i.* The only act which is faulty is the tension of the cords. Although they approach, they remain festooned and slack, flapping more or less according to the force of the inspiratory or expiratory current of air. If under these conditions the patient is requested to increase the effort necessary to produce a sound, the vocal cords, instead of becoming stretched as they approach, close suddenly, as though by a spring, and then stick together as it were all along, so that not only is no sound produced but the impeded respiration requires a great inspiratory effort, like the sigh, to restore matters to their former condition.

The patient passes his days reading, and in writing veritable mémoires describing his different impressions. On February 15th, he wrote that he had pronounced the words "No, do you want any," and then that he was unable to continue, the throat being contracted, and as though it were obstructed by an obstacle. His respiration was also more impeded than before.

After several applications of faradism of the crico-thyroid muscles and along the course of the superior laryngeal nerve, he was able to emit a few sounds, then some vowels, though without precision, and intonation only occurred at the end of expiration. The same thing happened when he was made to bend his head forcibly, or when the inferior border of the cricoid was raised. But these exercises fatigued him very much, although he performed them willingly enough, being convinced that they promoted his cure.

On March 30th he pronounced the vowels easily enough, consonants with more difficulty. On April 30th he could speak and read in a loud voice, though not without fatigue. After ten minutes' reading he was out of breath and was obliged to stop to recover himself. He avoided speaking spontaneously.

It was discovered by the laryngoscope that the vocal cords were well stretched, but they did not close completely in the middle when the patient pronounced the different vowels, thus allowing a large quantity of air to escape unused.

On June 18th, 1881, Ch— quitted the hospital, speaking spontaneously and fluently without difficulty. He only experienced dryness of the throat after a long conversation.

The treatment consisted of faradization, and from May 6, subcutaneous injections of a milligramme of sulphate of strychnine: plates of copper round his throat.

After leaving Geneva, Ch— found employment at Lyons. On September 11th, 1882, he was found unconscious in his bed. Bleeding restored him, but on waking he was again mute, and paralysed on the left side. He was taken into the wards of Dr. Raymond Tripier at the Hôtel Dieu, where he remained for eight months and underwent constant treatment by tepid baths, electricity, tonics and bromides. The patient states that on laryngoscopic examination the vocal cords were found in the same condition as that discovered by M. Revilliod.

On leaving the hospital he resumed his irregular life, and again had stifling sensations and vomiting (of bile and of blood!). His sleep was disturbed by visions and nightmares.

In January, 1883, he went to Valentia to recover some debts; and the next day he was found asleep at his hotel. He was taken to the hospital, where on waking he was again found to be mute and paralysed on the left side.

Then he returned to Geneva and entered the wards of Dr. Revilliod, enjoying the full integrity of his intellect and all his functions, but absolutely mute. The laryngoscope afforded the same indications as on the first occasion. On June 4th, a fresh attack of cataleptic sleep. Speech returned a few day later, and he left on July 21st.

The patient is unwilling to enter into the details of events which occurred in 1884 and 1885. As far as can be learned he had in 1884 five nervous attacks in a month and a half resembling the first (in 1869) though incomplete. In one he was bled. Twice he attempted suicide. The last attack of mutism and paralysis lasted four months, during a journey to Havre. He entered the Salpêtrière on November 8th, 1885.

On admission, he still dragged the left leg a little, and the mutism was complete. He had nightmares, and hallucinations during his delirious attacks, sometimes terrible sometimes agreeable, and the latter were accompanied by involuntary emissions. In the course of last year, touching his forehead produced the sensation of an aura which at the present time can be produced by pressure in the left iliac fossa, circumferential zone above the knee, and on the scalp of the same side. Exploration of the sensibility reveals on the left side apart from the three hysterogenic zones, an analgesia over the left half of head, trunk and thigh; pricking is perceived as a touch. In the leg anæsthesia is complete; in the foot, simple analgesia. On the right side sensibility is intact excepting the hand, where there is analgesia on the palmar face. The left arm was amputated in 1871.

Hearing is a little diminished on the left; there is no retraction of the visual field, nor achromatopsia. There is almost no sense of smell in the left nostril. He has noticed for several years that when he has a coryza there is dryness of the left nostril, whereas the other has an habitual running.

There was complete absence of reflex in the soft palate, of the pharynx and larynx; anæsthesia is absolute. It was even possible to touch the vocal cords with a laryngeal sound without producing reflex action. On examining the larynx the vocal cords were widely spread apart in a position of deep inspiration. If the patient was told to make the sounds, i, e, the vocal cords were seen to rapidly approach, but leaving between them an ellipsoid space due to the faulty action of the thyro-arytenoids, tensor and adductor, muscles. But no sound of any sort is produced. When he was told to pronounce certain consonants, the patient was able by his lips to produce a slight noise, purely labial. In producing a forced expiration, a sort of noise is similarly produced, but it does not correspond to any vowel sound.

Ch— has had four attacks of hemiplegia accompanied by aphasia, always with preservation of intelligence. When the patient is questioned he does not attempt to make movements of his lips to express what he wants. He seizes pen and paper with alacrity, and replies in a high-flown style, often humorous, which denotes an intelligence far above the average. When requested to produce the movements of the lips necessary for the pronunciation of words, or consonants, he attempts the movements, but neither word nor consonant is pronounced. The same thing happens with whistling: he screws up and protrudes his lips, but no sound issues.

The movements of the tongue were quite free and there was no trouble of deglutition. The patient is also very positive on this point, that there has never been any deviation of the mouth or tongue after any of the attacks. On waking it only seemed to him as though he had something in his throat which prevented him from speaking.

Ch— left the hospital at the end of November, still mute. A few days afterwards speech suddenly returned to him without known cause, though for several days he stammered. After former attacks speech had not suddenly returned to him: he had commenced by stammering, repeating twice the same syllable, if the word was at all long or complex. He said that it seemed as though air was wanting to finish the ends of words.

From the daily papers we have learned that Ch— was found a few days afterwards in a cataleptic sleep at his hotel.

CASE II (communicated by M. Charcot). M. S—, Félix, of Madrid, 26 years of age. Hereditary antecedents unknown. Has had a delicate childhood, and frequently subject to chest pains and epistaxes, one of the latter being so severe as to require plugging of the nares. In his youth he suffered from stomach-aches and indefinable ailments of a neuropathic order. The patient has constantly been in difficulties, and his uncle is a great worry to him on account of his constant remonstrances.

In 1880, according to the statement of his Spanish doctor, the patient had syphilis, though he denies it himself absolutely. However, he underwent specific treatment, and it was after a thermal course at one of the sulphur bath places that he had his first convulsive fit. Since that time (three years ago) he has had frequent "attacks" with loss of consciousness, of which he usually receives no warning. These fits were regarded as epileptic fits having a syphilitic origin. A very energetic specific treatment was instituted, but the crises only became longer, more violent, and more frequent. Lately these attacks have been followed by loss of speech, the aphasia lasting a few days and then the normal condition returns.

It was under these circumstances that M. S— presented himself at M. Charcot's out-patients'. He had been dumb since the last attack. These attacks were rather sudden, but he has never bitten his tongue nor passed urine involuntarily. The patient had a bright, intelligent look. The tongue was easily moved in all directions; no deviation of face. He could perform the movements for whistling and blowing; deglutition was not impeded in any way; but he was unable to pronounce a word, a cry, or even a sound. When spoken to, he comprehended perfectly, immediately took a pen and wrote very good answers in French, although he is Spanish, without the least embarrassment. This characteristic circumstance was suspicious of hysteria. M. Charcot made the patient undress and discovered a right hemianalgesia. There was a certain degree of hyperæsthesia in the dorso-lumbar region, but no true hysterogenic points, neither in the testicles, groins, nor iliac fossæ; no pharyngeal reflex. Laryngoscopic examination was not made. Examination of the eyes by M. Parinaud, revealed a very pronounced retraction of the visual field with spasm of the accommodation.

The right upper extremity was affected with chorea, like post-hemiplegic chorea.

The patient was treated with tonics, bromides, and hydrotherapy, and speech returned a few days later, though he still stuttered a little.

A month later, November 10th, the right hemianalgesia still existed, and also hemichorea of the right upper and lower extremities. The chorea of the lower limb was specially marked when the patient was sitting down.

Here are some specimens of the patient's replies when he departed a few days later. "I have - - - I have just done." "Yes, yes, I speak a little better." "Wh - - - what?" Given a journal to read: "All - - - all the preparations are - - -, are made for - - -, for the conference - - - -, it is reported on good auth - - - authority," &c. The same results occurred when given a Spanish journal to read. In a few weeks' time all symptoms had completely disappeared.

Case III (communicated by M. Charcot). Bill—, Antoinette, 21 years old, was admitted into the Salpêtrière under the care of Professor Charcot. She comes of a family of musicians; her mother died of hemiplegia at forty-nine. The patient has had typhoid fever. At the age of nineteen, after a fright (brokers came to levy a distraint) she was attacked with chorea which lasted six months, then by dumbness which lasted for eight days and was followed by stammering. The mutism reappeared at intervals after attacks which were accompanied by stifling sensations, constrictions of the throat, sensation of a ball, pains in the legs, which the patient likened to cramps, with swelling. Then hiccup came on with respiratory spasms, but she has not had attacks of hysteria major. She had never had stammering or dumbness before the fright. Left anæsthesia. No laryngoscopic examinations.

Case IV. Larch—, Syndonie, 19 years old, was admitted into the Salpêtrière under Professor Charcot on April 11th, 1885.

No personal or hereditary antecedents of importance, though the patient had often complained of pains in the right ovarian region.

On April 9th, at 10.30 p.m., she experienced a great fright (entered a room where a young girl had died). That night she was disturbed by nightmares. Next morning at 6 o'clock she let the slop-pail, which she was carrying downstairs, suddenly fall out of her right hand: paresis of the right upper extremity. She went upstairs and went to bed. At 10 o'clock the doctor who was called in discovered that she had completely lost the power of speech; she could neither read nor write.

On admission into the hospital the mutism was complete, though the patient could understand what was said to her; at least, she replied by signs to simple questions. The labial commissure was slightly raised during repose; more marked when she laughed. Tongue slightly deviated to right, but she could blow. Sensation deficient on right side. Taste and smell intact. Audition less on right than on left side: ticking of a watch heard at 9 centimetres on right, 34 on left. Retraction of right visual field; no dyschromatopsia.

Reflex of soft palate not good, fairly marked pharyngeal anæsthesia. On laryngoscopic examination the mucous membrane of the larynx was found healthy; vocal cords in complete state of abduction. If the patient was told to cry out or make the sound é, the vocal cords closed incompletely, leaving an open ellipsoid space (deficient tension of the thyro-arytenoid). No sound was emitted; the patient could not even speak in a low voice. Mutism was absolute. There was then no trace of paresis of right arm.

On April 24th, without any treatment, the retraction of the visual field had disappeared; sense of hearing improved; tension of the vocal cords was more complete; patient could say, "And then - - -, no."

May 6th, the patient could pronounce a few words. There was then no deviation of the mouth.

This case was the subject of some discussion, and at the time of admission Professor Charcot was not inclined to admit that the case was one of hysteria, because of the deviation of the tongue and mouth. The case is therefore published with reserve, although it seems to us to come within the category of hysterical manifestation.

The patient left the hospital a few months later, not cured.

CASE V. Gué— came into the Salpêtrière under the care of Professor Charcot.

A man 30 years of age. His first nervous attack occurred in September, 1882. Since January, 1885, the attacks had always been followed by transitory aphasia. These attacks, which were very violent, were classic (aura, loss of consciousness, tonic and clonic periods, &c.). When the patient regains consciousness he is unable to speak; he makes a sort of clucking noise to emphasise the gestures by which he expresses what he thinks or writes. He thoroughly understands what is asked him, and writes his answers correctly. This condition lasts for a longer or shorter time, which seems to bear relation to the severity of the attack; the duration averages four to five minutes.

This condition is accompanied by subjective phenomena, constriction of throat, &c., and in proportion as these disappear the patient recovers his speech.

During the state of mutism the reflex sensibility of the palate is preserved, and otherwise his condition is normal.

Sometimes the mutism has lasted for a longer time, several hours, several days. He had a very violent fit on February 24th, 1885, with spasms and attacks of suffocation, after which the aphasia lasted for six days. On several occasions the mutism has been dispersed by a fresh attack. At other times speech has returned spontaneously; he feels as though "something had given way in the throat."

Case VI. Lip—, a sculptor, æt. 20, came into the Salpêtrière under Professor Charcot. On June 16th, while in a restaurant, he was seized with aphasia, and at the same time with deafness, hearing nothing that was said to him. This deaf-mutism came on after reading a letter in which his father reproached him for his conduct and refused him money. On his arrival at the hospital he could not hear when spoken to quietly, but could understand when the question was shouted into his ear. He would reply very clearly by writing either in French or Polish to questions addressed to him by writing or shouting in his ear. No paralysis or troubles of sensibility. Movements of tongue and lips good; intelligence intact.

The mutism was not as complete as on the day when he lost his speech; he could pronounce a and e. The following days he seemed to be affected with motor amnesia. Varsovia, written down before him in French or in Sclave, was not pronounced satisfactorily: he said Vavic and Vava instead of Varchava, although he showed by writing that he clearly understood the word Varsovia. He replied in writing without the least hesitation.

These phenomena lasted for about a fortnight, then the speech returned and the deafness began to improve.

I can only give a brief summary of the next case, of hysterical aphasia in a child of eleven. The history is given at length in the thesis of Dr. Peugniez, a pupil of Dr. Charcot ('On Hysteria in Children,' Paris Thesis, 1885).

Case VII. Marie D—, 11 years old, was admitted into Professor Charcot's wards April 21st, 1885.

Her father had frequently had convulsions; the brother of her grandfather was hemiplegic; mother healthy; maternal cousin in an asylum. Brother had had convulsions.

The hysterical phenomena dated from the year 1884. In the early part of February, 1885, convulsive fits, contracture, &c. The voice got gradually weaker from this time, and the patient became aphasic. For three months she had only been able to pronounce a few words: Ah, mamma, I, pa - - - -.

Affections of taste, smell; retraction of visual field; achromatopsia. The patient replied to all questions, "Ah, Oh." On May 11th, after a severe fright, she cried out, "Wicked woman, I am afraid," and from this moment the speech returned.

Case VIII (published by Dr. Thermes in the 'France Méd., 1879, p. 290.'). Mdlle. X—, æt. 21. On February 15th, 1876, after exposure to damp cold—at least, according to the patient's account—she was taken with a fit of coughing, and soon after the voice became modified both in quality and intensity. Laryngoscopic examination (by Isambert) did not reveal any organic lesion, nor inflammatory condition, and the diagnosis was "paralysis of the vocal cords from defective innervation of the muscles of the larynx, and particularly of the crico-thyroids." Consequently the induced current was advised, and applied by Isambert himself. But instead of the usual amelioration, as expected, the aphonia rapidly degenerated into a mutism. Many varied medicaments were employed, but without effect.

During treatment at the thermo-resinous baths we had the opportunity of examining Mdlle. X—, and certain objective and subjective symptoms caused us to suspect the case to be one of mutism grafted on to hysteria of a non-convulsive form; or rather, a case of hysteria, the manifestation of which had invaded the laryngeal region, and particularly the tensor muscles of the vocal cords; a paralysis of the laryngeal portion of the pneumogastric, or paralysis of the motor filaments of the superior laryngeal.

The laryngoscopic examination then made (February, 1877) by Krishaber revealed that the left vocal cord was immobile, that the free borders occupied the median line and divided the glottic space like the perpendicular in an isosceles triangle. The corresponding arytenoid did not perform movements of rotation on its axis. The left vocal cord seemed shorter than the other, because of its laxity and because it was hidden by the arytenoid. The pharynx was slightly hyperæmic.

Prescription, hydrotherapy. At the first application, cry of surprise; the mutism was changed into incomplete aphonia. After a dozen local and general douches, the aphonia gradually disappeared, and a fortnight after the first douche the voice resumed its normal character and intensity.

Under the influence of a fall a convulsive attack occurred, on coming out of which the voice was again lost and the mutism again became complete. This happened in 1877.

The family applied to a quack doctor. At this time (February, 1878) the mutism was still complete. Hydrotherapy, as on the first occasion, produced the same result. Mdlle X— cried out and instantly regained her voice, but only for a moment. However, incomplete aphonia succeeded the mutism. She was able to whisper, the words being weak and low, but she could be well understood. Amelioration progressed to cure, and the patient at the time the case was published had not relapsed for ten months.

Case IX (Lionville et Debove, 'Progrès Médical,' February 26th, 1876). A girl of 18, hysterical but generally of good health. Her mother had attacks of hysteria major. A sister, thirteen years old, had frequent attacks, and for two months she had been affected with trembling, which several doctors had qualified as hysterical chorea. Father very nervous.

Until the last few years the hysteria had only been manifested by incomplete attacks. For eighteen months the patient had been painfully impressed by the quarrels and violent scenes between her father and mother; and it was to this cause that the patient, probably with reason, attributed her symptoms. About this time, in fact, she became aphonic, not being able to speak above a whisper, and in the course of two months the aphonia grew into mutism. In the house where she lived they named her "the mute." She communicated with those around her by means of a slate, which she habitually carried. The patient came several times into hospital. All those who examined her were agreed in the diagnosis of hysterical paralysis of the vocal cords. Different methods of treatment were adopted without success.

November 10th, 1875, she was brought to the Hôtel Dieu. She had no globus hystericus, no hemianæsthesia, no affection of the organs of special sense. Ovaries, especially the left, were tender on pressure; but, briefly, apart from the laryngeal troubles and the ovarian pain, the patient presented nothing abnormal.

The laryngeal paralysis is not simply a paralysis of movement, it is also a paralysis of sensation. Not the least pharyngeal reflex. Laryngoscopic examination, by Dr. Moura, revealed a paralysis of the vocal cords; these made an almost imperceptible movement when the patient tried to emit a sound.

Pressure over the ovary brought on attacks of dry cough, and a few stifled cries. The patient was able to articulate these words, in an almost imperceptible voice: "You hurt me." The following days, the compression was continued (five to ten minutes each time), and intonation became more and more distinct; she first ceased to be aphonic, then mute; she became able to speak, though in a low voice, hissing out her words.

Case X (Debove, 'Soc. Méd. des Hôp.,' November 10th, 1882). X— had been attacked on different occasions with delirium, irregular contortions of the face, &c. At certain times X— ceased to be convulsed, but was unable to speak; he corresponded with those around him by means of writing, and thus replied to questions. The fit came to an end, and sleep was induced by strong doses of chloral and morphine.

Case XI (Sevestre, 'Soc. Méd. des Hôp.,' 1882). Halz—, æt. 22, was admitted on April 14th into the wards of M. Sevestre for paralysis of the right arm which had come on suddenly the night before. He had previously had, in 1870 and 1874, two sudden attacks of unconsciousness; in 1877 transitory affections of vision, fugitive amauroses, which reappeared in 1880. Two years before, after one of these attacks of blindness, he had become aphasic for eight days; the speech returning, then the sight disappeared, and so on for several times.

On the 12th of April he had an attack of aphasia, which remained till the next day when he suddenly recovered speech, but then perceived that his left arm was powerless. On the 14th this paralysis was found to be accompanied with incomplete left hemianæsthesia. The following day the paralysis disappeared. No dyschromatopsia.

From the 14th to 18th of April, the patient continued to present this alternation of transitory phenomena.

Case XII (Sevestre, *ibid.*). G—, Léon, æt. 25, was subject to fits which could be arrested by pressure on the testicle. After one of these attacks, the patient was affected with a contracture occupying all the right side of the body; at the same time he was quite unable to speak, though his intelligence was perfect. After several days the speech gradually returned and the contracture disappeared.

Case XIII (Sevestre, *ibid.*). In one of the hospital attendants who consulted M. Sevestre for abdominal pains, a right hemianæsthesia was discovered; skin, conjunctiva, nasal mucous membrane were all insensitive. The patient stated that, about three months after the onset of this hemianæsthesia, one morning on getting up he had fallen to the ground, without loss of consciousness, but had been unable to speak for forty-eight hours.

Case XIV (Wilks, 'Diseases of the Nervous System,' 1883, p. 463). A girl æt. 22, who had kept her bed for more than a year on account of an affection of the spinal cord. Six months before taking to bed speech had failed her from time to time, and for a year she had been unable to pronounce a single word. She had replied by movements of the head and writing on a slate. Wilks, when consulted about the case believed it to be one of hysteria, and promised recovery if the patient would come into the hospital. After at first refusing, she yielded, and Wilks, addressing her with severity, threatened to make her imposture public. They took away her slate; she then attempted to move her lips as though she were talking. After several efforts, and the application of electricity, they were able at the end of a week to make her say "yes" and "no" in a low voice. The voice returned shortly afterwards, and the paralysis of the limbs also completely disappeared.

Case XV (Wilks, *ibid.* p. 465). A woman of 28, who had kept her bed for four and a half years. She had had nausea, and pains in the legs, and one day on getting out of bed she had lost the use of her legs. During the four years the symptoms had often varied. Paralysis of the hands fifteen months before. For ten months she had been unable to speak; the loss of voice had been sudden; she communicated with those around her by means of a slate. All treatment had been without success. She came into Dr. Wilks' wards on April 7th, 1886. As in the preceding case, she was cured by moral persuasion and electricity. During the application of the faradic current on the 24th, she cried out, "Oh, dear! yes." She was then able to speak slowly, and the recovery of speech was finally complete. The paralysis of the legs disappeared more slowly.

Case XVI (Case II. in the paper by Revilloid, 'Revue de la Suisse Romande,' 1883). A man, aged 48, admitted into the State hospital as a deaf mute with paralysis of the left side.

He could neither read nor write. Complete paralysis of movement and sensation on the left side, excepting in the face, which although insensitive was not deviated. The right arm was affected with almost continuous rhythmical choreiform movements. The leg was quiet. If any part of the right side of the body was tickled the right limb responded with a very pronounced epileptoid clonic trembling. Slight percussion of the patella tendon produced the same result. Vision almost lost on the left side, normal on the right. Complete deafness on both sides. Absolute mutism.

After tonic treatment and electrisation for a fortnight it was observed that the spontaneous tremor of the right arm was diminished. Voluntary movement on that side had slightly returned. One fine day, after an application of electricity, the patient shouted with joy, and laughed violently. Little by little the hearing returned. It was evident that when they shouted in his ear he heard, and then he was able to whisper a few words in a low voice. At the same time the movements and sensibility returned in the left side. In short, after a month's stay in the hospital, the patient was able to talk in a low voice, distinctly enough to give information.

After having had some epileptiform fits, he had been hemiplegic since 1869, and had been deaf and dumb since 1878.

CASE XVII (Revilliod, Case III in the same paper). A woman of 47, who without being actually hysterical, had suffered almost continually from manifestations of this neurosis, intractable vomiting, cough, and finally mutism with sternal and spinal pains. The mutism had returned on four occasions, each time lasting not less than two months, and sometimes for six months, at which times the patient could not open the mouth or put out the tongue.

Neither the loss nor the recovery of voice took place suddenly.

CASE XVIII (H. A. Johnson, Chicago, 'New York Med. Journ.,' Nov. 14th, 1885, *Paralysis of the Larynx*). H. B—, an unmarried girl æt. 24. No change in the structure or form of the larynx. Vocal cords in a cadaveric position. General health good, menstruation normal. Iron and strychnine were prescribed for her, and to live as much as possible in the open air. Faradic and interrupted galvanic currents were applied. None of these measures produced any improvement in the condition of the organ. After several months she departed for the East, and thence to Europe, where she consulted a large number of laryngologists, who prescribed the same treatment with strychnine, electricity, and tonics. After having visited California and the Southern States, the patient again returned to Europe, and passed the winter in Egypt. On her return she placed herself under the care of Dr. Hughlings Jackson, of London, who had the good fortune to hear her speak after five years silence. For three years she had been unable to speak even in a low voice, or to whisper. The vocal cords had remained in the condition described until her return from England. At this time she spoke at times in a loud voice, though only sometimes. On examination it was then found that during efforts at phonation, the vocal apophyses approached each other, but that there still remained a triangular opening behind; in other words, that there was paralysis of the arytenoid muscles, leaving a space through which the air escaped, rendering phonation difficult, and producing complete aphonia at times. From this time, that is for several years now, there had been periods of a few days, and occasionally of a week or more, when the patient could not speak except in a whisper. She was and had always been in good health, though she was of a lymphatic temperament, and easily tired. The larynx had been frequently examined in recent years without finding any modification in the state of the organ.

There could be no reasonable doubt but that the case was one of hysterical aphonia, which resisted all treatment until her visit to Dr. Hughlings Jackson.

Dr. Jackson's treatment had not differed much from those already tried. No trace was found of derangement of the uterine or other organs.

Case XIX (communicated by Dr. Chauffard). L—, Léonie, a servant, æt. 28, entered the Hôpital de la Pitié on March 27th, 1885. Mother very nervous, father hypochondriac. Two years previously the patient had had severe disappointments, then a miscarriage. It was about this time that the voice began to change its character.

On admission there was complete aphonia; the patient could scarcely whisper. No pain on pressure over the larynx, pronounced laryngeal anæsthesia. Signs of commencing phthisis. Patient was very nervous, cried without motive, and got into violent passions.

Hysterogenic points below and external to the left nipple, and in the corresponding ovarian region. Complete hemianæsthesia on the right side.

Laryngoscopic examination revealed no lesion, neither paralysis nor contracture. Application of the mirror was easy; vocal cords pale, perfectly mobile.

Shortly after admission, absolute mutism came on. On the third day electricity was applied; after the second application, the patient shouted out loudly, and on the following days the voice and speech returned; a certain effort was necessary; articulation did not become clear till the end of several days.

Case XX (Demme, 'Wiener med. Blätter,' December 18th, 1884). The author was performing the operation of dividing the tendo Achillis for club-foot on a little girl of six without an anæsthetic. Before the operation the child had been merry, playing with her doll, chatting with her father and mother. At the moment of section of the tendon she uttered a piercing cry, and from that moment could not speak a word. That lasted eight days, during which, having regained her spirits, she replied by signs when spoken to. On the morning of the ninth day she said "Mamma," and repeated it thirty or forty times. By the fourteenth day her vocabulary was enriched by the words "Papa, béb, schlassen, tiniken." By the eighteenth day she could say others, and then her normal state returned.

A perusal of the cases here reported at some length, shows that within a little the cases of hysterical mutism are identical, and present the following principal characters: sudden onset; impossibility of speaking or crying out; perfect preservation of the intelligence; return of speech, accompanied by stuttering which lasts a certain time.

1. The onset is in general sudden; after a fright, or some emotion the patient is deprived of speech. We say, generally, because in certain cases (see VIII, XVII, XIX) aphonia has existed a certain time prior to the loss of speech. In one of M. Revilliod's cases, he says that phonation diminished little by little before it was abolished.

It often happens that on return to consciousness after an hysterical seizure absolute mutism is discovered, with or without other paralysis. At other times, the loss of speech comes on suddenly without appreciable cause.

2. It is impossible for the patient to cry out or emit a single sound. He is aphonic; but he is also aphasic, for he cannot articulate words in a low voice.

Perhaps I may be allowed to say a few words on the subject of the distinction between aphonia and aphasia.

Hysterical paralyses of the larynx are very frequent; certain authors consider them as the most frequent symptom in the category of hysteria. It is some of these cases which furnish a means of easy and always surprising success to the doctor, of instantaneous cure of the patient, occasionally by the simple application of the mirror. The features are quite characteristic: sudden onset in neurotic subjects, most frequently bilateral, and involving the tensor and adductor muscles, much more rarely the abductors. According to the muscles attacked, and the degree of the paralysis, the aphonia is more or less complete. There is extinction or hoarseness of voice, impossibility of speaking in a loud voice, though whispering remains. The patient can make himself understood by speaking in a low voice. It is phonation which is wanting; there is no aphasia nor disturbance of intellect.

It is a fact now well established by numerous observations in the physiology of phonation that the larynx takes no part, nor do the vocal cords vibrate, in whispering or speaking in a low voice. The air glides through the larynx in the same manner as it does through the trachea or bronchial tubes, without the intrinsic muscles imparting any movement to the vocal cords. Rosapelly ('Travaux du labor. de Marey,' 1876),[1] Boudet de Paris ('Acad. des Sciences,' 1879), and other physiologists have shown experimentally by means of a simultaneous registration of the vibrations of the larynx and the movements of the lips and tongue, that the first-named organ is not brought into play in the production of consonants or even vowels, in the whispering voice.

I should be less concerned to discuss this point if Prof. Revilliod had not sought to explain by a simple paralysis of one of the muscles of the larynx the troubles observed in the patient who forms the subject of Case I. Ch— passed several months in the wards of the distinguished Professor at Geneva, for the same symptoms which brought him to the Salpêtrière. The laryngoscope revealed a faulty tension of the vocal cords. There existed also a certain degree of anæsthesia of the isthmus of the glottis and of the ventricle, troubles dependent on a

[1] *Vide* 'Progrès Médical,' Nos. 7 et 9, 1886.

paralysis of the superior laryngeal. The patient was absolutely mute on admission.

The way in which Dr. Revilliod interprets these phenomena is as follows: "The anæsthesia in the distribution of the superior laryngeal of itself tends to show that this sort of mutism is due to a paralysis of this nerve, albeit one often observes mutism without anæsthesia, and anæsthesia without mutism. . . . . However, this symptomatic triad (crico-thyroid paralysis, anæsthesia of the isthmus of the larynx, sternal pain during vocal effort) courts the supposition that the superior laryngeal may be alone attacked by hysteria, and that this nerve enjoys the unfortunate privilege of being easily affected by this malady; so that when, in a case of mutism, the laryngoscope reveals an absence of tension of the vocal cords, coincident with the integrity of their movements of abduction and adduction,—that is, when paralysis of the superior laryngeal is combined with a normal state of the recurrent—we should be authorised in admitting the hysterical nature of the affection."

I am unable to agree with these conclusions. That crico-thyroid paralysis, coincident with integrity of the functions of the adductors and abductors, indicates a hysterical origin of the malady is often correct, although there are several other causes which may give rise to faulty tension. That this lesion explains a more or less complete degree of aphonia is also true, but paralysis of the superior laryngeal cannot explain the mutism; for speech in a low voice subsists when the larynx alone is attacked, and the loud voice alone is wanting.

In the case quoted by Dr. Revilliod the mutism was complete, as I myself observed, though when I examined this patient the laryngeal paralysis was less localised, the crico-thyroid was attacked, but so also were the thyro-arytenoids. The mutism was as absolute as before.

Further, in opposition to this interpretation, those cases may be quoted where a laryngeal paralysis involving other muscles besides the crico-thyroid exist, together with the mutism.

In Jarvis's case (XVIII) there was paralysis of the arytenoid. In that of Dr. Thermes, Krishaber noted a paralysis of one abductor. In certain cases, as in this last one,

one may see varieties of the laryngeal troubles supervene in the course of the malady without any modification in the mutism.

There is nothing peculiar about the aphonia in these complex cases. The laryngoscope reveals paralysis of the tensor and adductor muscles, crico-thyroid, thyro-arytenoid, arytenoid; but the other muscles fulfil their functions; the vocal cords open and close as far as the median line when the patient is instructed to attempt phonation.

There is also a more or less complete anæsthesia of the pharynx or even of the larynx. But this anæsthesia has nothing special in relation to the aphonia or the mutism. It is frequently found in hysterical subjects who have no affection either of phonation or speech.

Thus, in hysterical mutism we find both aphonia *and motor aphasia*. This, in fact, is one of the most characteristic features of the affection. In simple hysterical aphonia, paralysis of a group of the laryngeal muscles is a very frequent occurrence. On the other hand, in mutism it is relatively rare. And what confirms the central, the psychical nature of this neurotic manifestation, is that the laryngeal muscles are not always affected with weakness, and that when they are more or less involved the functional trouble resulting from this paresis or paralysis does not afford us an explanation of the phenomena collectively.

3. The intelligence is completely preserved. On being asked a question, the patient (this is a very characteristic feature), conscious of his incapacity, does not make a lot of useless attempts at articulation, but immediately takes a pen or pencil and gives a very clear and precise reply.

This, I repeat, is a very characteristic feature. On more than one occasion M. Charcot has recognised the hysterical nature of the mutism solely from the manner in which the patients conduct themselves when interrogated. The opinion of M. Legoux must not, I think, be accepted too rigorously. He believes that the aphasia is not an element in the diagnosis of hysteria, though he allows that there are undoubted signs of hysteria which enable us to give this symptom its true significance. I certainly do not believe that one is able to dispose in a dogmatic fashion of all the difficulties in the diagnosis of nervous affections, or to identify at first sight every case of hysterical origin. But I hold that this collection of symptoms [syndrôme] by its special and differential characters, should at once evoke a suspicion of its nature in the mind of an attentive observer, though one ought not to omit the further investigation of the patient as to anæsthesia, hysterogenic zones, antecedents, &c.

Yet, as a matter of fact, this form of aphasia does not at all resemble that due to organic causes. In the latter case the patient makes an effort to pronounce and to repeat the word he wants, to stammer it out in an unintelligible fashion, or to reply by some other or some invariable word. There is nothing of the sort here, no word-blindness, no word-deafness; intelligence is perfect. Reply follows question immediately, if the patient knows how to write. At a stage when speech is returning, when the aphonia is less complete, this difference is less apparent. Sometimes the patient has difficulty in pronouncing the word because he stutters, though he can write correctly enough, showing the integrity of his intelligence and his writing faculty. Now, in certain cases of aphasia due to an organic lesion this dissociation may be detected—abolition of speech, preservation of writing faculty. But it never exists in such a striking way, and combined with the vivacity of intelligence which characterises the hysterical mute.

4. The recovery of speech is rapid in most of the cases, but it does not arrive *ad integrum* all in a moment. There is a stammering or hesitation in the speech during a period which may vary from a few days to a few weeks. Chauffat (Case I) remarked this on himself, and the same occurrence may be noticed in Case II.

It is unnecessary to add that other evidences of hysteria may be discovered either in the patient or the antecedents. Frequently there is anæsthesia or hysterogenic zones; one patient may have vomiting, another deafness. Such symptoms help to confirm the diagnosis. When hemiplegia comes on at the same time as the aphasia it creates some embarrassment in certain cases, but in the hysteric the deviation of mouth and tongue, and facial paralysis, are wanting. It was the presence, albeit transitory, of this symptom which alone caused us to regard the case of S— (Case IV) as doubtful.

It is easy to reproduce hysterical mutism by means of hypnotic suggestion. If during the somnambulic period you converse with the patient, then, lowering the voice, say to her, "I do not hear." "Eh?" "But you cannot speak then?" the patient soon becomes aphasic and aphonic. Being unable to cry out or to speak, she becomes impatient at not being able to reply to questions, and if she can write, seizes a piece of paper and writes hastily, though without embarrassment, a few lines which convey her thoughts: "I am unable to speak. Dear me! You see that I cannot." This is exactly what occurs in the patients we have tried; but I am only able to mention, in passing, these researches which ought to form the object of a special work.

INDEX.

For Product Safety Concerns and Information please contact our EU representative GPSR@taylorandfrancis.com
Taylor & Francis Verlag GmbH, Kaufingerstraße 24, 80331 München, Germany

www.ingramcontent.com/pod-product-compliance
Lightning Source LLC
LaVergne TN
LVHW011101300926
849160LV00008B/246
* 9 7 8 0 4 1 5 7 3 1 9 2 8 *